Front Cover

सौः

SAUḤ

Heart (hṛdayabīja)
or emanation (sṛṣṭi) mantra

The phoneme 'SA' symbolises
the thirty-one tattva from Earth to Māyā.
The phoneme 'AU' symbolises
Śuddhavidyā, Īśvara and Sadāśiva.
The phoneme 'AḤ' symbolises
Śiva and Śakti.
'SAUḤ' thus includes all the tattva.

"As the great banyan tree
lies in the form of potency in its seed,
even so this universe with all
the mobile and immobile beings
lies in the seminal mantra (SAUḤ),
the very heart of the Supreme."

"Those who are devoted
to hṛdayabīja, the very import of Trika,
even when they do not realise
its full virility, are the very Lord,
in a veiled form, having
entered the human body."

Abhinavagupta, Parātrīśikāvivaraṇa,
Jaideva Singh, Page 244-245

The Hero's Contemplation

The Hero's Contemplation

This English language edition first published in Great Britain by YogaWords Ltd 2011
Originally published by 'Connaissances et Savoirs' under the title 'La Contemplation du héros' 2011

ISBN 978-1-906756-10-9
British Library Cataloguing-in-Publication Data
A catalogue record for this book is available from the British Library

Printed in the EU by Graficas, Spain
This book has been printed on paper that is sourced and harvested from sustainable forests and is FSC accredited

YogaWords Ltd, 32 Clarendon Road, London N8 0DJ

www.yogawords.com

Christian Pisano

The Hero's Contemplation
- Vīrasamāveśa -

Yoga in the Light of the Teachings of Śrī B.K.S. Iyengar
and Non-Dual Kashmir Śaivism

Foreword by Śrī B.K.S. Iyengar

Introduction by Dr Mark S.G. Dyczkowski

Translated from French by Ian Sanderson

YOGAWORDS

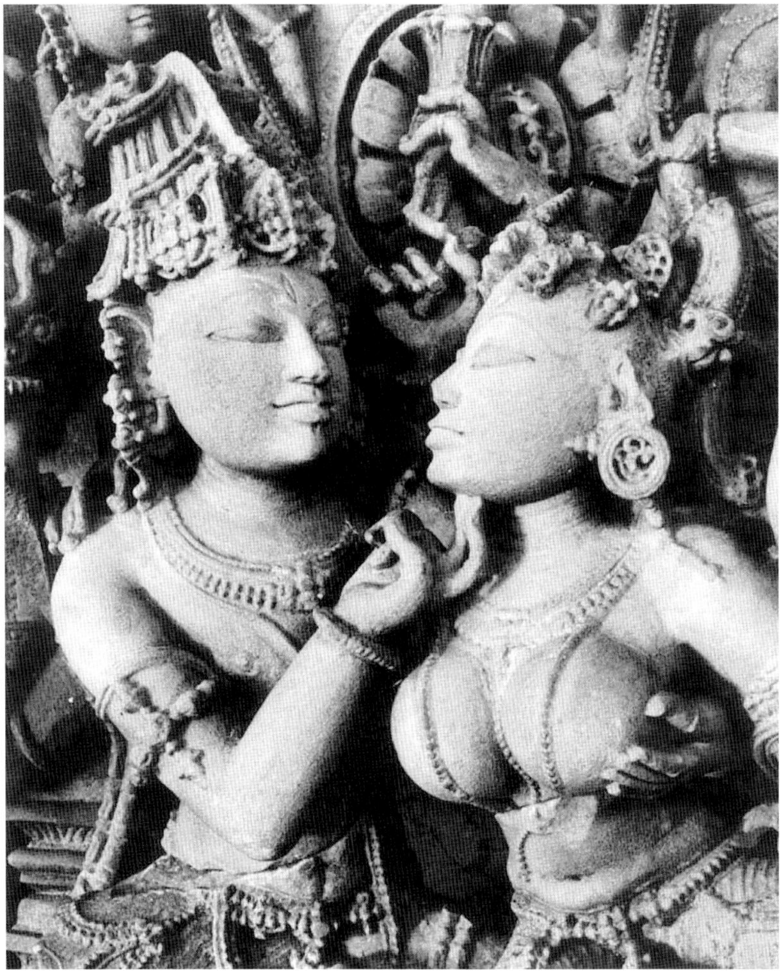

Śiva and Pārvatī

10th century

(Tewar, Jabalpur, Madhya Pradesh)

…to my father Giovanni, to my mother Francesca,

…to the real author of this book, my wife June,
expression of the supreme Śakti,

…to my brothers Franco, Victor, Sébastien and Antoine

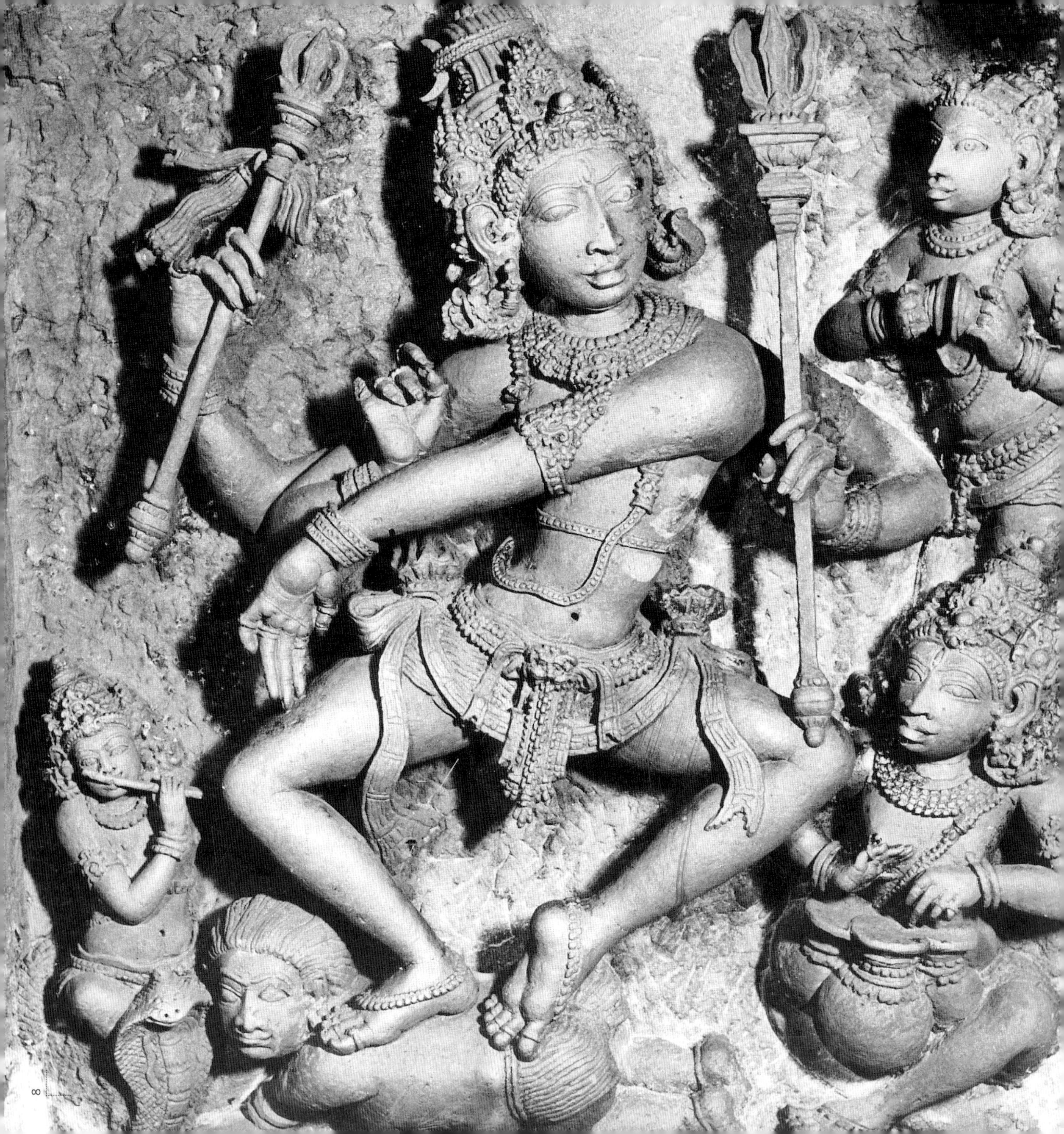

ॐ नमः शिवाय गुरवे
सच्चिदानन्दमूर्तये ।
निष्प्रपञ्चाय शान्ताय
निरालम्बाय तेजसे ॥

Om namaḥ Śivāya gurave
saccidānanda-mūrtaye,
niṣprapañcāya śāntāya
nirālambāya tejase.

Salutations to Śiva the Guru,
Who assumes the forms of Reality,
Consciousness and Bliss,
Who is ever present and full of peace,
Totally independent and all illuminating.

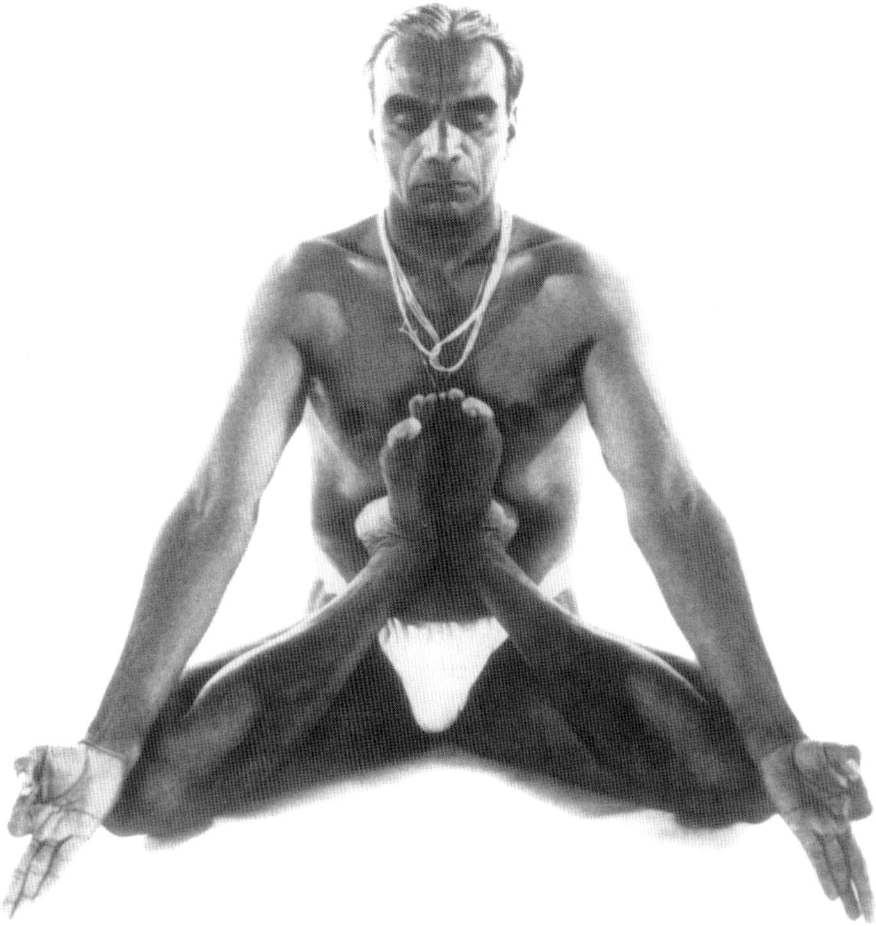

I bow before my Guru,
Yogācārya Śrī Bellur Krishnamāchār Sundararāja Iyengar,
Mahāsiddha amongst Siddha, whose playground is the universe.

Praise to the Guru who,
out of compassion for my ignorance, initiated me to Yoga.

I pay homage to the Guruparamparā, Geetajī and Prashāntjī
who are like the sun's rays.

Glory to the Guru, light of Consciousness,
mirror of my own Presence!

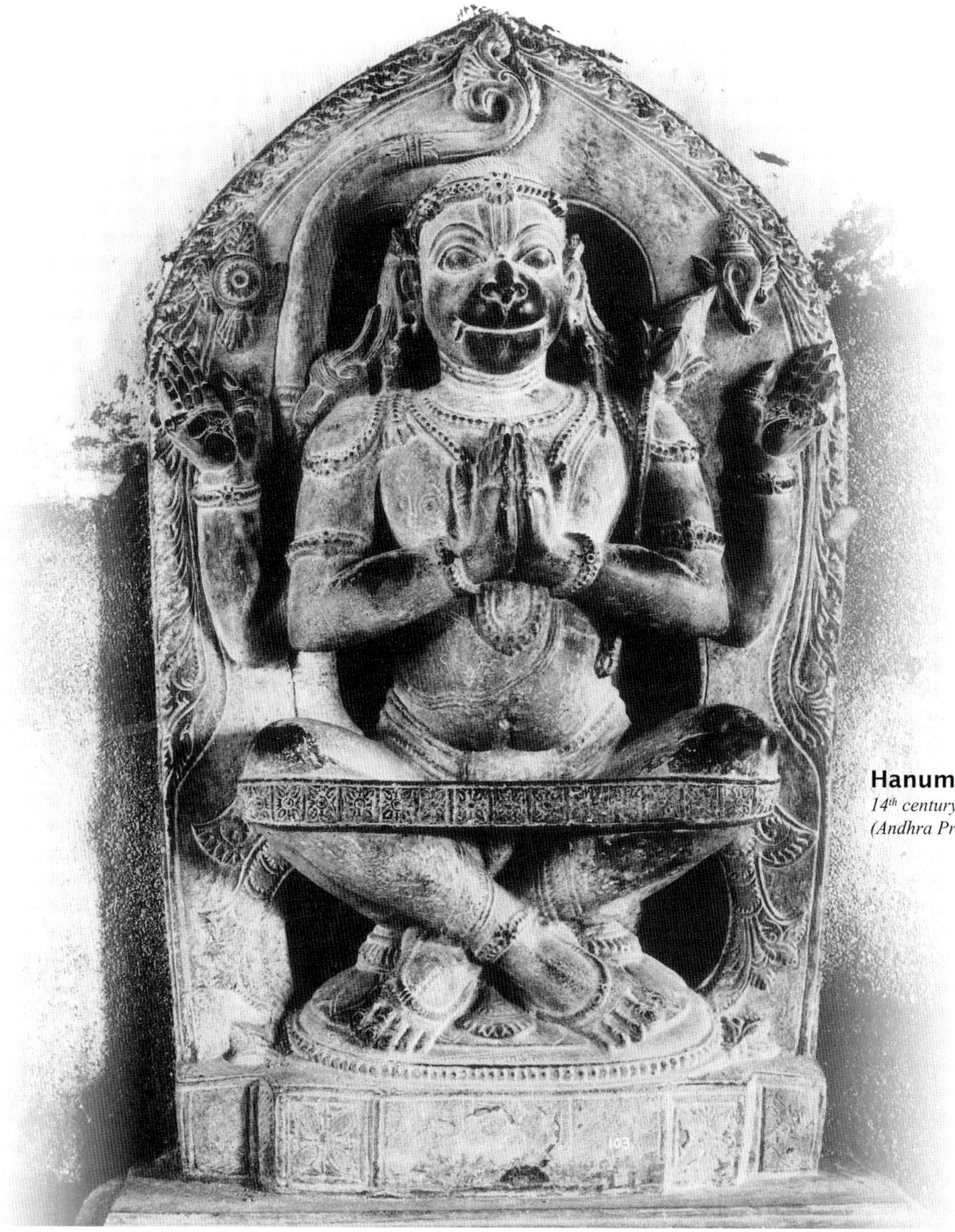

Hanumān
14th century
(Andhra Pradesh)

Foreword by Yogācārya Śrī B.K.S. Iyengar

I was delighted to read 'The Hero's Contemplation' (Vīrasamāveśa) written by Christian Pisano on the 'quest of the impossible'.

Because the intelligence of the average intellectual is veiled by external knowledge that is itself acquired through the 'gates' of the senses of perception, this quickly influences the mind and Consciousness and thus makes us dependent on the senses of perception.

Christian Pisano investigates what Reality is not! Through the expression of the 'real', he explores the facets of our bodies, containing the five elements (earth, water, fire, air and ether), with their atomic qualities (odour, taste, form, touch and vibration/sound), the mind, intelligence and Consciousness. He explains through Yoga how these are channelled in transforming one's mind, intelligence and Consciousness so that they submerge in the 'Sea of the Soul'.

At the end of the book, he narrates on the importance of āsana in establishing total firmness in the body - the element of Earth, the Shrine of the Soul - which is the foundation of knowing all the contents of nature (Prakṛti). When one understands the contents of the body (nature) very well and it is felt fully and totally, then the so-called Infinite surfaces and beams forth the 'Light of the Soul' to dwell in its splendour.

Christian Pisano has presented his thoughts as pointers towards the unalloyed and untainted bliss that shines from the quest of the impossible.

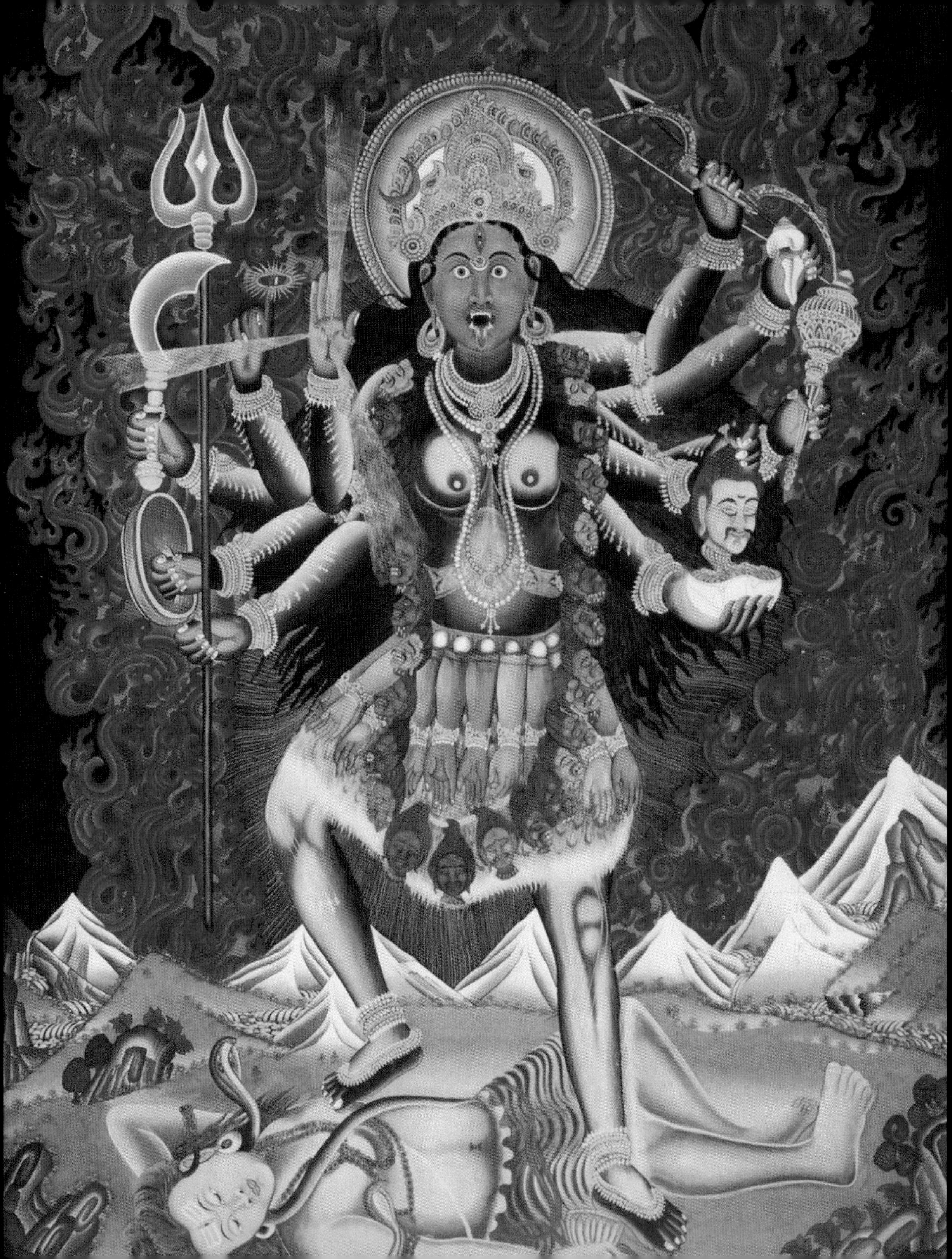

Introduction by Dr Mark S.G. Dyczkowski

A Brief History of Śaiva Tantra and Kashmir Śaivism

Fundamentally all Hindus believe in the existence of one ultimate, supreme reality to which they pray and contemplate as deity. In this sense they are monotheists. However, unlike the monotheism of the Jews, Christians and Muslims, they accept that the One Deity can assume many forms. Indeed, even in the most casual encounter with Hinduism we see that there are many deities, and as we get to know it more we soon discover that there is virtually an unlimited proliferation of divine forms. We find them out in the millions of villages in India, the towns and cities, out in the countryside, the mountains, valleys and plains. While many are just of local importance and are known to just the local inhabitants, some emerge as the Great Goddesses and Gods of Hinduism. These are the deities whose worship, mythology and teachings are recorded in scriptures revealed in Sanskrit. Although there is a great deal of sacred literature and a vast oral religious culture in the many vernaculars of the vast Indian subcontinent, the scriptures in Sanskrit are generally accorded a special status as the prime authorities. The first, and for most Hindus nowadays, the most authoritative, are the Vedas. They are made up of hymns intoned to the Vedic deities, revealed to the inspired Vedic seers over a number of centuries, possibly beginning as far as back as 1500 BC or even earlier.

With the passage of time, the Vedic religion gave way to the form of Hinduism we have today and from which it is variously derived, sometimes more, sometimes less directly. The Epics - the Mahābhārata and Rāmāyaṇa - were redacted perhaps from around the 2nd or 3rd centuries BC and new corpuses of sacred scriptures came to be revealed. One major group are the Purāṇas, traditionally said to be eighteen. Their original nuclei were the histories and genealogies of the kings and great souls, and extensive, detailed cosmologies. In addition, many Purāṇas contain long sections on a range of 'secular' including medicine, astrology, geography, the measurements of the body, quality of gems and more. What came to be their major concern was the rich and astonishingly extensive mythology of the great Hindu deities - Śiva, Viṣṇu and forms of the Great Goddess, Durgā, Kālī and others, and many other deities besides. The Purāṇas relate themselves to the four Vedas very closely. They are sometimes said to be the 'fifth Veda'. The Vedas are śruti - 'what has been heard', in relation to which the Purāṇas are smṛti - 'what has been recollected'. The earliest prototypes of the Purāṇas may indeed go back to late Vedic times, but it seems that they began to be redacted on a large scale from around the 4th or 5th centuries AD onwards. New ones continued to be written and additions to existing ones made right up to relatively recent times. Parallel to this great revelation were the Tantras. These felt themselves to be independent of the Vedas, although they respected them as revelation. Their main concern was to elaborate great ritual systems centred on the worship of the Great Gods, Śiva and Viṣṇu and forms of the Great Goddess. The fire sacrifice, that is, the worship and propitiation of deities by making offerings to the fire, which is the basic format of Vedic ritual, was taught in the Tantras but for this they revealed thousands of new Mantras, major and minor, which were not Vedic. In addition they taught another ritual format which is more basic called 'pūjā', that is, the worship of deities in iconic or aniconic representations, especially the Śiva Liṅga for Śaivites and the Śāligram (fossil ammonite) for Vaiṣṇavas, and, even more important, in maṇḍalas. These then are the Tantras of which the Śaiva ones contain the scriptures that are the major scriptural authorities of the Kashmiri Śaivism we shall examine in what follows.

Kashmiri Śaivism is a modern name for a form of Śaivism taught and elaborated by Kashmiri teachers in their works written in Sanskrit, most of which were produced during a period ranging from about the middle of the 9th century into the 13th century of the Common Era. The first amongst them was Vasugupta, who was followed by Kallaṭa Bhaṭṭa and Somānanda, then in succeeding generations, Utpaladeva and, the greatest of them all, Abhinavagupta (c. 975-1075 AD). After his distinguished disciple Kṣemarāja, the next, and last, great teacher was Jayaratha who lived some hundred and fifty years later. Other teachers emerged in the subsequent centuries but they were relatively minor figures. The early teachers formulated a new and highly sophisticated non-dualist Śaiva theology and metaphysics. This they applied to a rich and extensive exegesis of the Tantras that were their scriptural authorities, foremost amongst them were the Tantras of the Trika and Krama schools. In order to understand the nature of these Tantras and the schools associated with them, we need to have a basic understanding of what Tantras are and what they contain.

The Tantras are scriptures in Sanskrit that began to be revealed around the 6th century of the Common Era. The earliest were probably Śaiva, that is, Tantras that teach the supremacy of forms of Śiva and the Goddess, His consort and embodiment of His divine power. Tantras were produced in huge numbers in the centuries that followed by all major religions and schools of the period,

◀ **Kālī** *Kālasaṃkarṣiṇī She who devours time*
(Illustration by Romio Bahadur Shrestha)

including Buddhist which began to be produced around the same time as the Śaiva, and then, subsequently, Vaiṣṇava and Jaina. Hindu Tantras continued to be produced until recent times despite a major break in the religious traditions of which they were the scriptural authorities due to the dominant Muslim presence in the Indian subcontinent from around the 12th century onwards.

Tantras are very numerous and some very long. They belong to various schools that are distinguished from one another largely according to the deity and its attendant pantheon of which they describe the method of worship and other features of their cult, including yogic practices. The Śaiva Tantras of the early period, that is, prior to the 12th century, which were known to the Kashmiri masters may be roughly divided, for the purpose of this introduction, into two major categories. These are the Siddhānta Tantras that centre on the benign form of Śiva called Sadāśiva, the Ever Auspicious, and the Bhairava Tantras that centre on the fierce form of Śiva called Bhairava, the Terrific One. The Siddhānta Tantras, more commonly called Āgamas, became the scriptural authorities for the common public Śaiva rites that largely focused in the worship of the Śiva Liṅgas. This form of Śaivism largely died out in the North of India after the 13th century. It survived and developed in the South where the Siddhānta Āgamas grew in number and size and are still venerated to this day as the sources of the rites performed in many of the large Śaiva temple complexes of South India. There they were integrated with the recitation of Vedic hymns to Śiva's Vedic precursor, the god Rudra, and other Vedic rites. The melodious recitation of Vedic hymns of this sort were probably the manner in which Śiva Liṅgas were worshipped prior to the advent of the Tantras, which prescribed their own Mantras and ritual procedures. A surviving example may well be a rite called Rudrābhiṣeka (the Consecration of Rudra), which is still the most common way to worship the Śiva Liṅga throughout India, in which the Mantras are entirely drawn from Vedic hymns to Rudra, Śiva's Vedic precursor. The Siddhānta Āgamas we have at present do indeed devote a great deal of space to describing different forms of Liṅgas, their installation and worship. This does not seem to be such a major concern in the earliest period of their formation. The fact that Liṅga worship is largely done with Vedic Mantras raises the question whether Liṅga worship may not have been the focus of other forms of pre-Tantric Śaivism. This possibility becomes a virtual certainty when we consider the practice of the earliest documented form of sectarian Śaivism, namely, the Pāśupata. These votaries of Śiva Paśupati (Lord of the Beasts) took the vow to wander around India as ascetics, stopping at sacred sites to worship Śiva Liṅgas. Many of these they installed themselves and so contributed considerably to the spread of Śaivism in the subcontinent.

The Siddhānta Āgamas that exist nowadays, mostly in South Indian manuscripts, are extensively concerned with temple architecture and the rituals performed in them. However, surprisingly, none of the manuscripts that have been recovered in Nepal and references to them in the Kashmiri sources, all of which predate the 11th century, are at all concerned with these matters. Although we do find in the early Siddhānta sources that have been recovered in the north of the Indian subcontinent, the usual concern with ritual (which we will have occasion to discuss further ahead), it is performed by single individuals or small groups in their homes or private places, not in public temples. Apart from these rites, beginning with those of initiation, they deal with cosmology, metaphysical principles and soteriological concerns, including rules and regulations for spiritual disciplines for individual practice, originally mostly for renouncing ascetics and which were subsequently adapted to the householder's needs and way of life.

The world-views of the Siddhānta Āgamas are generally forms of tempered dualism. Their earliest commentators, who were Kashmiri, formulated what they perceived to be their basic view. They teach that there are three fundamental realities. The supreme reality is Śiva. He is one and essentially pure, divine consciousness. Endowed with all the attributes of Deity, He possesses the power - Śakti - through which He performs the five functions of creating, sustaining and destroying the world and those of obscuring Himself and bestowing grace, whereby He reveals Himself. The second reality consists of innumerable individual souls (aṇu). Like Śiva, they too are eternal consciousness, but unlike Him, until they are liberated by His grace, they are in a state of bondage which, although it ends, has no beginning. Once liberated, they are just like Śiva. The only difference between them and Śiva is that Śiva has never been subject to bondage. Although both Śiva and the individual souls are essentially pure consciousness, the latter, in the fettered state, are enveloped by Mala. Mala, which literally means 'dirt' or 'impurity', obscures the innate purity (i.e. divine, pure conscious nature) of the soul and separates it from Śiva. This third reality is also eternal but, unlike the other two, is an insentient substance. This has two aspects. On the one hand it is the substance from which the mental, cognitive and material world is generated. On the other, it covers the soul's consciousness making it ignorant of its true nature and liable to the binding constraints of the world of Māyā that has evolved out of that same impurity and the consequences of its actions, Karma. It is said to be like a cataract that covers the eye or the husk that envelops a grain of rice. Just as the cataract is removed by surgery and the husk by threshing the rice, similarly, the teacher, who is identified with Śiva, frees his disciple's soul from Mala by initiation. Once the covering has been removed and the soul has been purified in this way, nothing separates it from Śiva and so is conjoined to Him. Thus Śiva graces the soul through ritual action and reveals Himself to him. Now all the individual needs to do is maintain this state of purity. He must patiently wait for the exhaustion of the Karma that keeps him in the body to experience its consequences. Thus, in order to avoid accumulating more Karma, he takes care to observe all the precepts - injunctions and prohibitions - he was taught when he took initiation, worship the Deity regularly daily and observe the prescribed feast days.

The earliest independent works based on the Siddhānta Āgamas were commentaries and short independent treatises written by Sadyojyotis. Sadyojyotis was a Kashmiri who lived sometime before Somānanda who, around the middle or second half of the 9th century, was the first to systematically expound non-dualist Śaiva philosophy in his treatise the Śivadṛṣṭi - the Vision of Śiva. Sadyojyotis was followed in the next few generations by a number of Kashmiri Siddhāntins who continued his work of commenting on the Āgamas and expounding the metaphysics of dualist Śaivism. After the 12th century the Siddhānta gradually died out in the North of India, continuing in the temples, monasteries and households of the South. There, new schools of the Siddhānta developed and the Kashmiri teachers were forgotten. The transition was accompanied by a considerable growth of the Āgamas, both in number and extent. Moreover, a vast literature in Tamil developed which practically superseded the Sanskrit Siddhānta. Although commentaries on Āgamas and treatises on Siddhānta metaphysics were written in Tamil, much of it was devotional in character rather than liturgical.

The principle god of the Siddhānta Āgamas is, as we have already noted, Sadāśiva. He is a benign form of Śiva who is visualised as white, covered with ashes and with the faces of Vedic forms of Śiva. Turned towards the five directions, they utter all the scriptures of which the most excellent are, of course, the Śaiva Āgamas, which are spoken by the middle, upper face. He is mostly worshipped in a Liṅga, but may also be worshipped in a Maṇḍala. His female counterpart is clearly present, but is largely represented in abstract terms as his energy of Speech, usually with the same name in the feminine of the aspect of the god she accompanies. He is also often worshipped alone, invariably with vegetarian offerings. The ghosts (bhūta), demonic supernatural beings, both male and female spirits that are part of the god's host (gaṇa), are carefully segregated from him and propitiated separately in a circle (maṇḍala) or seat (pīṭha) where substitutes for animal sacrifice (bali) are offered to them.

Bhairava, Sadāśiva's dark, wrathful counterpart is the god of the rest of the early Śaiva Tantras. Accordingly, these Tantras are collectively called Bhairava Tantras. Although Bhairava retains the primary position of the supreme deity - and hence these scriptures are rightly termed Śaiva - he tends to be overshadowed by his consort, the goddess, and the hoards of female beings associated with her, generically called Yoginīs. There are many forms of the goddess, as there are of Bhairava. A well-known example is Kālī, of which there are a great many varieties. These goddesses and Yoginīs, like Bhairava, who is fierce and strangely antinomian, are commonly worshipped with liquor, meat and bodily fluids. The cults of the Bhairava Tantras, each of which had a primary Tantra and associated corpus of revealed scripture, are largely centred on the worship of goddesses. As the embodiment of Bhairava's divine power, their votaries considered them to be more powerful than their counterparts in the tamer, milder cults centred on Sadāśiva. Moreover, for this reason, they were kept secret. Their practice was private in sharp contrast with the Siddhānta's worship of Śiva, which served as the public, outer form. Entrance into these cults and access to their Tantras and practice was through special extra initiations that could be taken by Śaivites who were mostly already initiates into the common, exoteric form.

The same pattern was maintained within the ambit of the esoteric cults and their Tantras. As the stream of the Bhairava current flowed on, as it were, higher teachings would be revealed, that is, greater secrets that required higher initiations. The most secret were considered to be those most centred on the goddess and her attendant Yoginīs. These were understood to belong to 'families' or 'clans'- Kulas. A Kula was in the initial stages of these developments linked to one of eight Mothers (mātṛkā) who were embodiments of the powers of major gods. Thus, for example, the first was Brahmaṇī, the consort and energy of the god Brahmā. Another was Māheśvarī, the energy of Maheśvara, and so on. Ultimately, Kula Tantras developed in their own right as an independent category of scripture called the 'Kulāgama'. This development took place in stages as the Yoginī cult came to the fore in consonance with the progressively heightened prominence of Bhairava's consort who assumed varied identities. It was also reflected in the typology of the Tantras themselves.

The Bhairava Tantras reflected on themselves as belonging to four main groups or types called 'pīṭha'[1]. These are the Mantra-, Vidyā-, Mudrā- and Maṇḍala- pīṭhas. The last two soon became largely defunct categories. The first two concern us. Mantras are used to invoke male deities of whom they are the sonic form. Similarly, Vidyās invoke the female deities they embody. The Tantras of these two types are indeed distinguishable by the relative prominence of the god and the goddess, respectively. The most substantial representative, and possibly the earliest one, of the Mantrapīṭha of the great Bhairava current of Śaiva scriptures is the Svacchandabhairava Tantra. As its name implies, the main deity of this Tantra is a form of Śiva called Svacchanda Bhairava. Even though he is a Bhairava, that is, a fierce form of Śiva, he retains much of the mildness of Sadāśiva, a feature reflected in his homonym - Aghora - the 'Non-fierce One'. Like Sadāśiva, he has five faces and can be worshipped alone. His form is then black, not ash white, as is Sadāśiva. Svacchanda Bhairava is white, however, when he appears along with his consort Aghoreśvarī, also called Vyādhibhakṣiṇī 'She Who Devours Disease'. Unlike the Great Goddesses of the Vidyāpīṭha, who are powerful independent deities

1 *The term 'pīṭha' is well known as a word denoting a major type of sacred place where a goddess resides and is worshipped. In this sense the word can be translated as 'seat'. In this context 'pīṭha' means 'a collection of scriptures' (śāstrasamūha).*

in their own right, she is simply a female replica of her male counterpart and is hardly more than a supporting figure.
Compared to the rambling style of many of the Tantras (which may well be a sign that they were compiled by a number of initiates over time), the cult of the Svacchandabhairava Tantra is systematically expounded in a relatively well-ordered fashion. In many respects the cult of the SvT resembles those of the Siddhāntāgamas more than those of the Bhairava Tantras of the Vidyāpīṭha. For example, the acquisition of magical and yogic powers (siddhi) and worldly benefits is a major concern of the Tantras of the Vidyāpīṭha. As in the Siddhāntāgamas, they are less important for the SvT, which is primarily focused on the detailed exposition of the regular (nitya) and occasional rites (naimittika) rather than the magical ones aimed at fulfilling particular aims (kāmya). More significantly, Yoginīs are absent in the SvT except in the last two chapters, which are evidently late additions. The cult of Svacchanda Bhairava had a significant influence on all the major traditions of the Bhairava Tantras, supplying them, when required, with a mild form of Bhairava. The SvT also served as a source that channelled into the Bhairava Tantras the basic cosmology and related Mantras common to the Siddhānta in general, and with them the major rites, especially the standard form of the rites of initiation.
The intermediate character of Svacchanda Bhairava's nature and his cult, that is, between the mild Sadāśiva of the Siddhānta and the fierce Bhairavas of the Tantras of the Vidyāpīṭha, is also apparent in his variant forms. Thus he is also represented as wearing bone ornaments and carrying a skull. He is visualised along with his consort surrounded in the eight directions by cremation grounds and attendant Bhairavas. Here we find ourselves in the culture of the cremation ground which pervades, in varying degrees and forms, the cults of the Vidyāpīṭha and Kaula Tantras. Sanderson sees in the Bhairavas of the Bhairava Tantras the common model for the famous Kāpālika - Skull-bearing ascetics[2]. These ascetics imitate the god who carries the skull of the upper head of Brahmā, the creator, which he severed to punish him for the sin of looking lustfully at his daughter. Bhairava carries the skull as a penance known as the Great Vow (mahāvrata). By imitating the god, the Kāpālika purifies himself, just as Bhairava did, of the worst of sins - brahminicide[3]. This is most clearly evident in the Tantras of the Vidyāpīṭha, but can also be noticed in the mild Bhairava cult of the Mantrapīṭha[4]. Sanderson explains that the Śaiva who entered the ritual universe of the Vidyāpīṭha:

...was consecrated in the cults of deities who presided in their maṇḍalas over predominantly female pantheons, and who passed as he ascended from Bhairavas with consorts, to goddesses above Bhairavas, to the terrible Solitary Heroines (ekavīrā) of the cults of Kālī... The initiate gained access to the powers of these deities by adopting the observance of the Kāpālikas. ...intoxicated with alcohol, he alternated periods of night-wandering (niśāṭana) with worship (pūjā) in which he invoked and gratified the deities of the maṇḍala into which he had been initiated. This gratification required the participation of a dūtī, a consecrated consort, with whom he was to copulate in order to produce the mingled sexual fluids which, with blood and other impurities of the body, provided the offerings irresistible to this class of deities[5].

As the Tantras grew in number and the Tantric schools with them, each school reflected on the others in relationship to itself as, of course, the highest. All the Tantras are considered to be revelation, as are the Vedas, although not of equal authority. From the perspective of the schools, the Kashmiri Śaiva teachers considered the most secret to be the most elevated Tantras. Their schools are arranged in a hierarchy reflected in the serial order of progressively higher initiations corresponding to deepening levels of secrecy and, as it happens, their internal doctrinal development. This reflects, to some extent, their chronological order which we can observe as the upward progression through time carries over elements of the

2 *Cf. Dyczkowski 1988: 29-30.*

3 *Lorenzen 1991 (second edition) remains the most authoritative work on the Kāpālikas. For the myth, see, for example, the Kūrmapurāṇa, 2/31ff. See also Dyczkowski 1988: 26 ff. Kṣemarāja in his commentary on the SvT explains that the adept pursues this vow in order to effect this imitation so that identity with the supreme Bhairava will guarantee the efficacy of his ritual performance (Arraj 1988: 51, note 1).*

4 *Amongst the (kāmya) rites of the SvT that serve to attain yogic and magical power we find one that is designated as Kāpālika practice, alerting us to the possibility of this influence (albeit well sanitised) on the earliest strata of the formation of this important Tantra of the Mantrapīṭha. Concerning a section in chapter six of the SvT (book six pp. 148-155) Arraj (1988: 187-8) notes that it: "presents eight rites that promise to subjugate another to the adept's will (vaśikaraṇam). In each rite, the adept prepares potions according to different recipes (sic). Notably, the text apparantly designates one of these procedures as a Kāpālika practice [(SvT 6/33) although Kṣemarāja dissimilates this possibility]. This label, at least in passing, therefore, links these procedures to the adept's main formula service, and possibly furnishes the only direct evidence for the provenance of the Bhairava source [of the SvT]."*

5 *Sanderson 1988: 670-1.*

preceding traditions into the subsequent, more secret ones.
It is not possible to say exactly when the first Tantras were revealed, but there can be little doubt that it was not prior to the 6th century and probably not much before the middle of the 7th. By the 9th century when the first exegetical and independent works were written by the Śaiva teachers of Kashmir, first by dualist Siddhāntins and then by the non-dualist, this progression had probably fully worked itself out. From the perspective of the non-dualist, so-called Kashmiri Śaivites, as championed by the great Abhinavagupta (c. 975-1050 CE), the first in the series were the Siddhāntāgamas. These are followed by the Bhairava Tantras, first of the Mantrapīṭha and then the Vidyāpīṭha.
Ascending from the Mantrapīṭha into the Vidyāpīṭha we first come to the Yāmala class of Tantras. The Brahmāyāmala is one of its earliest and most excellent representatives[6] and which some scholars believe to have been a scripture of the Kāpālikas[7]. This Tantra, some 12,000 verses long, although preserved solely in Nepalese manuscripts and lost for centuries in the rest of the subcontinent, still enjoys considerable prestige for many contemporary Śaiva ascetics who know nothing more about it than just its name. The extent of its spread and influence can be gauged by the status accorded to it in early Tamil literature as the best of the Yāmala Tantras[8]. The ascendance of the feminine, and with it the development of the Yoginī cult, is apparent in the BY. Although the main deity of the BY is Kāpāla Bhairava, it is the Vidyā of his consort, Caṇḍā Kāpālinī, which is considered to be the main one thus making way for the feminine in a male milieu. She is said to emanate from the god as his energy and deploys herself in the eight directions around him in the form of his surrounding eight goddesses[9].
As an example of the ethos of the BY, we may cite a typical rite described in it[10] in which Kāpālīśa Bhairava appears as Manthāna Bhairava, the Churning Bhairava. He is worshipped in a cremation ground by the adept of the BY, the avadhūta[11], in the midst of the eight Yoginīs mentioned above to each of whom is offered a skull full of blood. Surrounding them are eight more Yoginīs with their consorts[12]. Along with his female companion (sakhi), the avadhūta consumes the remnants of the offerings of meat together with wine and a mixture of male and female sexual fluids (picu)[13]. Manthāna Bhairava is in the middle, 'brilliant like pure crystal'. After the initial offering to the Yoginīs, the avadhūta baths and then commences his practice proper. Terrible noises are heard in the air as he takes

6 *See Dyczkowski 1988: 115 for a brief note on the Yāmalas and the BY in particular.*

7 *Nagaswami reports the following statement by a commentator on the Takkayāgapparaṇi by Oṭṭakkūtar (12th cent. CE), which is acclaimed as the best Tamil literary work of the Chola period: "The Yāmalāchāryas are those who are well versed in the Sakala Pañchakas which are liquor, fish, flesh, sign (sic) and sexual union (Madhu, Matsya, Māmsa, Mudrā (sic) and Maithunā). This information is available in the Āgama Śāstras (sic) of the Mahāvratin." (Nagaswami 1982: 33)*

8 *Nagaswami (1982: 33) notes that Oṭṭakkūtar's work is: "remarkable for the information it provides on the followers of the Yāmala Tantra in their worship of Kālī." Perhaps Oṭṭakkūtar was referring to the followers of the cult of the JY. We know that the Kālīkrama that developed out of it was well known in the South in the 12th century. In his work Oṭṭakkūtar describes a fabulous temple to the goddess which is said to house, along with the eighteen Purāṇas, the main Yāmalas, of which the first is the BY, along with ninty-one secondary ones (Nagaswami 1982: 34).*

9 *Sanderson 1988: 672. The Vidyā of Caṇḍā Kāpālinī is: (OṂ) HŪṂ CAṆḌE KĀPĀLINĪ SVĀHĀ. The nine syllables of the Vidyā are presided over by the nine deities who are the main object of daily worship. These are Kāpālīśabhairava (HŪṂ), his four goddesses (also called Yoginīs), Raktā (CAṂ), Karālā (ḌE), Caṇḍākṣī (KĀ) and Mahocchuṣmā (PĀ) and their four attendant powers (dūtī) - Karālī (LI), Danturā (NI), Bhīmavaktrā (SVĀ) and Mahābalā (HĀ). The goddesses, also called Yoginīs, are set in the eight directions around Kāpālīśa Bhairava as follows: 1) East: Raktā; 2) South: Karālinī; 3) West: Caṇḍākṣī; 4) North: Mahocchuṣmā; 5) Southeast: Karālyā; 6) Southwest: Danturā; 7) Northwest: Bhīmavaktrā; 8) Northeast: Mahābalā: BY 30/21ab, 23-25ab. These Yoginīs appear throughout the BY, but refer especially to chapters 29 and 30 where their maṇḍala is described.*

10 *This is found in chapter forty-six of the BY where the 'practice with regards to the Churning (Bhairava)' is described.*

11 *The word avadhūta literally means 'one who has shaken off (worldly desires)'.*

12 *These eight are, effectively, the BY's version of the Eight Mothers (aṣṭamātṛkā). The first four of these couples are commonly found amongst the seven or eight Mothers mentioned above as presiding over the clans (gotra) or families (kula) to which initiates belong. They are: 1) Mahendrī and Maheśa in the east; 2) Brahmī and Brahmā in the southeast; 3) Vaiṣnavī and Viṣṇu in the south; 4) Kaumārī and Kumāra in the southwest; 5) Vivaśvatī and Vivaśva in the west; 6) Vāyavī and Vāyava in the northwest; 7) Bhairavī and Yogeśa in the north; 8) Guhyaśakti alone (?) in the northeast.*

13 *Concerning the term picu from which the BY derives its other name, i.e. Picumata, see Dyczkowski 1988: 115.*

a sword consecrated to the god from the middle of the maṇḍala. He offers garlands to the god and repeats the Mantra noted above as he 'churns' his partner in sexual union on the sacrificial ground. Clearly, the text is referring in this way to sexual union with his companion. Frightening sounds are heard everywhere and the Yoginīs approach him from all directions. He makes an offering to them of wine and mixed sexual fluids, male and female, in a skull in the centre of the maṇḍala and continues 'churning'. Hot coals rain down from the sky, the earth quakes, lightning falls from the sky and horrifying ghosts emerge out of the ground. He offers them the same liquid offering and, seeing the sword he is holding, they bow to him. He continues 'churning'. Then gods and demons come to him followed by six Yoginīs. Each time he makes the offering and resumes his 'churning', strengthened by the voice of the god who tells him not to fear as long as he is engaged in this way. Then, invoking the deity requesting the attainment of all the accomplishments (siddhi), he begins the 'Great Churning'. This produces an embodiment of the Poison of Death (kālakūṭa), who is overcome in the same way. After similar apparitions associated with the mythical churning of the cosmic ocean, the avadhūta offers a skull bowl full of sexual fluids (picu) to the god and the goddess. The goddess Aghorī, that is, Caṇḍākāpālinī, finally appears before him, to whom, along with Aghora (that is, Svacchanda Bhairava), the form of Kāpāleśvara that manifests with her, he makes the same liquid offering. Pleased, she feeds him and his companions with milk from her breast and thus he finally becomes omniscient and attains oneness with Śiva.

The Siddhayogeśvarīmata is one of the earliest, if not the earliest Tantra of the Vidyāpīṭha. It links itself in at least two places to the SvT of the Mantrapīṭha, which thus probably pre-dates it[14]. Although it may pre-date the BY, from the perspective of the Kashmiri Śaiva teachers, it is higher, and hence follows after. Indeed, the school which came to be called Trika, that begins with it, is for them the highest one. This is, of course, true for the Trika Tantras that continued to be revealed throughout the period of these developments and which came to reflect on themselves as constituting the highest school and culmination of the others. A few thousand verses of the SYM have been recovered in manuscripts. This is certainly just a fragment of the original, which may have been even longer than the BY.

The SYM came to be seen as the first of a triad (trika) of Tantras of the school, along with the (A)nāmakamata, which has been lost, and the Mālinīvijayottara (the Highest Triumph of the (Goddess) Mālinī). Unlike the SYM, which was a long rambling revelation, the MVT is a compact, dense treatise, which considers itself to be the essence of the teachings of the SYM. The very name of the MVT implies this. Siddhayogeśvarī, which literally means the Mistress of Accomplished Yoga, is more of an epithet of the goddess than a proper name. The deity of the SYM and thereafter of the Trika is Parā, the Supreme, called Mālinī or, more generically, Rudraśakti. The cult of the SYM, which is the foundation of all the subsequent Trika Tantras, from which the name of the school is derived, is centred on a triad (trika) of goddesses who are worshipped as aspects of Mālinī. Called Parā, Parāparā and Aparā, each is seated on her own Bhairava that lies prone on one of the tips of the three prongs of Śiva's Trident. The SYM tells us that they are white, red and black, respectively, because they embody the three divinised qualities (guṇa) (here understood to be energies) of Nature (prakṛti). The SYM teaches that the Trident Maṇḍala should be worshipped, as is the Maṇḍala of the Lord of the Skull, in a cremation ground. There the adept goes on a moonless night and traces a simple circle surrounding a trident with the ashes of a human corpse. In a nearby pyre he makes offerings of blood he draws from his body to the Trident, repeating the Mantras of the triadic goddess. As he does so, the Tantra tells us, the stars light up and grow larger. The sky begins to rumble and as the sounds grow louder the lights in the sky turn into burning coals that start to rain down on him as the earth trembles and shakes. Soon the rain of fire turns into hoards of screaming, ferocious Yoginīs. The Tantra admonishes him not to waver in his vow to repeat the Mantras without ceasing. This he must continue to do at all cost, even as the Yoginīs stream with tremendous force into his body. If he is successful, he will experience, with great joy and wonder, the pervasive presence (vyāpti) of the Goddess Supreme (Parā), first in the Maṇḍala and then throughout the universe and his body.

Even more dramatic are the rites and visionary experiences of the Kālī Tantras. Here we enter a world populated by immensely varied and powerful forms of Kālī. Devouring and consuming, they dance frenetically in battlefields and cremation grounds indulging in wild orgies in the night of the New Moon, shrouded in the darkness of Māyā. A Tantra describes the scene in the terrible cremation ground called Karavīra where Bhairava, also called Rudra, is the fire (dāhaka) that consumes the worlds and their gods, countless Yamas (gods of death), death (itself) and diseases. There the hoards of Kālīs and their Bhairavas are practising ritual orgies (cakrācāra), in violently passionate union (haṭhamelāpa) they are intent on the Primordial Sacrifice of sexual union (ādyayāga). Some sit together engrossed in drinking liquor (vīrapāna). Others eat burning coals, some the Sun, others the Moon (soma), holding hands with one another as they eat and drink. Some hold corpses, others meditate quietly or, in couples, are engaged in worshiping Maṇḍalas[15].

14 SYM 32/6 and 32/13. Törzsök 1999: p. vii, note 31.

15 Summary of KuKauM 15/68cd-76ab.

As we progress through the cults of the Vidyāpīṭha and observe them develop in their Tantras[16], we notice that they tend to be more internalised and thereby domesticated, that is, accessible to initiated householders. From the body we progress inwards to the senses, mind, vital breath and finally consciousness. As we move further inward the imagination develops from the creation of images to the contemplation of consciousness. As we make these transitions we enter the innermost realm of mystical experience. As we ascend, the representations of inner, progressively more elevated states of consciousness become more vivid. The inner Path is marked by the outer forms of the Kāpālika's practice, which supply a wide and rich range of symbols that can both represent inner states and supply ideal frames for outer rites and their internal representation. One could cite many examples. The following is drawn from an unknown Tantra quoted by Abhinavagupta in his Tantrāloka:

(The body) is the support of all the gods, the cremation ground frightening with the funeral pyre (citi) (of consciousness (citi), which destroys all things). Attended by Siddhas and Yoginīs, it is their awesome playground wherein all embodied forms come to an end. Full of the countless pyres (of the senses) and pervaded by the halos of their rays, the flux of the darkness (of duality) is destroyed and, free of all thought-constructs, it is the sole abode of bliss. Entering this (body), the cremation ground of emptiness, who does not achieve perfection?[17]

The Kāpālika's Vow, the Great Vow of Knowledge to wander in the sacred sites repeating without ceasing the Mantra which is this Knowledge, seeking the perfect Yoginī with which to couple and receive from her the food of eternal life, is understood as the profound, continuous contemplation of the Yoni. The Yoni is the Goddess's Womb, the Abode of the Crevice. It encompasses all the universe, every sacred place, but now it is no longer outside. The adept finds it within himself. There he delights in its touch as he experiences the Supreme Goddess Kuṇḍalinī in the Wheel of Passion within the body, gross and subtle, and, above all, in consciousness, where Śiva and Śakti unite. There he drinks the juices of their union at every level of Being and attains Eternal Life.

So we read this beautiful prayer in a Kubjikā Tantra:

Salutations to the wealth of touch (sparśalakṣmī), the supreme (goddess) who, contemplated by means of the Wheel of Passion (raticakra), sports (performing) the Vow which is perpetually intent on the (Yoni which is the) Abode of the Crevice in which time and timelessness have been eradicated. (This is the Vow) which is the manifestation of self-realisation that takes place once one has abandoned the abode divided by the diversity of oneness and duality. (This is the Vow) which is the manifestation of one's own (innate) vibration (svaghūrma), once drunk the supreme nectar of the juice of each state of being[18].

As we advance inward we leave the realms of name and form to discover the unconfined expanse of Infinite Being, that is, the pure consciousness of Deity which precedes them and is their source. Ultimately, all representation ceases, all that remains is the pure abstract contemplation of emptiness. Thus we are taught in the Netra Tantra:

One must not meditate on anything above, below, in the centre, in front, behind or on either side. One should not contemplate anything within the body or outside it. Do not fix your attention on the sky, nor below (on the earth). Neither close the eyes nor gaze fixedly. Think not of the support, the supported or the supportless, nor of the senses, or of the gross elements or sound, taste and touch, etc. Having abandoned (everything) in this way be established in contemplation (samādhi) and become one. That is said to be the supreme state of Śiva, the supreme soul. Having attained that unmanifest (nirābhāsa) plane, one no longer falls from it[19].

This was the situation when Vasugupta appears on the scene in Kashmir around the middle of the 9th century. To him Lord Śiva revealed the Śivasūtra - the Aphorisms of Śiva - with which Kashmiri Śaivism in the modern sense of the term begins. Through less than a hundred short, pithy statements - sūtras - Śiva Himself lays the foundations of Kashmiri Śaiva practice. The Aphorisms introduce us into a wonderful world of mystical experience to which we are invited to enter by the assiduous practice of the many forms

16 *Sanderson (1988: 137) has provided what has become a classic formulation of this progressive ascent as follows. The terms will become clear in the following pages.*

Tantras of Kālī
Śakti-tantras
Vidyāpīṭha
Bhairava-tantra
Trika-tantras
Yāmala-tantras
Mantrapīṭha
Śaiva Siddhānta

Sanderson writes: Whatever is above and to the left sees whatever is below and to the right as a lower revelation. [...] As we ascend through these levels, from the Mantrapīṭha to the Yāmala-tantras and thence to the Trika and the Kālī cult, we find the feminine rises stage by stage from subordination to complete autonomy.

17 *TĀ 29/183-185. See Dyczkowski 1985: 144*

18 *CMSS 1/3.*

19 *NT 8/41-45.*

of meditation taught in the Aphorisms. These wonderfully rich and inspiring meditations imply an equally rich view of reality that remained to be made explicit. This was done to some extent in the fifty-one verses of the Stanzas of Vibration possibly written by Vasugupta himself, but more likely by his disciple Kallaṭa Bhaṭṭa. Here we find an exposition of a number of essential features of Kashmiri Śaiva metaphysics and practice. Śiva (also called Śaṅkara) is all that exists. He is full of countless energies through which He does and becomes everything by expanding out into His cosmic form and to then withdraw it into the emptiness of His transcendental nature. Thus the first verse exclaims:

We salute that Śaṅkara Who is the source of the power of the Wheel of Energies by Whose expansion and contraction, the universe is absorbed and comes into being.

The commentators at first understood this 'expansion and contraction' to be the outpouring and withdrawal of Śiva's energies for 'all this universe is His powers and the Great God (Śiva) is their possessor'. Nonetheless, it was clear to all of them that it is Śiva Who 'expands and contracts', which the Stanzas equate with the opening and closing of His eyes. Thus right from the start the stage was set to understand this activity as the universal activity of consciousness, of which each act of perception of each perceiver is the microcosmic counterpart. But, as we shall see, this connection with consciousness and a theory of consciousness which supports it was yet to be worked out. Even so, the author of the Stanzas did understand that there is a vital connection between this universal activity and perception. This he explained using a model of perception drawn from the earlier dualist Siddhānta, which in its turn was inspired by the Sāmkhya, which preceded the development of the Tantras by several centuries. Whereas Kallaṭa maintains that there is only one reality, according to this view, there are two. One is the perceiver, who is pure consciousness. The other is the object in all its forms, ranging from the gross external, through to the mental. These Kallaṭa understood to be the agent and the product of his action[20]. He agreed that the latter - the object, which is the product of the agent - is perishable and transitory, whereas the former is not. But although they are opposites, this did not mean, according to him, that they are separate realities. The one reality is Śiva and these are the polarities of His being with which the opposites are conjoined. However, the relationship between them continued to be understood in the same, earlier terms. The perceiver and agent is pure consciousness that impels the activity of the body, senses and mind, through which it perceives and acts. This is because it possesses an 'inner strength' which is inherent in its own nature. Kallaṭa teaches that we have forgotten that we are the perceivers and agents and that we already possess this inner spiritual strength and its immense might. This same power flows through all the states of waking, dreaming and deep sleep, it infuses energy into Mantras and awakens the vital forces that lead the individual soul up into the higher states of consciousness along the ascending Path of the channel of Suṣumṇā that extends along the axis of the subtle body. What must be done then is to 'catch hold' of one's Self, that is, our own pure conscious nature, and regain possession of that strength which we already essentially possess. There is little talk of 'power' - Śakti - in this early phase of the development of the teachings.

The Sāmkhya taught much the same. The individual soul, which is one out of countless others, stimulates the activity of the sphere of objectivity, sensorial, mental and externally objective. The Sāmkhya in those early days of Indian philosophy did not know much about the nature of this power, only that consciousness had the capacity to do this[21]. The Siddhāntins, who took over the Sāmkhya model, adding to it Śiva as a third and highest reality, explored this capacity further and understood it to be the 'strength' of consciousness. By this time the concept of Śakti had been sufficiently understood to recognise that the activity of the sphere of objectivity is that of its many 'powers', physical, sensorial and mental. Indeed, the non-dualist schools understood the sphere of objectivity to be that of Śiva's Śakti, with which He is one. This the dualist Siddhāntins do not do. The 'strength' of consciousness impels the energies of objectivity, like a strong man who applies the power of his muscles to lift a heavy weight. In the same way, the senses are impelled to act by the 'strength' of the Self. They are not impelled to do this by the will alone because, clearly, there may be an intention or desire, but that can only be fulfilled if there is the capacity to do so. Thus the Stanzas teach how to 'catch hold' of this inner 'strength' by attending to the impulse which impels the senses. Again following the Siddhānta model, he teaches that this can only be done by the removal of the impurity that obscures the soul - the impurity which belongs to the sphere of objectivity. Ultimately Kallaṭa develops beyond the dualist model because it does not allow the possibility of freedom from the binding activity of objectivity. He discovers that the distinction between the two - subject and object, freedom and bondage - is in their location as it were, within oneness. The capacity - śakti - to act is experienced by the ignorant within the sphere of objectivity - the outer world, body, senses and mind. The Yogi, who looks inwards, discerns instead that it is within consciousness, the agent and perceiver.

20 SK 14.

21 Note that the word 'śakti' is commonly translated as 'energy' and even when it is translated with the word 'power', this 'power' is understood to be on the model of energy, like electricity. Although 'śakti' did come to be understood this way in India also, the original sense was power as 'capacity'. Thus, for example, the powers of the will, knowledge and action are the capacity to will, know and act.

That is its true place, its 'own path'. The well-known theory of Karma declares that we are bound by our actions - Karma. Kallaṭa agrees with this view, which is common to all schools of Indian thought, but adds an important proviso. What is binding is not action in itself, it is the mistake that activity is taking place outside consciousness, that is, the perceiver and the doer. Thus, he declares that the power to act is binding when it operates in the individual soul who is bound by his or her mistaken identification with the body, senses and mind, which are objective. Their activity in reality takes place within consciousness. Indeed, it is the activity of consciousness. He who recognises this, sees Śakti (in this case in the form of the power of action) on her 'own path', and is not bound. On the contrary, Śakti's activity is liberating, indeed, it came to be understood as the freedom (svātantrya) of consciousness to act spontaneously and freely.

This then is the central concept of Spanda, from which the Stanzas drew their name and came to be the designation of one of the major branches of Kashmiri Śaivism. It is so important that we can build part of our brief presentation of the development and schools of Kashmiri Śaivism around it. The word 'spanda' literally means 'pulsation' or 'vibration'. It is the activity of divine consciousness which is said to 'subtle' because, unlike gross action, it is not measured in time. On the contrary, as the universal activity of Śiva, Who is consciousness, it is the source of time, as it is of all things. Kallaṭa teaches that as all things arise out of Śiva consciousness and return to it, it cannot be obscured by them or by His universal activity. Activity is the very essence of all that exists. The entire universe expands and contracts as it rises out of the pure infinite consciousness of Śiva and returns to it. Within it, everything is in motion, from the vast galaxies right down to the tiniest pulse of subatomic particles. This activity, Kashmiri Śaivism maintains, is not the activity of some insentient matter or energy. It is the activity Śiva's consciousness.

In India the highest and most sacred reality is consciousness. All theistic schools, whether dualist or non-dualist, whoever be the supreme God, Śiva or Viṣṇu, or the supreme Goddess, Durgā, Kālī, or any other, all agree that the Deity's essential nature is consciousness. Consciousness in this theistic perspective is not just sacred, it is personal. This central insight illumines Kashmiri Śaivism. Consciousness, which is also our own most authentic and essential nature, is the vital link that connects us to God and the universe, which is His wonderful activity. Accordingly, the core of both the world view and practice of all schools of Kashmiri Śaivism is consciousness. The Śiva Sūtras and the Stanzas of Vibration (Spanda Kārikā), along with their commentaries, constitute the first of these schools which draws its name from its central teaching, that is, Spanda - the activity of Śiva consciousness. The next one is called Pratyabhijñā, which means 'Recognition'. This name is also derived from its central teaching, that is, the recognition of one's own fundamental identity with Śiva and that all that exists in any form is the manifestation of the power of His absolute freedom. In a strangely parallel fashion it is also the name of the work which expounds it, namely, the Stanzas of Recognition (Pratyabhijñā Kārikā). This too, like the Stanzas of Vibration, was the work of a great disciple - Utpaladeva - of the founder, Somānanda. We now turn to this school of Kashmiri as we follow the thread of the teachings concerning Śiva and consciousness.

Somānanda may have been a young contemporary of Vasugupta, or at least of his student Kallaṭa. Somānanda considered his teachings to be grounded in the Tantras and proudly professed it, but the language and perspective is not so much mystical, as is that of the Śivasūtras, it is more philosophical. It is a philosophy that does emerge as an explication of the metaphysics implicitly sustaining the kind of practices we have observed, but it is best understood as development in the history of Indian philosophy, rather than religion, even though the distinction between the two often disappears in what might be called a theology of Śaivism. In his great work, the Śivadṛṣṭi, the Vision of Śiva, Somānanda expounds the view, and sustains it with reasoned argument, that everything is Śiva. Above all Śiva is every one of us. Like an actor, Śiva assumes countless roles. As Somānanda puts it, a king may freely choose, if he so wishes, to play the part of a common foot soldier. Somānanda invokes Śiva accordingly at the very beginning of his work thus:

May Śiva who has penetrated my own (limited embodied) Self, concealing Himself by Himself pay homage to his (all) extensive Self by means of His own power.

According to Somānanda, Śiva is our own true Self and everything that exists because He is the one pure consciousness which, although it rests within itself, and so does not change, is engaged in making all things manifest. This takes place through each act of perception, which is the activity of consciousness. This is its power to act and know, which, together with its omnipotent will, make up the freedom of consciousness to be all things without being subject to change or limitation. There can be no differences, divisions or distinctions within consciousness. We do refer to 'my consciousness' and distinguish it from 'your consciousness', but this difference pertains to the psychophysical organism with which it is mistakenly identified. All predication of things as 'this' or 'that' relates to objectivity. Consciousness is purely subjective. It cannot be defined as 'this' or 'that'. Moreover, according to this idealist view, an object is an object because it is known by a subject. It can have no independent existence apart from consciousness, whereas consciousness does not require another consciousness to know it. If consciousness were to be known as an object, it would no longer be consciousness. We have seen that this basic axiom, which we can easily ascertain from our own experience, justifies the dualist view of the Sāmkhya and Śaiva Siddhānta. Somānanda avoids this dualism by understanding that consciousness could not perceive, or indeed act, if there were nothing to see or act upon. But the object of perception and action cannot be separate from consciousness. Otherwise how could consciousness know it and act upon it? There can be no relationship between two totally different realities. So Somānanda concludes that the one consciousness is both subject and object. The object known by consciousness is consciousness itself. The jar, he declares, knows its perceiver, as it were, by being known to him. The object is always known to be such as it is by a perceiver. They know each other in the sense that the perceiver knows himself to be the perceiver of the jar and the jar knows itself to be the object of the perceiver's perception. The knowledge of the former is grounded in itself and that of the latter in the other. Thus, the perceiver knows that he knows, whereas the jar does not. Moreover, as perception is an activity the perceiver is its agent. The jar is the product of action applied to its material cause by an agent. The potter has made the jar from clay. All phenomena are, like the jar, products generated from a cause. Dualists consider the material from which phenomena are made to be, as it were, the stuff of objectivity, which is both physical, from which outer objects are made, and mental, from which inner mental objects are made. This, they say, is inert, devoid of consciousness. The Sāmkhya does not believe in a creator God and so maintains that the jar is produced by the clay and by the potter who is himself, as it were, psychophysical clay, with the difference that he is illumined by consciousness whereas the physical clay is not. The dualist Siddhānta, who are theists, maintain that the Deity acts through the potter. Somānanda maintains that for this to be possible the three - Deity, potter and clay - must be one and the same consciousness in these three forms. This is because, as is the case with perception, if they were to be separate realities they could not interact. Thus, in terms of causality, consciousness is at once the causal agent (the potter), the material cause (the clay), activity (of the potter's wheel, hands, etc.) and the effect (the jar) they produce.

Somānanda has much more to say in his rich and complex work but these few points are sufficient to illustrate the seeds he sowed that developed from the Vision of Śiva in the Doctrine of Recognition (pratyabhijñā) forged by Utpaladeva, Somānanda's disciple. Utpaladeva extends the insight of his teacher by analysing thoroughly the nature of consciousness, perception and the manifestations of consciousness as each particular that appears within it. Moreover, he establishes his view on sound philosophical ground by defending it against opponents, in particular the Buddhists, who deny the existence of a permanent consciousness or indeed anything else. This means that both an unchanging consciousness and the world are illusory. They are mistaken notions, that is, thought constructs, without any reference beyond themselves. Accordingly, Utpaladeva frames his exposition as a debate with the Buddhists in order to establish both the existence of a permanent consciousness, which he identifies with Śiva and the Self, and the reality of the world. He achieves this by expanding Somānanda's vision by explicating his implicit, incompletely formulated insights and filling them out with his own. Thus he seeks to establish what he calls a New Path which he defines as the 'Discovery of Śakti'. This is what he means by the 'recognition' of the identity of Śiva, whom we learn about from the scriptures, with consciousness, the Self and the world. Utpaladeva gives the example of a young woman who hears about the fine qualities of a prince and falls in love with him, even though she has never seen him. One day she is walking in the market place with her female companions and the prince happens to be there. Although she sees him, she feels nothing for him until one of her friends tells her that he is the prince she has heard so much about and then she immediately feels love for him. The prince is, of course, Śiva, the woman, the fettered soul, and her companions are the powers of consciousness. By discovering that we see, act and will by the power of consciousness and that the world around us, like our thoughts and feelings, are all manifestations that appear within consciousness by virtue of its inscrutable, miraculous power, we recognise that consciousness is Śiva and that He is who we really are.

Utpaladeva's metaphysics and theology was adopted by subsequent Kashmiri Śaivites, following the lead of the greatest of them, Abhinavagupta, as the underlying implicit view of the Tantras. The Buddhists considered their Tantras to be direct continuations of the earlier forms of Buddhism, especially those of the Mahāyāna, the Great Vehicle. Thus they could refer to the preceding Buddhist philosophy directly to support and explain the teachings of the Buddhist Tantras. Although later Hindu Tantric schools did view their Tantras in an analogous way as being continuations of the Vedic scriptures (especially the Upaniṣads) and the philosophies that took them as their authorities, early Hindu Tantric schools (i.e. those prior to the 12th century), Śaiva, Vaiṣṇava and Śākta, did not. All of them in varying degrees and with their own modifications, great and small, came to adopt Utpaladeva's philosophy. Some did this *in toto*, for example, the Śrīvidyā tradition of the goddess Tripurā, very well known for its distinctive Cakra with many triangles. Others adapted it to their own metaphysics and/or in just some branches of their traditions. An example is the Vaiṣṇava Lakṣmī Tantra, which draws very extensively from the Pratyabhijñā, although many other Vaiṣṇava Tantras of these schools (the Pañcarātra) hardly do so at all. Clearly, as the Pratyabhijñā was only formulated in the 10th century by Utpaladeva, Tantras and their corresponding schools did not do so prior to this time. The Muslim invasion of northern India and Kashmir in particular brought about huge changes in the political, cultural and religious environment. Hindu patronage that supported Hinduism in all its forms, including Tantric, weakened considerably as political power passed into Muslim hands. As a result the Kashmiri Śaiva tradition was almost lost in Kashmir and ceased to exert its direct influence outside. However, the Śrīvidyā tradition continued to flourish in the south of

India far from the Muslim domination in the north. Through that, Kashmiri Śaivism, which supplied its theoretical framework, survived as the dominant, most sophisticated philosophy of the non-dualist Śākta Tantrism. This philosophy was essentially Utpaladeva's Pratyabhijñā, to which we now briefly turn.

Utpaladeva's Doctrine of Recognition is based on a few central concepts embodied in the technical terms that denote them, which we will examine. The first of these is the term 'prakāśa', which literally means light. Universal consciousness is Mahāprakāśa, the Great Light, which illumines all things. This idea, which is clearly derived from a primary, direct experience of ultimate reality, is already found in the oldest Upaniṣads which date back to the last centuries BC. So it is not new. What is new is the systematic application of this analogy to perception and the manifestation of phenomena. The light of consciousness illumines every perceiver, perception and the object of perception. Indeed, they are aspects of its shining, what Utpaladeva calls 'spuraṇa' or 'sphurattā', the effulgent pulse of the light of consciousness. This is Spanda, the dynamism of the activity of consciousness, which emits, sustains and withdraws all things. All that appears in any form in the three domains of the perceiver, act of perception and their object, is a configuration of countless, one could say atomic, manifestations. The term for them is ābhāsa, which is derived from the root bhā - to shine. These 'shinings', that is, manifestations, come together and separate in countless ways every moment to make up the beautiful radiant picture of experience which is the effulgent pulse - sphurattā - of the light of consciousness. This takes place spontaneously by virtue of the freedom of consciousness. This freedom is the universal power of consciousness, which contains all its countless powers. The term for this freedom is 'svātantrya', which literally means 'self-dependence'. It is the opposite of 'parātantrya', which means 'dependence on another'. The autonomy of consciousness, as Utpaladeva understands it, is not just its detachment or independence from all that is not consciousness, as the dualists believe, it is a positive power or capacity 'to do the impossible' (atighaṭakāritva). And what could be more 'impossible' and miraculous than the shining of the Light as all things without it thereby suffering any change or limitation. Other non-dualist schools, the Hindu Advaita Vedānta, and non-dualist Buddhists, safeguard the oneness of reality by teaching that the world of multiplicity and duality is an illusion which cannot, therefore, impinge on the oneness of ultimate reality. This view does not suit the Tantric Śaivite Utpaladeva who, with great devotion, views the world as Śiva's creation. Śiva's 'independence' is His freedom to will, know and act in every way without compromising His identity as pure, transcendental consciousness, on the one hand, and the world, including every soul that inhabits it, on the other.

This leads to another fundamental concept and term Utpaladeva uses for the first time, namely, 'vimarśa'. This term and its common synonyms, āmarśa, pratyavamarśa and parāmarśa, are derived from the root mṛś, which means to reflect, cogitate, discern, contemplate and the like. I translate the word as 'reflective awareness'. I use the word 'awareness' to distinguish it from the consciousness of which it is the awareness. Several schools of thought in India maintain that a 'pure' consciousness exists which is not 'sullied', as it were, by objectivity. Utpaladeva also teaches this, but whereas other schools maintain that this is possible only when consciousness is not in contact with an object, Utpaladeva says that consciousness is always 'pure' because it itself manifests as the object. There is nothing separate from consciousness that can sully it. Only the one pure Light shines as all things. The other schools say that this not possible because, obviously, objects are perceived. According to the dualists they belong to the sphere of objectivity, which is a separate reality. Non-dualist Vedānta, that also maintains, like Utpaladeva, that there is no separate reality, affirms instead that objectivity is an illusion. We have seen that Utpaladeva maintains that Light has the power, its inherent freedom, to do this. And this is its power to reflect on itself, which the other schools would say is impossible, for that would reduce consciousness to an object. But this is indeed its freedom 'to do the impossible'. The Light of consciousness views its countless manifestations within itself as itself. Thus this 'awareness' is 'reflective' in both senses of the word. One is that it 'reflects' on the manifestations of its own Light and knows what they are as 'this' and 'that', object, perceiver or perception. This specific and specifying knowledge is embodied in thought constructs and within the realm in which individual perceivers 'reflect on', that is, perceive their objects. The Light also 'reflects' back on itself. The direct experience Śiva, the light of consciousness, has of Himself as all things is His awareness that reflects back onto Himself. Śiva's reflective awareness is His freedom, namely, His independence of all causes and conditions with respect to His being all things. It is also the effluent pulse of His cosmic manifestation and radiance of the Light that thereby illumines itself. In short, the reflective awareness, freedom and the effulgent radiance of the Light are its power - Śakti, the discovery of which is 'recognition'. How is that? The reflective awareness of the Light is the pure 'I' consciousness of the supreme subjectivity that Śiva has of Himself as the transcendental 'I am' and its immanent aspects - 'I am all this universe' and 'all this universe is me'. This is the supreme subject's supreme subjectivity. The limited form of subjectivity that results due to ignorance of this higher subjectivity and mistaken identification with the body senses and mind, and the ignorance which envelops individual consciousness, is essentially this same subjectivity. However, the contraction of consciousness brought about in this way subjects it to the trammels of the body and personality, which are really objective, not subjective, and so are ultimately, inevitably destined to come to an end.

Finally, it's important to note that this reflective awareness at all levels of subjectivity and its corresponding levels of objectivity is understood to be Speech. This is a very important dimension of reflective awareness. From the very beginnings of Indian thought, Speech was considered to be the source of all creation. The early Vedic Indians believed that the world was created through the performance of the Vedic sacrifice. The Vedic sacrifice consists essentially of the offering of food in the sacrificial fire to the Vedic gods. The offerings and associated ritual actions are accompanied by the intonation of hymns from the Vedas, the earliest parts of which are probably not less than 4,000 years old. The hymns and all else that forms a part of the Vedic scriptures are called Mantras, a word which literally means 'invocation'. The sound of the recitation of Vedic Mantras has an awesome numenous quality which is so powerful and inwardly penetrating that it is not surprising that the Vedic Indians believed that the universe was created through them. We have observed several examples of the basic idea that the world is a manifestation of an originally unmanifest potential, whether it be understood, as the dualists do, of the physical-cum-mental 'substance' of objectivity or, as non-dualists do, of consciousness. The earliest example of this fundamental idea that the world is a manifestation, in the sense of an actualisation, of an original potential hidden in some ultimate reality, is the Vedic belief that the world is generated by the intonation of the Vedas. The silence that precedes them and which abides, one could say, as their fundamental sustaining ground, is where the Vedas rest in their original unmanifest form. The Brahman, a well-known word that came to mean the Absolute in Vedic times, originally denoted the invocation of the Vedic Mantras. Those who uttered them are called Brahmins. Thus the Vedic Absolute was implicitly understood, amongst other things, from the earliest times, as the essence of the Vedas. And the Vedas are Speech. Accordingly, a famous Vedic hymn praises the beauty of the goddess Speech who is portrayed as a young woman whose clothes hang loose so as to reveal some of her body and hide the rest. The image illustrates how, as the Vedas say, a quarter of Speech is here 'below' and three quarters 'above'.

Speculation concerning the nature of Speech developed extensively from many aspects. One of the major results was a sophisticated theory of language expounded by a great grammarian and philosopher called Bhartṛhari who probably lived in the 4th or 5th century AD. He maintained that the Brahman - the Absolute - is the Word - Śabda. This word Absolute - the Śabda Brahman - is the one reality, that is, all things that can be expressed by language of which it is the sum total contained within it as innumerable energies or potencies (śaktis)[22]. Bhartṛhari understands this original language to be Sanskrit and its complex grammar to be, therefore, the very structure of reality. According to him, the summation of these (female) potencies are the (female) Speech of the (male) Śabda Brahman by virtue of which It knows Itself to the speaker (i.e. agent) and knower of Speech. Thus Bhartṛhari states that Speech (vāc - a feminine word like 'śakti') reflects on itself and uses (although just in one place) a form of the term vimarśa that, as we have seen, Utpaladeva uses extensively. There can be no doubt that he has taken it from Bhartṛhari. Indeed, he even quotes the verse in which Bhartṛhari defines it as the power of Speech. Bhartṛhari taught that there are three levels of Speech. The grossest is audible, Corporeal (vaikhari) Speech. Next, subtler than that, is the Middle (madhyamā) Speech through which thoughts are inwardly articulated in the intellect. The third, which he considered the highest, is the Speech of Vision (paśyantī). This is the reflective awareness to which he referred that 'sees' the inner contents of consciousness, that is, the energies of the Word, which it views with the intent to combine them to form the array of phenomena, physical and mental, their interrelationships, activities and the rest that constitute the universe of words and meanings. Utpaladeva accepts this formulation but adds another level that he calls Supreme Speech. This is a very significant development in this philosophy of language. Supreme Speech according to Utpaladeva is the pure awareness of 'I am' of the light of consciousness. Thus manifestation is not just the 'shining' of the Light we have examined, it is also a kind of 'speaking'. The innermost utterance of 'I am' flows out through the three levels of Speech into outer expression. When it is Śiva Who speaks, the 'meanings' (artha) of His words are the 'things' (artha) of the outer physical world and the inner mental one. This notion not only serves as the basis of the theory of the nature of things (ontology) and how we know them (epistemology), it also serves to explain the nature and power of Mantras.

Here then is an example of the application of Utpaladeva's Doctrine of Recognition to the explanation (hermeneutics) of the teachings of the Tantras. Much of the teachings of the Tantras of all schools is concerned with Mantra. The Tantras which, as we have seen, began to be revealed around the 6th century AD, developed in all their schools, for at least five centuries, independently of the Vedas. Although they retained practically all the fundamental underlying presuppositions of the Vedic world, above all the power of Speech, they applied them in a novel way, and almost entirely new Mantras, which like the earlier Vedic Mantras, are believed to be so potent that the universe is created through them. Kashmiri Śaivites, applying Utpaladeva's philosophy, could now explain why and how this happens.

So we have seen that the first school of Kashmiri Śaivism taught the Doctrine of Vibration - Spanda, and the second, the Doctrine of Recognition - Pratyabhijñā. We now turn to the remaining two,

22 It is interesting to note in passing that here we have one of the earliest uses of the term 'śakti' and certainly its first detailed philosophical exposition.

namely, Krama and Trika. It is most convenient to deal with Trika first. This came to be understood as encompassing all of the Kashmiri Śaiva schools. So much so that Trika is virtually a synonym of Kashmiri Śaivism. Trika, like Krama, differ from the first two schools in that they are in a literal sense originally Tantric. By this I mean that they began and grew in their first stages of development as traditions taught and transmitted through their own Tantras. Therefore in their case we cannot refer to original authors, we talk instead of lineages of teachers beginning with the Deity who revealed the Tantra and imparted the initiation taught in these Tantras to the first teachers, who then imparted them to their disciples.

We may contrast this situation with the Śiva Sūtras. These too, as we have seen, are revelation, but do not present themselves as a Tantra of any particular school. Indeed, it is hard to determine the scriptural sources that may have inspired them. It is most likely that this was a uniquely original revelation, nonetheless, the Aphorisms were soon, if not from the beginning, understood to be Trika teachings. At this early stage of development of Kashmiri Śaivism, its connection with Trika is apparently made clear and explicit (according to later Kashmiri Śaivites), not by Vasugupta, as one would expect (as the Śiva Sūtras are revelation), but by Somānanda who wrote a philosophical treatise. Somānanda tells us with great reverence at the end of his work how the teachings of non-dual Śaivism that he expounds belong to the lineage of the Tryambaka, who received them from Śrīkaṇṭha, a form of Śiva, through his 'mind born' son Durvāsa. Tryambaka transmitted them through his spiritual daughter who founded a lineage called Ardhatryambaka (Half Tryambaka), through which it flowed on down to Somānanda. These teachings, not directly scriptural, although from an original divine source, came to be identified with the Trika teachings taught in the Tantras of the Trika school, namely, the Siddhayogeśvarīmata, and other Tantras mentioned above. The early mystical revelations of the Śiva Sūtras and the soteriological and philosophical reflections of the Stanzas of Vibration were also implicitly connected to the Trika school by the latter Kashmiri Śaiva teachers. There was no explicit justification for this association, but by the time we reach Kṣemarāja, Abhinavagupta's disciple and last in the series of commentators, it is fully accepted. Thus Kṣemarāja understood the Sūtras, and hence the Stanzas, which he saw to be directly derived from them, to be 'the secret of the secret doctrines' (rahasyopaniṣad) taught by the Siddhas (accomplished Tantric Yogis) and Yoginīs. Kṣemarāja was a fully initiated Trika Śaivite who considered Trika to be the most elevated Tantric school. This means, from these Śaivites' perspective, that it is the most secret. Thus Kṣemarāja is referring to the Sūtras and Stanzas as Trika works. Within this Trika framework he, like his teacher Abhinavagupta, perceives another 'most secret' tradition, namely the Krama, which we shall have occasion to examine further ahead. To what extent later Kashmiri Śaivites projected their preference for Trika Śaivism onto the earlier teachings is hard to say. There can be no doubt, however, that for Abhinavagupta, who was four generations on from Vasugupta, this was certainly true. A vast range of Tantric traditions flourished in Kashmir at this time. It was, as it still is, essential to follow one teacher who is venerated as the best and belonging to one school considered to be the highest. Even so, Trika Śaivites were encouraged to learn from everybody. Abhinavagupta quotes a Tantra as saying:

Just as a bee, greedy for honey, goes from flower to flower, so a disciple, desirous of knowledge, goes from teacher to teacher. If he has a Master devoid of power how can he ever attain knowledge and liberation? O Goddess, how can a tree without roots bear flowers or fruit?

Abhinavagupta himself was the prime example of the 'greedy bee'. He tells us that he studied at the feet of numerous teachers, even Buddhist and Vaiṣṇava. He learnt Pratyabhijñā from Lakṣmaṇagupta, a direct disciple of Utpaladeva, and contributed long complex commentaries to Utpaladeva's work. From other teachers he studied literary criticism and dramaturgy. He wrote extensive and authoritative commentaries on the Dhvanyālocana (the Reflections on Suggestion) by the Kashmiri Ānandavardhana, one of the greatest works on Sanskrit poetics. He also wrote a long commentary on the Nāṭyaśāstra, the root text on Sanskrit Drama. His most extensive contribution, however, was to Trika Śaivism. He received initiation into Trika from Śambhunātha, who, we are told, came from Jālandhara, which may have been in the Punjab. Śambhunātha received it from Sumati who lived in the Deccan (dakṣiṇapatha)[23]. Abhinavagupta believed Trika to be the highest spiritual tradition in India. In accord with a system of ranking found in the Tantras themselves, he believed all the scriptures, starting from the Vedas, to have been revealed by Śiva. Revelation is a process of a progressively heightening vision of ultimate truth that manifests in the teachings of the scriptures of progressively elevated schools. The progression is such that what follows accepts the authority of what precedes and so contains it in a higher revelation. In this way, the teachings of the highest school include those of the others. Abhinavagupta, entreated by his disciples and inspired by the Deity, took up the task of expounding the teachings

23 *The Jain Somadeva confirms that Trika was known in South India during the 10th century. Somadeva identifies the followers of the Trika school as Kaulas who worship Śiva in the company of their Tantric consorts by offering him meat and wine. As one would expect, Somadeva was very critical of Trika Kaulas. "If liberation," he says, "were the result of loose, undisciplined life, then thugs and butchers would surely sooner attain to it than these Kaulas!" (The Yaśastilaka and Indian Culture by K.K. Handiqui, Sholapur, 1949, p. 204). We discuss the Trika's Kaula identity below.*

of this full integral Trika, which he called Anuttara Trika Kula. Abhinavagupta expounds the teachings of Anuttara Trika Kula in several important and very rich texts of which the main one is his great Tantrāloka, the Light of the Tantras - certainly one of the most important books ever written in India and one of the most extensive and rich works of any Tantric school. At the beginning of his work, Abhinavagupta defines it as a liturgical manual (paddhati) of the Anuttara Trika Kula[24] and he writes it in order that he and others may worship Śiva[25]. Moreover, he claims that there is nothing in it that is not contained in some way in the Mālinīvijayottara Tantra, which teaches the essence of Trika which is, in the manner just explained, the essence of all the Śaiva Tantras[26]. In this way, identifying, on the one hand, all preceding forms of Kashmiri Śaivism with Trika, as well as entire teachings of the Śaiva scriptures, on the other, Abhinavagupta's exposition of his Anuttara Trika is a synthesis. His Tantrāloka is 'a compendium of the essence of the whole of the Trika teachings'[27] and, from that perspective, of all Tantric Śaivism.

This does not mean that whatever is said in all the Śaiva traditions is all correct. Indeed, Abhinavagupta dedicates a good deal of space in his Tantrāloka to refute what he considers to be wrong views, including those of other Śaivites. He even sometimes rejects the view of one Śaiva scripture in preference for another. But how can there be inconsistencies, yes - even mistakes, in the scriptures? From Abhinavagupta's integral perspective they are not really inconsistencies or mistakes, simply incomplete revelation which attains fullness progressively as we ascend through the hierarchy of revelation. Lower revelations are completed, not contradicted, by higher ones. The view is (somewhat idealised) that scriptures at the initial level teach dualism (bheda), those above them unity-in-difference (bhedābheda), and then, non-dualism. These are the Śiva, Rudra and Bhairava Tantras respectively. From this perspective, the Trika scriptures, which emerge from the Bhairava Tantras, teach the most complete non-dualism because it includes the others. Indeed, this is one of the reasons why it is called Trika - the Triad - because it includes all views, dualist, dual-cum-non-dualist and non-dualist. These are the triad of domains of the Individual Soul (Nara), Śakti and Śiva, governed by the three goddesses Aparā (the Lower One), Parāparā (Higher-cum-Lower One) and Parā (the Supreme) respectively.

We have some idea about Trika. What does Abhinavagupta mean by Kula? The most literal, non-technical sense of the word 'kula' is 'family'. In this context a 'kula' is the spiritual family of a teacher or deity. A person can belong to this or that Kula, as do the teachings transmitted through it. Thus a Kula in this sense can be named after the original deity who taught it. While this could be a general way of referring to a lineage or school, the term is reserved for those that are associated with the Bhairava Tantras. We noted that the earliest Kulas mentioned in the Bhairava Tantras are associated with eight Mother Goddesses (Mātṛkā) who are symbolically arranged in the eight directions. Accordingly, they drew their names from those of the goddesses. Originally, and probably just one of many ways of enriching the variety of iconic forms and the assembly (maṇḍala) of the pantheon, the teachings of the Kulas came to be understood as the most secret of the esoteric Bhairava Tantras. Teaching the most secret modality (prakriyā) of the tantric modality of practice (tantraprakriyā), they came to assume an extensive identity of their own, first within the Bhairava Tantras and then, as we have noted already, they ultimately developed independently of them.

A major figure in this development was a Yogi called Matsyendranātha who lived, perhaps, around the 8th century, when he first appears in the Tantras as the recipient of Kula teachings. By this time, they were already well represented in the Bhairava Tantras and a number of Kulas had developed. They were generally focused on the worship of goddesses; the most extensive centred on the worship of forms of Kālī, to which we shall return. These were most developed in a class of Bhairava Tantras called Mata Tantras, which were the immediate precursors of Kula Tantras in their own right. This development was traditionally linked with the figure of Matsyendranātha. He is of such great importance in this respect that the Kashmiri teachers, including Abhinavagupta himself, considered him to be the founder of Kaulism (kulāvatāraka), although this cannot be literally true. We have seen that the outer rites of the Bhairava Tantra that were dedicated to fierce deities and often performed in cremation grounds, involved sexual intercourse and the consumption of meat and wine. It appears from the texts we have received attributed to Matsyendranātha that he reformed these practices by internalising them and detaching them from the worship of specific deities. He represents the highest reality as an abstract energy called Kula, and Bhairava as the transcendental possessor of that power, as the abstract 'non-Kula' - Akula - beyond it as its source. This was the revelation of, we might say, the non-sectarian Matsyendranātha. At the same time he was considered to be the first teacher in this Age of Strife (kaliyuga) of all forms of Kaulism and so, as such, the developing Kulas, centred

24 TĀ 1/14.

25 TĀ 1/21.

26 TĀ 1/18.

27 nikhilaṣaḍardhaśāstrasārasaṃgrahabhūtagrantha - commentary on TĀ 1/1.

on the worship of goddesses, came to adopt him as their original founder. He was understood to have imparted the original, generic Kula teachings he received from the Deity to his disciples, who in turn went on to teach others that founded particular Kulas.

We can see from the name that Abhinavagupta's version of Trika is a Kula. This is not the case in the earliest Tantras that taught Trika doctrine. The Siddhayogeśvarīmata, which is considered to be the prime authority from which the Mālinīvijayottara says it is derived, is the oldest Trika Tantra. It is also one of the oldest Bhairava Tantras. At that early stage of development of the Bhairava Tantras, Kulas had not yet formed. By Abhinavagupta's time, Trika was understood to be the highest at the end of series of types that included Kula[28]. Trika itself was a Kula as the name of a text Abhinavagupta quotes - the Trikakula[29] - testifies. However, the Mālinīvijayottara, which was probably redacted before this identification had been fully made, does not think of Trika as a Kula. Instead, we find that it teaches Kula practice (kulācāra) separately. We have seen that the term Kula was used in the early Śaiva Tantras to denote the most secret teachings, and this is how it appears in the Mālinīvijayottara. This too is how Abhinava presents Kula teachings as part of his Anuttara Trika Kula, that is, as a modality (prakriyā) of practice, along with the Tantric one (tantraprakriyā), for some adepts who are fit for it, which he does in a separate chapter of the Tantrāloka. At the same time, this modality of practice, which involves, as we said, the offering and consumption of meat, wine and sexual fluids, recurs throughout the Tantrāloka, although generally in the context of expositions of the inner transformations of consciousness and the vital breath. In this way, the Anuttara Trika of the Tantrāloka reflects the Trika schools of the scriptures, where we are told that Kula pervades them like oil in the sesame seed, scent in the flower or the soul in the body.

Abhinava's expanded Trika mirrors the Tantras in another way. At the most basic level of the Tantric modality, Abhinava incorporates Siddhānta-like ritual and cosmology which he mostly draws from the Svacchandabhairava Tantra, a Bhairava Tantra which is very similar in these respects to the Siddhānta in general. At the highest most secret level of the Kula modality, he illumines Trika with the Kālī Kula teachings, as had already taken place in the Tantras of some branches of the Trika. My teacher, Swami Lakshmanjoo from Kashmir, used to say that 'Śakti is the secret of Śaivism'. He was referring in particular to Kālī. Dark goddesses already appear in the Vedic corpus, for example, the goddess Kālarātri (Dark Night) and Nairṛti (the Nefarious One). What became names of Kālī are said in the Katha Upaniṣad to be those of seven flaming tongues of Agni, the god Fire. Kālī is known to the Baudhāyanagṛhyasūtra as Bhadrakālī. There we are told that, like the earlier Kālarātri, she should be worshipped before going to sleep at the head of the bedstead for sound, untroubled sleep. But although the Dark Goddess was known to the Sanskrit sources, and may well have been a popular folk goddess, She appears in the Bhairava Tantras suddenly, as it were, with great force, in the Jayadrathayāmala. This great seminal revelation, as yet unpublished, is divided into four sections of about six thousand verses each. Written in chronological order, very probably in Kashmir, they document the early developments of what came to be the Kālī Kula. The Kālī Kula, also called Kālī Krama, emerged in the Kashmiri Śaivism as one of its schools, which we refer to in English as the Krama system.[30]

The word 'krama' means most literally 'sequence', 'progression', 'process' or 'series'. The primary sense can be applied to the 'sequence' of teachers and hence means 'lineage of teachers' (gurukrama). It can also mean the 'sequence of deities' (devatākrama) worshipped in a liturgy or those that constitute a hierarchy in a pantheon. The same word is also used to mean a 'liturgy' in the sense that a liturgy is a series - krama - of ritual actions that accompany the sequence of Mantras used to invoke a series of deities. Finally, in the most subtle extension of the term krama, it refers to the sequence of subtle centres and states that mark the stations of development of the inner energies of the body, gross and subtle, senses, vital breath and consciousness. Thus, by extension, 'krama' came to mean a particular tradition with its lineage, deities, rites, Mantras, Yogic practices and states. Although this term is used to mean a 'liturgy' in general, it came to be specifically reserved for Kula schools. Accordingly we can refer to the Kālī Kula as the Kālī Krama.[31]

28 *Jayaratha in his commentary on the TĀ quotes an unknown source as saying: 'Śaiva (scripture is greater) than the Veda, then that of the left, then the right, then Kula, then Mata and then Trika which is the most excellent. Again, a teacher who knows the supreme reality needs to be initiated into the Bhairava (Tantras), then into Kula, Kaula and (then finally) also Trika.' Commentary on TĀ 1/18.*

29 *Abhinava quotes from a text called Trikakula quoted in TĀ 26/20, 28/15,51 and 31/60.*

30 *In the Sanskrit sources we find various names for the 'Krama system'. The most common are Kramanaya (Krama Doctrine), Mahānaya (the Great Doctrine), Kramadarśana (Krama Philosophy), Kramārtha (Krama Teaching) and Mahārtha (the Great Teaching).*

31 *See Dyczkowski 1985 pp. 75-77.*

The Jayadrathayāmala is a Bhairava Tantra of the Mata variety that presents an astonishing variety of Kālīs. In a way, one could say that the Yoginīs that proliferate in immense numbers in other schools of the Bhairava Tantras are here called Kālīs, or at least, are a particular type of Yoginī. Yoginīs are the most prominent members of the immense hoard of Bhairava's attendants in the various schools of the Bhairava Tantras of the Vidyāpīṭha. Amongst them some rise to prominence and become Great Goddesses endowed with the attributes of Supreme Deity. One can think of the hoards of Yoginīs in this respect as a pleroma and source of feminine Divine Forms. Thus amongst these countless Kālīs a number of them emerged over time as Supreme Goddesses. The first of these is Kālasaṃkarṣiṇī (the Attractress of Time), followed later by Siddhalakṣmī and Guhyakālī. Kālasaṃkarṣiṇī was the Kālī of the Anuttara Trika in Kashmiri. The other two became popular in Nepal and are still worshipped there.

We have seen that the triad of Trika goddesses - Parā (the Supreme One), Parāparā (the Middling One) and Aparā (the Lower One) - are worshipped on the prongs of Śiva's Trident. This Trident is the centre of the Trika Maṇḍala which, like the main Maṇḍala of any Tantric system, is the primary focus of worship. Abhinavagupta follows the lead of a branch of Trika Tantras which acknowledge the supremity of the goddess Kālasaṃkarṣiṇī who, called Beyond the Supreme (Parātītā), is worshipped above Parā.[32] Kālī is the Goddess Who embodies the power of time (kāla). In the microcosmic psychophysical body, the cycles of time manifest in and through the breathing. The vital breath (prāṇa) is the first transformation of consciousness. Consciousness begins its descent into the manifestation of the universe of subjects and objects, as the Breath. Withdrawing first into itself, as it were, absolute consciousness leaves behind the emptiness of absence, which it then pours out into as the flow of the vital breath. This flow is the flux of the power of time. Kālasaṃkarṣiṇī (She Who Attracts Time) is the form of Kālī Who absorbs time into pure eternal consciousness by withdrawing the breath back into it. Abhinava quotes a Tantra that teaches how this is done:

The Attractress of Time (Kālasaṃkarṣiṇī), who resides in the face at the extremity of the nose[33], measures inhalation and exhalation constantly and so attracts (lit. drags - karṣati) the triple time into the heart[34]. By means of inhalations, she induces it to enter; by halting the breath, checks it; and by exhalation, consumes it. Rising up by the ascending breath[35], (she devours it ultimately) completely, in an instant. This power of the will who is called Supreme and awakens the three energies (of will, knowledge and action) is worthy of worship as she attracts all the vital breath which is the foundation of time[36].

The teachings of the Krama (i.e. Kālī Kula or Kālī Krama) flowed into Kashmiri Śaivism in two main forms. One was called the Great Teaching (Mahānaya) or the Great Reality (Mahārtha). It teaches in great detail the nature and function of the progressive unfolding - krama - of the energies of the transcendental Emptiness of pure consciousness. The universal pulsation of consciousness (sāmānyaspanda) manifests in this way as five cycles or particular pulses of power (viśeṣaspanda) represented by concentric circles. These circles symbolise the states of individualised consciousness from the subtlest, most subjective, to the grossest, most objective. They are 1) the centre of absolute consciousness which is cosmic motion transfigured into the inner revolving power of pure consciousness, 2) the circle of the Khecarī energies which constitute the individual subject, 3) the Gocarī energies of the inner mental organ, 4) the Dikcarī energies of the senses, and 5) the Bhūcarī energies of the outer objects of the senses[37].

The other form of the Krama, which is the one Abhinavagupta syncretises into his Anuttara Trika Kula, centres on the cycle (cakra

32 *See TĀ 3/89 and commentary, also ibid. 15/335cd. The main authority to which Abhinava repeatedly refers for this syncretism is the Devyāyāmala (also called Devīyāmala), especially the section in it that deals with the Sacrifice of the Warlocks (ḍāmarayāga). The passage quoted below is drawn from there.*

33 *Presumably the entrance to the nostrils is meant here.*

34 *The goddess induces time to pass constantly from the extremity of the nose to the heart and back. The three times (i.e. past, present and future) are the exhaled breath (prāṇa), inhaled breath (apāna) and the 'rising' breath (udāna) that ascends between them as Kuṇḍalinī.*

35 *According to Jayaratha this is a form of exhalation that flows through suṣumṇā passing through the causal forces.*

36 *TĀ 15/336-338.*

37 *There are three different texts called Mahānayaprakāśa – Light of the Great Teaching – which expound this form of the Krama, technically called the Five-fold Current (Pañcavāha). I have edited one of them, which is by Arṇa Siṃha, from the sole existing (Nepalese) manuscript and translated it into English. This can be downloaded from the website markdkashi.com. Here the interested reader will find a concise, detailed exposition of the Five-fold Current.*

- 'wheel') of Twelve Kālīs[38]. The cycle of Kālīs encompasses both the cycles of perception and time. The standard framework in which Kālī, the Goddess of Time, is worshipped are the cycles of emanation, persistence and withdrawal. To these is added a fourth state called the 'Inexplicable' (anākhya), which is Kālī Herself Who both contains all the cycles of time and is beyond them. The scriptures teach numerous variants based on this model. Treating each phase of emanation and the rest as a cycle or 'wheel' - cakra - in its own right, forms of Kālī are worshipped in them. From another perspective, but still temporal, the four 'wheels of Kālīs' represent other markers of time. These are the Sun, Moon and Fire (which is lit at fixed times of day), along with the Fourth, which is the perennial transcendental 'Inexplicable' Light that illumines and contains the other three. As we have seen, Kālī is the vital breath. Accordingly, these cycles flow with the breath, which measures the time of life. Here Abhinavagupta provides another dimension. Kālī, the energy of consciousness, is all this because She is the pure reflective awareness of Śiva's 'I' consciousness. As such, Kālī also flows from the perceiver out through the senses to their objects. Thus there are three polarities: the subject, means of knowledge, and object. All three arise, persist, fall away and enter the Fourth State, thus making twelve altogether. The practice requires attention to all these phases in every act of perception. The aim is to attain a state of pure awareness free of thought constructs. This seems difficult to do. Indeed, it is not easy, and is a gradual process whereby, as obscuring false notions of ourselves and the world recede, the underlying pure, divine consciousness becomes progressively clearer. As it does so we experience more and more intensely, and for longer periods of time, the presence of Infinite Being which reflects on its own nature in each moment of perception. We no longer experience ourselves as one amongst countless individuals experiencing many things. We recognise that our true identity and the fundamental nature of all things is the one self-reflective divine consciousness of Deity that Abhinavagupta calls Bhairava.

All Kashmiri Śaiva practice amounts to the development of this participation in the self-reflective awareness of Deity's Infinite Being. It is similar to the practice of mindfulness taught in Buddhism, and is indeed a way to 'be here now', but the focus is on God consciousness. The Kashmiri Masters, like all Śaivites, teach that we can only develop through Śiva's grace. Indeed, we must exert ourselves in our practice. But whether it be meditation, worship, āsana or any other spiritual discipline, it can only be successful if we are given this gift of grace.

Finally, we may ask ourselves what Kashmiri Śaivism and its Tantric precedents and subsequent developments have to do with āsana practice. The word 'āsana' means a 'seat', 'place where one sits', and 'sitting'. It also means 'abiding' in a certain place or position of the body and so, by extension, a posture. Nowadays, the practice of āsana, that is, the assumption of various bodily postures, is often equated with the practice of Yoga. In India, however, there are many varieties of Yoga. Indeed, so many, that the word practically means any kind of spiritual practice. So we can refer to the worship of a deity by means of any ritual procedure, simple or complex, as the Yoga of Worship and Devotion (Bhakti Yoga). The practice of regularly repeating Mantras is Mantra Yoga. The performance of selfless service to the teacher, the deity or other people is the Yoga of Action (Karma Yoga). The study of the teachings of the scriptures and our teachers is the Yoga of Knowledge (Jñāna Yoga). Then there is the practice of concentration, what we would call meditation. In the Bhagavadgītā this is called Rāja Yoga - the King of Yogas. There we are taught to sit straight in a comfortable posture - āsana - and concentrate the mind on the breathing and the centre between the eyebrows. This may be combined with concentrated attention to the utterance of OṂ and mindful attention of Deity.

This understanding of Yoga - as spiritual discipline in general - is the way it is taught by Kṛṣṇa in the Bhagavadgītā, the eighteen chapters of which are expositions of as many varieties of Yoga. The Gītā precedes the Tantras by several centuries, and although they focus primarily on ritual, as outlined above, they do teach Yoga and the figure of the Yogi as a Tantric initiate is prominent. Like the Gītā, they do not set Yoga apart from other practices they teach as a separate category. Even ritual is considered to be a form of Yoga, which one would not expect, although Yoga is also more specifically understood to be inner practice.

Another way to think of Yoga is as a specific and complete regime of practice. These Yogas generally have their own specific names. One of the earliest and best known is Patañjali's Aṣṭāṅga (Eight-limbed) Yoga which he teaches in his Yoga Sūtras. The eight limbs are 1) the observance of the rules of moral conduct (niyama), 2) desistance from prohibited, immoral action (yama), 3) seating posture (āsana), 4) breath control (prāṇāyāma), 5) withdrawing the attention from the activity of the senses (pratyāhāra), 6) fixing the attention (dhāraṇa), 7) meditation (dhyāna), and 8) perfect concentration (samādhi). The practice involves the development of detachment from objectivity which is always ultimately painful and disturbs the mind. As one develops in this practice through its eight stages, the mind becomes progressively more tranquil until, free of all activity, it ultimately comes to an end and the perfected Yogi achieves a state of pure eternal consciousness which is his essential nature free of transitory, painful and mortal objectivity.

Another well-known Yoga is Haṭha Yoga. The founder of this Yoga is said to be Gorakhanātha. There are many legends about Gorakhanātha in which he appears in the role of a great Yogi. He can fly and work all kinds of miracles, heal the sick and restore

38 *The Wheel of Twelve Kālīs is expounded in detail by Lilian Silburn in her book: Hymnes aux Kālī – La Roue des Énergies Divines, Paris – Éditions de Boccard, 1975.*

fertility to the infertile. He can even resuscitate the dead. He is very popular throughout India. Stories of his life and teachings attributed to him are in most of the major Indian languages. It is hard to say when he lived. The earliest dateable reference to Nātha Yogis belonging to the tradition he founded is in the 14th century. It is not likely that he lived more than hundred years before. This was a period of huge change in India. Muslims ruled in the North and armies swept through the country to strengthen their domination and extend it. The Islam brought with them teaches a ridged monotheism centred on a Deity who, Himself formless, does not tolerate representations of any form, yet alone sacred ones. Temples were laid waste and the followers of the Tantras were deprived of patronage. In return, enlightened Islam offered the mysticism of the Sufis with their profound devotion and elevated vision of Deity beyond the confines of the mind. In this changed situation Gorakhanātha reformed Kaula Tantrism divesting it of all but what was the most essential.

Traditionally, Gorakhanātha is said to be the disciple of Matsyendranātha who we have seen was a major figure in the development of Kaulism. As the latter lived around the 8th century and the former in the 13th, it is, of course, impossible that Gorakhanātha was literally a disciple of Matsyendranātha, but he can be seen to have received Kula teachings attributed to Matsyendranātha. His relationship with these teachings and Matsyendranātha is illustrated in a well-known legend, often narrated with numerous variants. The kernel of the story is that Matsyendranātha, although a great Yogi, had given in to the temptations of liquor and sex. Gorakhanātha, after much searching, found him on Candradvīpa - the Island of the Moon, surrounded by beautiful young women who were massaging his body and offering him wine to drink. Sharp words from the disciple brought the teacher to his senses, who taught Gorakhanātha a much cleaned-up version of the Kaula teachings. These Gorakhanātha promulgated as Haṭha Yoga, which developed over the centuries in many forms and continues to be influential in the teaching and practice of Yoga in India and the West. This reformed Kaulism lost virtually all its Kaula character apart from the most essential inner practice, which involves the awakening of Kuṇḍalinī (the inner spiritual energy within the subtle body) and Her passage up through centres of energy (cakra) arranged along the axis of the subtle body. At the summit of Her ascent is the Void of pure consciousness called variously Without Mind (Amanaska, Unmana), the Undivided (Akhaṇḍa), and the Nameless (Anāma).

In the works of the Haṭha Yogis we find the beginnings of Yoga that included substantial practice of āsana. A well-known work, by a member of Gorakhanāth's tradition, is the Haṭhayogapradīpikā - the Lamp of Haṭha Yoga. The Gheraṇḍasaṃhitā and Śivasaṃhitā are two other popular works, which although not affiliated to any particular school, teach Haṭha Yoga. These were all written after the 16th century and contain descriptions of some sixteen major āsanas. Patañjali does not describe any āsanas in his 3rd century Yogasūtra. Five are named by his commentator, Vyāsa, who was three or four centuries later. They are all simply seating positions for meditation that are, as Patañjali lays down, 'comfortable and stable'. The early Tantras, indeed, even the later ones, have virtually nothing to say about āsana in this sense. There a few exceptions such as one in the Buddhist Caṇḍamahāroṣaṇa Tantra (the Tantra of the Fierce Very Angry One). There we find a reference to sixty-four āsanas for sexual intercourse (kāmāsana) which are offered to the Deity like so many lamps. Otherwise, āsana in the Tantras is very important in another sense as the seat on which the Deity sits. The priest, the offerings and ritual utensils all have their seats, which are worshipped as cosmic beings. The Deity's seat, His or Her Throne, is the whole universe. When we sit to worship, our seat is the Tortoise that swims in the Cosmic Ocean and supports the universe. The body-mind, like a mirror, reflects it within itself, and so the Deity's seat is also the body. The Deity sits at the summit of the body and within the Heart, which is the very core of our being. These are also the seats of the Self, just as the seat of Kuṇḍalinī, which is the Self's vitality, is at the base of the spine.

Although, in this way, the symbolism of the seat - āsana - is very extensive in the Tantras, the modern perception and practice of āsana has developed in other contexts. One is Haṭha Yoga, which we have mentioned. Another is the gymnasium. The Malla Purāṇa is a late manual for the use of wrestlers - malla. It describes many wrestling holds and enumerates the weak points in the body (marma), which we also find in the works on Ayurveda, the Indian system of medicine. In addition, some āsanas are prescribed as a part of the wrestler's physical training. The Śrītattvanidhi is virtually an encyclopedia written by a Maharaja of Mysore in the 18th century. There we find an extensive section dealing with āsana in which over fifty are described. The book also includes drawings of them. Works exclusively dealing with Yoga as a total program of practice began to be written around the 15th century. Many of these are as yet unpublished. As we would expect, they include descriptions of āsanas, but they are usually limited in number. As we move into the modern period, we witness the rise of a number of great practitioners and teachers of Yoga, some of whom, like Iyengar developed further the application of āsana practice to therapy of the body and mind.

So, one may well ask, if the practice of āsana was unknown to the Tantras and the Kashmiri Masters, what do they have to do with one another? In fact they have much to do with one another. Many people (although certainly not Iyengar) understand āsana practice to be simply a sophisticated form of gymnastics of which the focus is not on toning muscle or gaining strength, rather the alignment of the body to its optimal form. Inevitably, if we don't pay attention, we strain parts of the body. Compressed internal organs do not perform their functions efficiently, leading to a range of diseases and disorders. Without proper exercise the effects of ageing increase. We are more liable to disease. Combined with a healthy diet, āsana practice keeps the weight of the body within the limits required for it to function properly. In these ways it also contributes to keeping the body beautiful and the physical benefits are manifold, as anyone who practises āsana knows well. Similarly, breathing exercises - prāṇāyāma - benefit one's health in many ways.

These benefits do not concern Kashmiri Śaivism. What does, is the most fundamental basis of āsana practice and prāṇāyāma, namely, Yoga. This the Kashmiri teachers understand to be the practice of self-awareness. This practice is couched in an understanding of reality which is uniquely suited to account for the deeper and most authentic benefits of āsana and prāṇāyāma. Let us see how. Consciousness manifests in two aspects, namely, the many perceivers on the one hand and their countless objects on the other. The body, senses, mind and vital breath are all objective in relation to the individual perceiver. At the same time, the individual perceiver is an object in relation to the supreme subjectivity of Śiva Who is pure, universal and divine consciousness. In our daily life we are generally engrossed in objectivity - the outer world and our inner mind, senses and body with which we unthinkingly identify. The embodied subjectivity that emerges in this way out of consciousness is the individual perceiver. Of course, it does possess a degree of subjectivity, that is, self-awareness, but it is much reduced with respect to fundamental consciousness and is largely submerged in objectivity. In this perspective, Yoga - which literally means 'union' - is the cultivation of self-awareness, thereby heightening the level of subjectivity until, by degrees, it expands to the full extent of the one supreme subjectivity of God consciousness with which it realises its identity and so unites. On the way, just as the individual subjectivity develops and expands out of the confines of being just one amongst countless others, so does the object. This is all the more so the closer it is, as it were, to the subject. As subjectivity develops, we rise along the scale of objectivity from the grossest insentience up through the body, senses, mind and the vital breath. As we rise, the content of the domain of individual objectivity develops from the particular to the universal and its specific contents dwindle away as we enter into the emptiness of contentless consciousness. From there, if we maintain awareness and do not fall into deep, dreamless sleep, we enter the sphere of pure subjectivity free of all identification with objectivity.

This does not mean that consciousness is empty and totally detached from objectivity as if it were a separate distinct reality. The emptiness of pure consciousness is its transcendental aspect. It is the profound awareness consciousness has of itself as the one unique reality. All that we experience is a manifestation of consciousness. The pure self-awareness centred solely on consciousness perceives this. It perceives that there is nothing but consciousness. This is its 'emptiness'. At the same time, without contradiction, consciousness, in its immanent aspect, is all things. This is its all-embracing 'fullness'. The 'emptiness' of consciousness is its 'fullness' and its 'fullness' is its 'emptiness'. This equation also works at the individual level, not just the universal. Every single thing is consciousness. Every single thing is both 'empty' and 'full'. Thus, as the Kashmiri teachers say: 'every single thing is everything' (sarvaṃ sarvātmakam). This is what we discover more and more as we develop in the practice of Yoga, that is, self-awareness. The perpetual change from moment to moment is the radiant pulse of the light of consciousness. Nothing in reality arises or falls away. Only the power of consciousness shines this way and that. From this perspective, āsana can be perceived as the pulse (in a sonic shape) of the body of vibration. Each āsana in the purity of its form, practised rightly, can become a maṇḍala in itself with awareness at the centre of the anatomical and organic body, the mental apparatus as the extension of that awareness. The same is true of the breath, the most intimate vitality of the organic body, senses and mind. We can enter, as it were, into the very being of the object through the body and breath consecrated with the awareness of the consciousness that sustains and generates it and into which it dissolves away. As we practise self-awareness and are freed of objectivity, the object progressively reveals its true, universal, conscious nature. This is why āsana and prāṇāyāma rightly practised, that is with centred self-awareness, not just concern with the correctness of posture (although that is also essential), elevates consciousness. The body and breath thus become a means to experience both the universal object and transcendental subjective consciousness. Both are wonderfully taught in the Vijñānabhairava which Pisano has most appropriately chosen as the guide to mindful āsana practice. Indeed, the majority of the 112 meditations taught there concern the body, senses and the breath.

The Vijñānabhairava teaches how to discover the Emptiness of the breath, the body, the senses and the outer world and abide within it. Emptiness is the Fullness of the plenitude of consciousness unobscured by the countless thoughts that limit our attention and experience to our small personal Self, which is mistakenly identified with our body, breath, senses and mind. Gripped by this false identification, the world around us is the place where we act to attain our goals, solve and avoid problems. Then, often after tremendous struggle, when we have achieved our goal, immediately another one appears on the horizon of our thoughts. And so we begin again. Indeed, we normally have more than one goal, sometimes very many, so we hardly notice that we have attained one engaged as we are in attaining the others. Emptiness is the opposite of all this struggle, frustration, narrow self-seeking, fear of loss and hope of gain, with their countless thoughts, efforts, joys and sorrows. The Vijñānabhairava teaches that Emptiness is fullness (24), the knowledge of the harmony of all things (64). It is a state of all pervasion (31) free of the body we experience as 'I am everywhere' (104). Perceived directly with the Void mind, free of thought constructs, all things are experienced as the Void (43). The mind is Void (122). The world is Void (134). The body is Void (46) and the senses are Voids (32). It is reality (50) where Deity is revealed (93, 119). The Supreme goddess shines there (54) revealing the god Bhairava's state (25, 35, 93). The Void is a state of perfect peace (27, 52). Supreme joy is the state of consciousness free of dichotomising thought constructs (46) and so is the experience of the One (48), the Absolute Self (108) which is the supreme state (111), the highest goal (34).

The Vijñānabhairava teaches how to use the body, senses, mind and breath in another way, not just for the affairs of our daily life, but as means to develop higher states of insight. We develop the habit of Emptiness, which is freedom from thought, by cultivating our power of awareness of the body and the rest as the Emptiness of Deity. For example, by paying attention to the breath, the places to which inhalation and exhalation ascend and from which they descend, where they meet, internally and externally (64), these are the two Voids (25). By paying attention to its movement as we fall asleep we enter into the world of dreams wakeful, master of them, not victims (55).

When the breath rests we experience the expansion of our inner energy. Attending to the centre between the two breaths, inhalation and exhalation, we experience the rise of the energy of Kuṇḍalinī, the vital force of the breath (26, 67). It ascends through the centres between the two breaths strung along the central channel, subtle as a lotus fibre (35), piercing the point between the eyebrows (31) and then up out of the body where it dissolves away (28-30). This is what happens if we breathe mindfully in the course of our āsana practice.

As we assume our āsanas, by practising awareness of the Void in the body and around it with the mind free of thoughts, we experience everything as the Void (43-45). Think of the body as empty enclosed by skin with nothing inside (48) or, if you can't manage to free your mind of its solidity, burn up the fortress of the body with the inner fire of the imagination (52). We experience the same universal Void by meditating on any point in the body as Void (44, 46), for example, within the skull (34). As an aid to this meditation prick any part of the body with a needle and concentrate on the emptiness there (93). Ask a friend to tickle you under the armpits, maintaining the same awareness. Then the laughter it induces will suddenly turn into the bliss of consciousness by which Reality is revealed (66).

Be aware as you do āsana practice that all the parts of the body are Void (50), as are the elements of which it constituted. As that awareness strengthens, they merge into one another, from gross to subtle, to ultimately dissolve away into Emptiness (54). These meditations free us from attachment to the body. When that is achieved we experience the presence of our true conscious nature everywhere, not just in the body (104). So we also experience other peoples' bodies as our own (107) because the same plenitude of consciousness resides in all bodies (100).

Āsana practice helps us develop our awareness and so experience Emptiness. The Vijñānabhairava teaches that if we maintain this awareness we attain the peaceful mental state of higher consciousness when we are seated on a moving vehicle or by moving the body slowly (83). Using the movement of the body - moving around and around until one falls - all agitation ceases and one experiences the peace of emptiness (111). Assuming a comfortable posture curve the arms and fix the mind on the Void under the armpits, it will merge in that (Void) and attain peace (79). Keeping the tongue in the centre of the wide open mouth one should fix the mind there (81). Sitting on a soft seat one should hold one's hands and feet without any support. By maintaining this position the individual mind will reach a state of supreme fullness of consciousness (78). Either sitting on a seat or lying on a bed one should meditate on the body as supportless. When the mind also becomes empty and supportless, in a moment one is liberated from the activity of the mind (82).

Freeing the body of supports is like freeing the mind from them. Freeing the mind from supports in this way also frees the body from them (119). Free the mind of supports (108) and don't allow thoughts to arise (108). In this way the mind is freed of agitation, by withdrawing it from whatever object it may wander to (129) or anything one may recall (119). Withdrawing in this way all thought and knowledge of objectivity, one becomes the Abode of the Void (120). We experience the same Void without withdrawing from objects by fixing our attention one-pointedly on one. In this way it gradually appears to be Void and so too the mind (122). All external objects depend on our knowledge of them. Therefore this world is Void (134). Imagine that this whole universe is Void. In that way one's mind is dissolved away into it and one merges into Emptiness (58).

Outer Space becomes one with Inner Space. Meditation on either or both leads to the same result. Both the body and the world are equally filled with the supreme bliss of the Emptiness of Consciousness (65). Contemplate simultaneously how one's body and the world consist of nothing but Consciousness, thus the mind is free of thoughts and we experience the supreme awakening (63). Fixing one's mind on the external space which is eternal, supportless, empty, all pervading and free from limitation, in this way one will be absorbed in non-space (128). Gaze with the same attitude into the dark night sky (87) or the variegated light of the sky during the day, or a space illumined by the light of a lamp (76). Just as outer and inner space are one so is outer and inner darkness. First close your eyes and meditate on the darkness in front, and then, opening your eyes, contemplate the dark form of Bhairava and so be one with His state of Emptiness (88).

Clearly, although āsana practice had not been systematically developed in the 8th or 9th century when the Vijñānabhairava was revealed, the essential principles that lie at the root of āsana practice as Yoga, had already been discovered and were being practised. It is very much to Pisano's credit that by his diligent study and practice of Śrī Iyengar's Yoga and the teachings of Kashmir Śaivism, he has been blessed with the insight that allows him to perceive the unity of these fundamental principles at the core of these two traditions, however different they may appear, at first sight, to be. May his work be of benefit to all.

Mark Dyczkowski

Diwali, Vārāṇasī, India, 5th November 2010

www.markdkashi.com

Abbreviations

BY: Brahmāyāmala
CMSS: Ciñcinīmatasārasamuccaya
KuKauM: Kulakaulinīmata
MVT: Mālinīvijayottara
NT: Netratanta
SK: Spandakārikā
SvT: Svacchandabhairava Tantra
SYM: Siddhayogeśvarīmata
TĀ: Tantrāloka

Bibliography

Dyczkowski 1985: The Doctrine of Vibration, State University of New York Press, Albany

Dyczkowski 1988: The Canon of the Śaivāgama and the Kubjikā Tantras of the Western Tradition, State University of New York Press, Albany

Handiqui K.K. 1949: The Yaśastilaka and Indian Culture, Sholapur

Lorenzen 1991 (second edition): The Kāpālikas and Kālāmukhas: Two Lost Śaiva Sects, Berkeley - University of California Press

Nagaswamy R. 1982: Tantric Cults of South India, Delhi - Agama Kal Prakashan

Sanderson 1988: "Śaivism and the Tantric Traditions" In The World's Religions edited by S.Sutherland et al, London - Routledge and Kegan Paul, pp. 660-704

Törzsök 1999: "The Doctrine of Magic Female Spirits" A Critical Edition of Selected Chapters of the Siddhayogeśvarīmata(tantra) with Annotated Translation and Analysis, PhD Thesis, The University of Oxford

Silburn L. 1975: Hymnes aux Kālī - La Roue des Énergies Divines, Paris - Éditions de Boccard

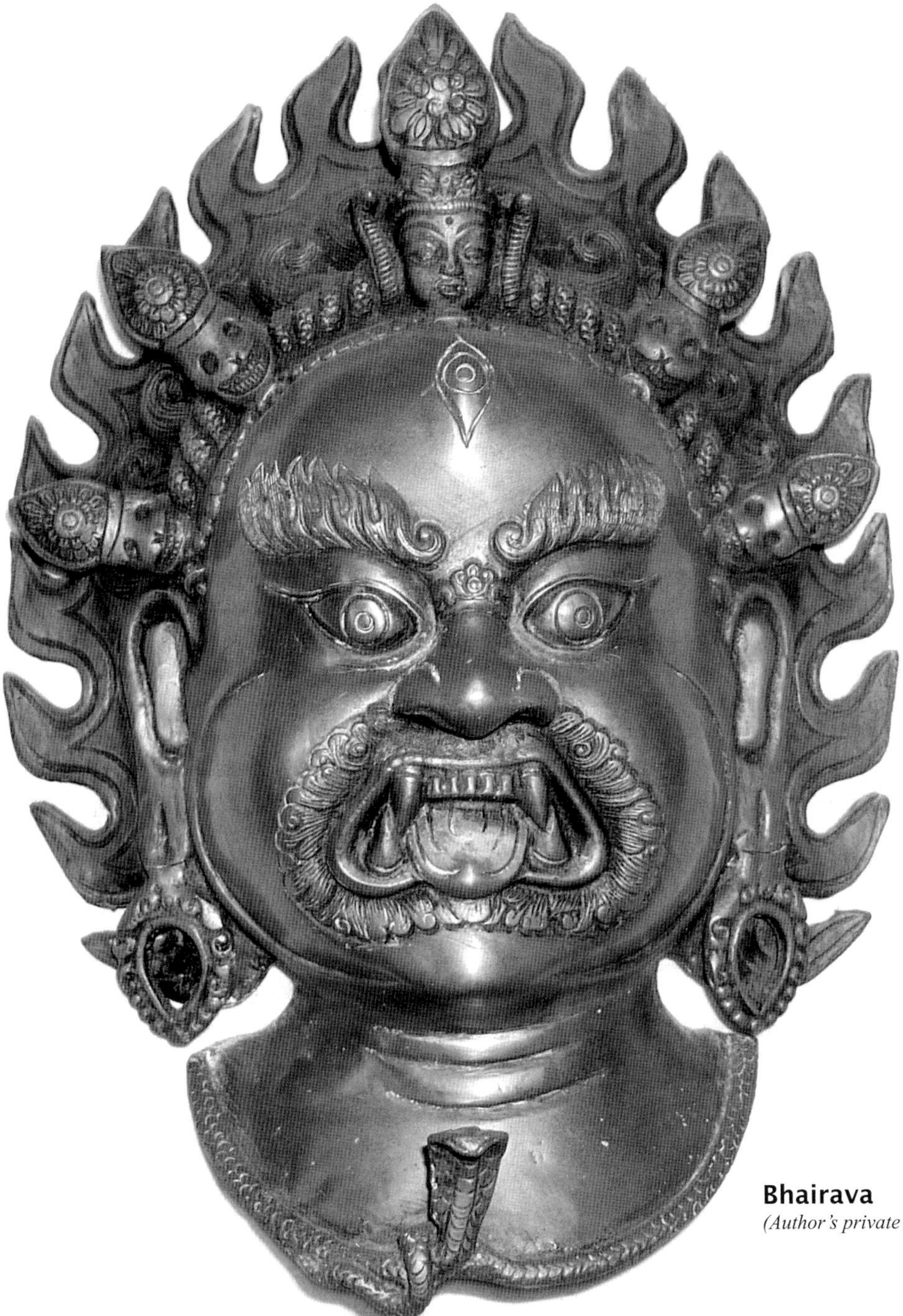

Bhairava
(Author's private collection)

Prelude

"Glory to Śaṅkara, glory to the omnipresence of the Lord's Consciousness,
which albeit manifests as diversity, is without duality.
Glory to this vibrant Reality, this undifferentiated mass of bliss,
whose form is the universe."
KṢEMARĀJA, ŚIVASŪTRAVIMARŚINĪ, INTRODUCTORY VERSES

"Abandoning themselves to the delight of the Great Banquet, where they drink
the intoxicating quintessence of nectar from the pots of undifferenced Energy,
the revellers make bold to masticate the sprouts of differentiating concepts."
MAHEŚVARĀNANDA, MAHĀRTHAMAÑJARĪ 58

"This sacrifice is only meant for those free of all doubts, who thus see everything
in the same light. Whatever the hero accomplishes in thought,
word or deed, through any activity requiring boldness and heroism
apt to reveal such essence is called sacrifice (Kula)".
ABHINAVAGUPTA, TANTRĀLOKA XXIX, 5-6

"Upon the death of the body, the supreme Lord remaining alone,
it is no longer a question of absorption.
For who can enter, where and how?"
ABHINAVAGUPTA, ĪŚVARAPRATYABHIJÑĀVIMARŚINĪ III, 2.11-12

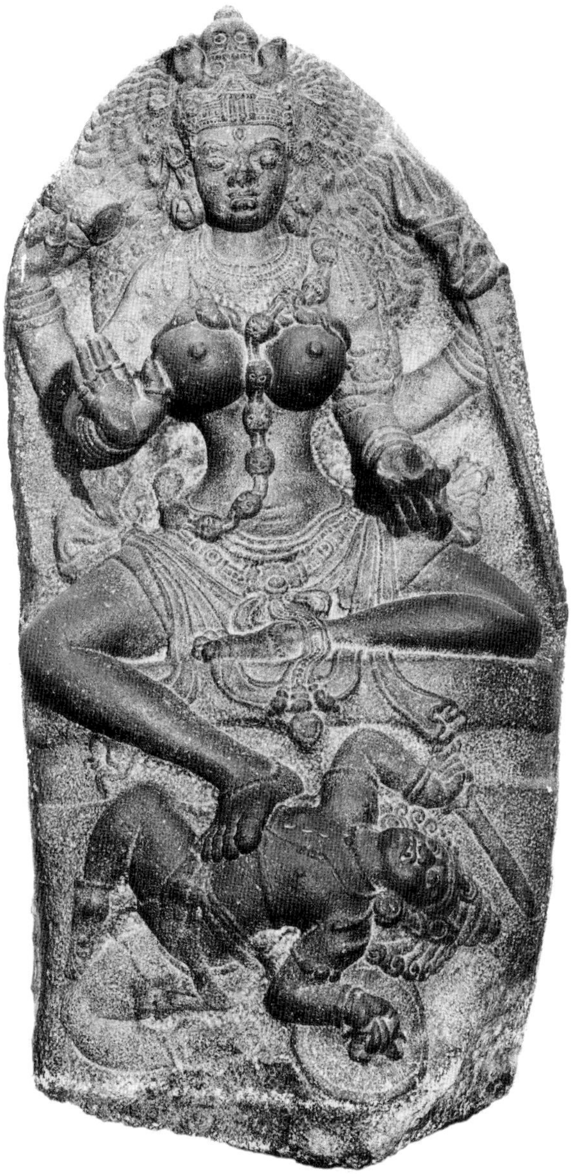

Durgā *10th century*
(Avani Koral, Karnataka, Bangalore Museum)

ACT I

Contemplation of the "vast and manifold glowing reddish net of māyā, made up of knots and holes, spread over all places."

ABHINAVAGUPTA, TANTRĀLOKA I, 7

"Be as you are, without worries,
Because the goal is already realised.
That is discrimination itself.
Who else other than the Self
could teach what to whom?"

MAHEŚVARĀNANDA,
MAHĀRTHAMAÑJARĪ 64

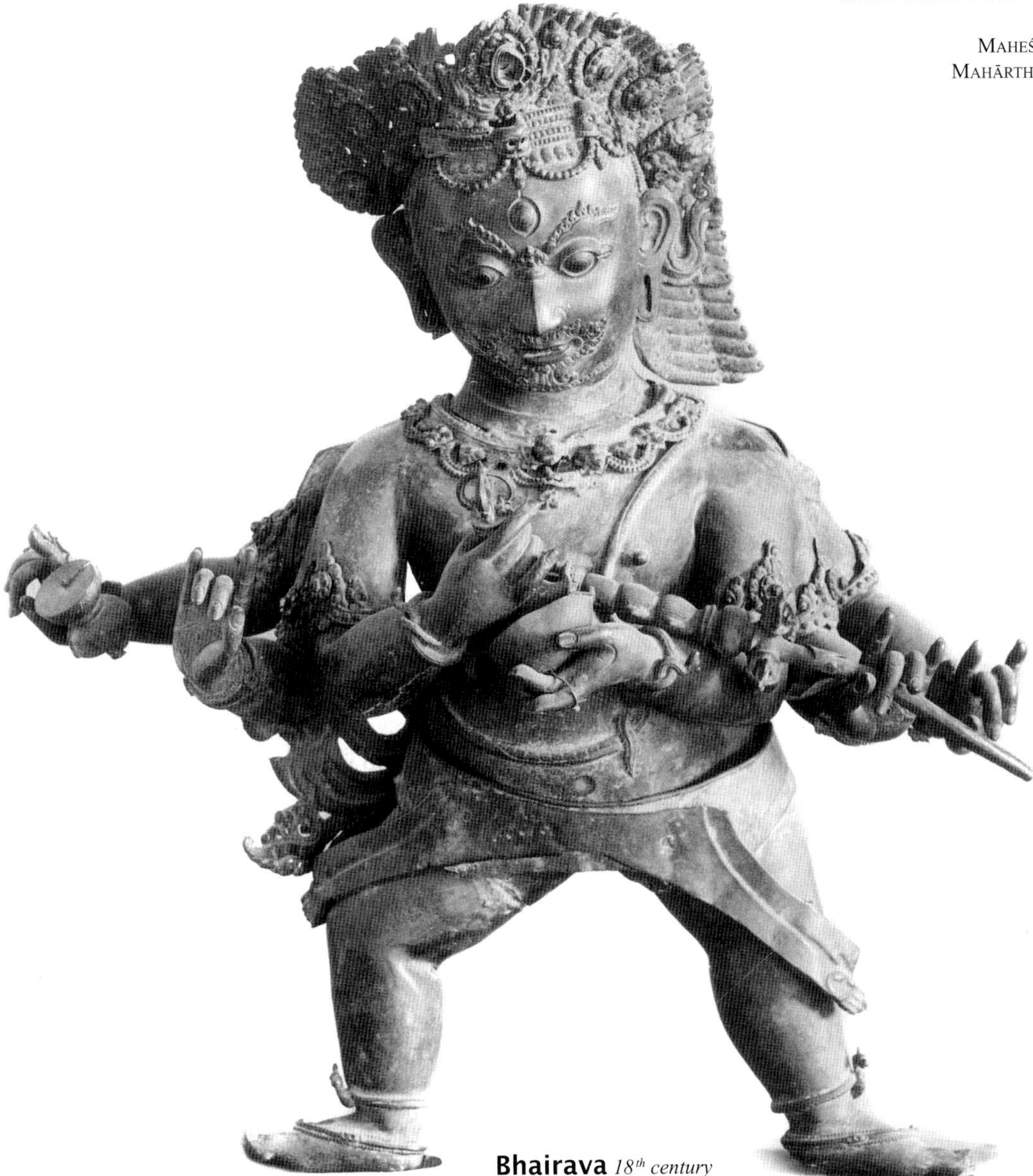

Bhairava *18th century*
(Bharat Kala Bhawan, Vārāṇasī)

1

Confessions of Ignorance

From the dull heights of my ignorance I pay homage to that by which I am able to recognise this nescience, the ever-incomprehensible Without-Equal. Had I any talent, my heart would have poured forth, like the great Abhinavagupta, Jñāneśvar, Kabīr or Tukārām in their hymns praising the Ultimate. If their talent had ever failed them, their mystical intoxication alone would have been enough. I have neither one nor the other.

Perhaps I'd have spoken of my childhood wonder as I laid on the grass, staring at the sky, savouring my first existential vertigo. Or when, in the depth of a Savoyard winter, as the sky snowed its thick white mystery of impenetrable silence, I too was snowing. Perhaps I'd have spoken of the joy of the world, riding behind my father on his moped, sitting enthroned like a king. Or of the rapturous bliss that filled me when my mother would bake a cake. Perhaps I'd have spoken of the magic of the ordinary, helping to fold the sheets, fascinated by the whiteness and texture of the fabric as it brushed against me in waves of freshness. Or of the infinitely calm peace that embraced me in a soft haze when I felt my mother's hands running through my hair, searching out the lice of tenderness. Perhaps I'd have sung of the intuitive resonance where boundaries vanish into a thousand silent names, into the sacred rhythm of absurd poetry.

Is it not this intuitive resonance (pratibhādhvani) of non-separation that is exalted in the art and rituals of yoga?

To speak of this luminous intuition, which is said to be closer and more intimate than our jugular vein or our next breath, I have summoned a whole army of concepts and their wicked mercenaries. Concepts are nothing but corpses that however well made up, are still just corpses! Like a decaying carcass that gives off a putrid smell, they reek of the pretensions of a dying knowledge. Their theories are no more reassuring than dykes of fear before the unknown, forever destroyed by the surge of life.

From this mental scaffolding, mummified by certitudes purchased from temple traders, shines a glowing incertitude that we know absolutely nothing, nor ever will. This incertitude transforms into the blinding certitude that we can never comprehend anything about the subject (pramātṛ), which is what is, and which can never be objectivised. This absence of knowledge, this 'I don't know', when thought collapses into itself, reveals a naked heart that depends upon nothing, but which encompasses everything. This is the essence of Yoga, which precedes all techniques, and from which stem all rituals of consecration.

"Because He pervades all things at the highest degree,
He, whose essence is conscious light, does not shine separately
from the lights of the sun, the moon or other objects.
Thus the expressions 'enlightenment'
and 'enlightened' are relatively true.
In fact nothing is separated from Consciousness
because there can be no duality
in Consciousness."
ABHINAVAGUPTA,
PARAMĀRTHACARCĀ 1-2

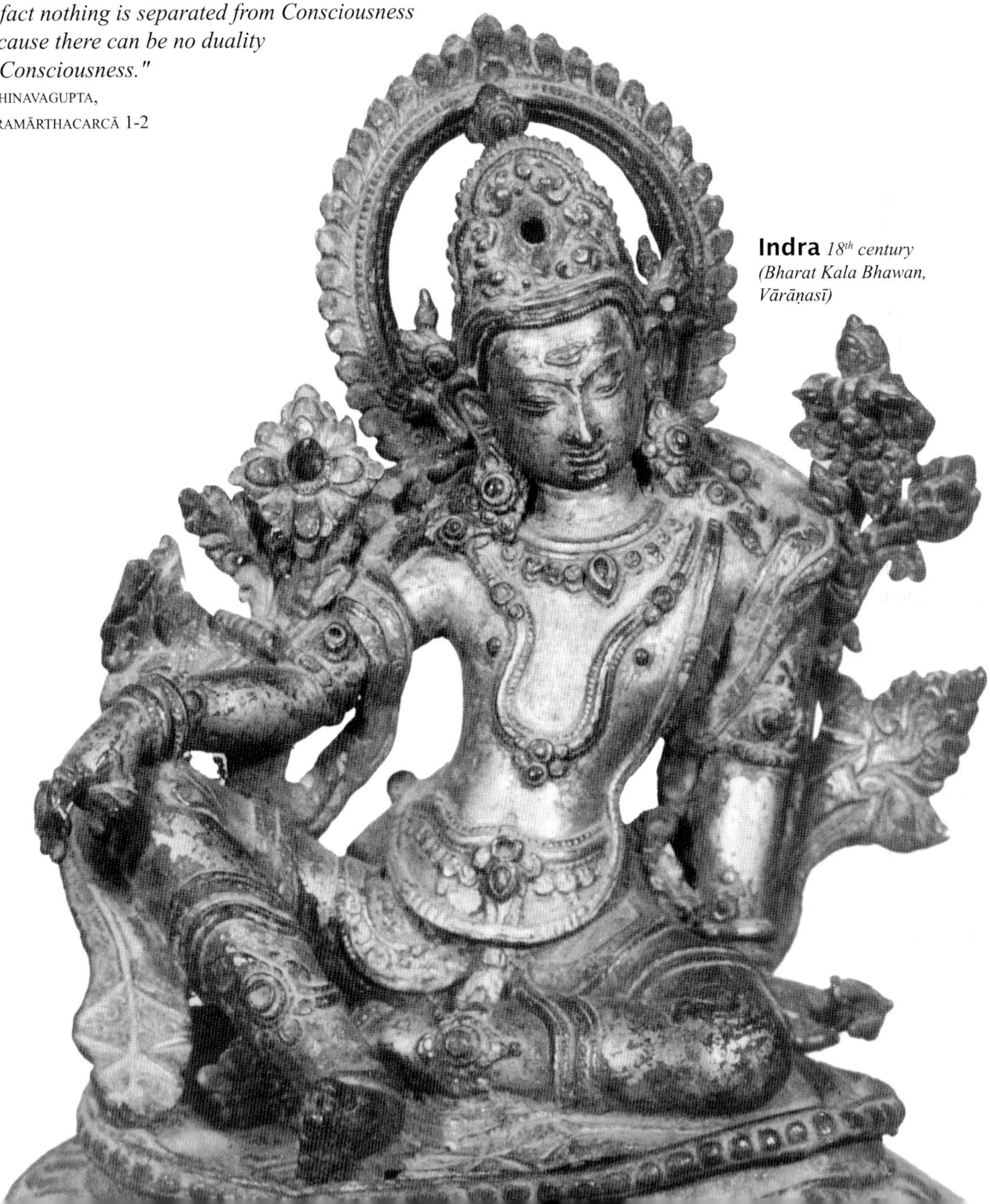

Indra *18th century (Bharat Kala Bhawan, Vārāṇasī)*

2

The Quest for the Impossible

Legends, born from the breath of dozing gods, murmur stories of raging madness within our daily lives. They have been gathered in the belly of the Earth and the depths of the Sky's eyes. They still have the fragrance of unspoken sorrows, as damp as an endless rainy day, and the burns of desert solitude. They have the mad enthusiasm of a child at play, lost in a charade invented in the instant. They have the sweetness of his abandonment when, tired, he surrenders into his mother's arms. They tell of a wandering dog, or of a heart too heavy like the clouds of a summer storm. They recount a desperate, never-ending wait on the platform of an abandoned railway station. They tell of intense suffering, as pristine and insurmountable as a glacier. They sing the joy of improbable weddings and their feasts, imagined in a moment as the eyes of two strangers meet.

They speak of humanity in exile and haunting nostalgia. They recount the epics of characters pulled out of anonymity, going through life in a wild saraband. Secret maps, forbidden roads, forgotten passages; they seek the way back to a home they never left. Their quest has a taste of the impossible, the inaccessible and the futile. Cursed vagabonds and wandering knights pursuing magical kingdoms, divine jewels and elixirs of immortality. They endure trials, all of them as futile and devoid of meaning as their courage, pushed on by an invincible desire for freedom and their insane faith. They reach sombre shores as dark and deep as a night of ink, at the antipodes of societies and their humanity. There they drink the dregs of their desperation, abandoned by everyone, fed to their inner monsters. And when Gilgamesh, deprived forever of immortality, had no choice but to return to his hometown of Uruk, a stranger among his own people, he could but cry: *"I've wandered through many a land, I've scaled solitary mountains, I've crossed many an ocean and I found no happiness. I've condemned myself to a life of misery and filled my flesh with pain."* But each kept one last irony, that of savouring the 'great marvel' and singing with Kabīr: *"I've seen a great marvel. Whosoever dies whilst living, makes death die."*

Those who return from this last kiss, this embrace with the goddess of the night, the great effacement, are left dumbfounded. Half-man, half-animal, half-god, half-demon, defying all definition, their eyes as intense as lightning and as deep as an unfathomable mystery. It is said they travel on the wind, command the elements and make the earth tremble with each step. Tigers among men, their roars awaken fear and wonder. All these Jasons of the elusive Golden Fleece, all these Don Quixotes lost in the aisles of a supermarket, are so much more than simply tales once told to children on long winter nights. They are an aftertaste of piercing interrogation.

Who is born? Who lives? Who dies? And is there really someone to be born and to die?

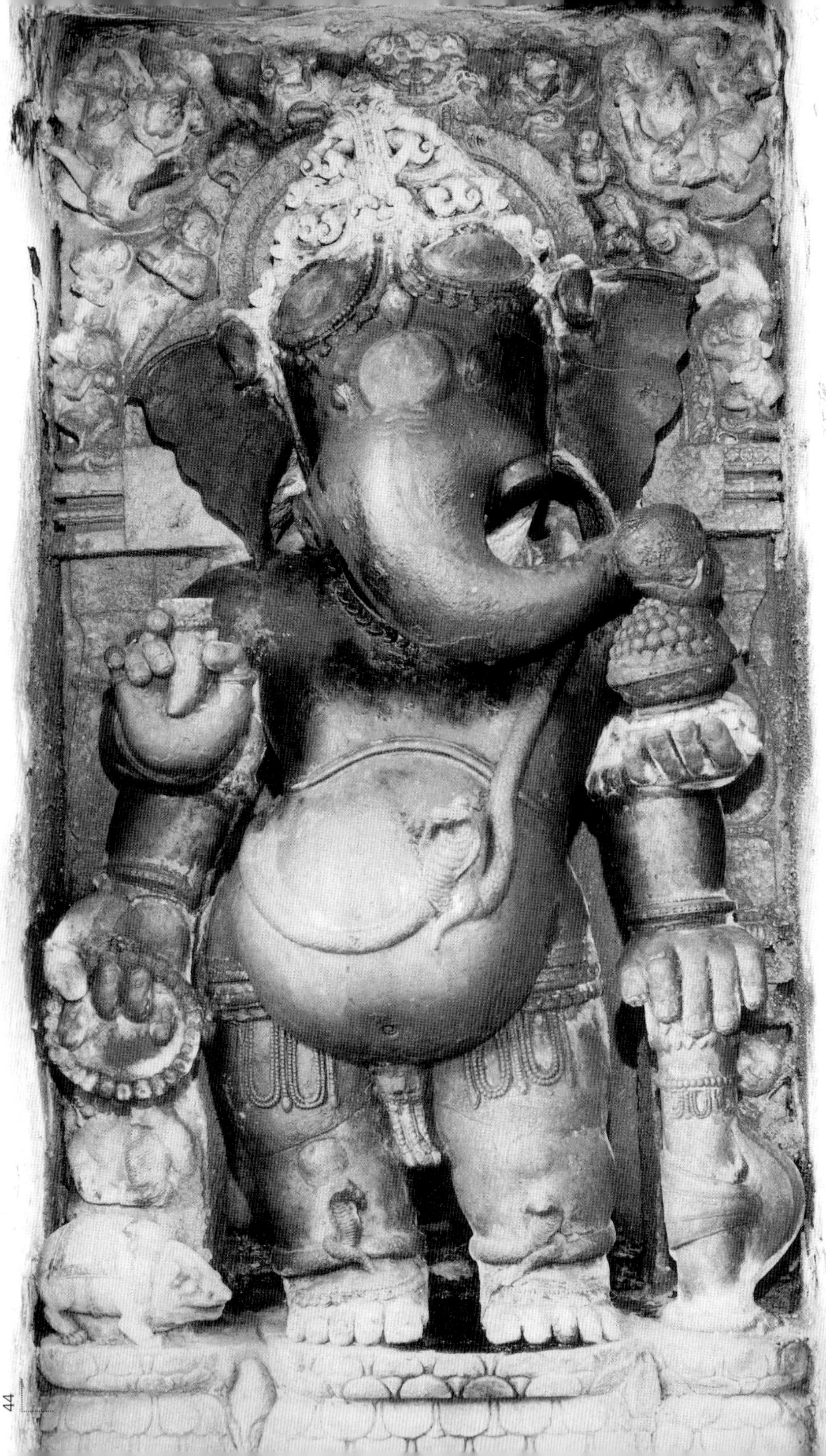

"In the absence of duality,
rest in God.
This is how the supreme Pūjā
is accomplished."

ABHINAVAGUPTA,
MAHOPADEŚAVIMŚATIKĀ 20

Lambodara *12th century*
(Sobhaneśvara Śiva Temple,
Niali, Orissa)

3

The Gift of the Lord of Tears

He haunts forbidden places and the frightening depths of darkness, bringing with him the odour of flesh burnt on the world's funeral pyre. He reigns over battlefields and makes pain and grinding teeth his temple. He wears darkness like a garland around his neck, punctuated with the skulls of our existence. His matted hair dances around him, like creepers of obscurity, to the sound of his fury where worlds collide and disappear. He howls with all his madness, and his cry pierces the hearts of men. It is the cry of their own deaths, their own nothingness.

"Master of the goddess of senses whose cry terrifies bound beings, he ends the whirl of saṃsāra. He is thus the Great Horrifier." Abhinavagupta, Tantrāloka I, 99-100

He dances frenetically, drunk with joy, dragging in his wake a procession of wandering souls of becoming, ogresses of pleasure, tormented spirits and all who have been banished. It is with great joy He drinks the poison of this creation, because for Him there exists nothing but the resplendent reality of His own Consciousness. We cannot pronounce His name, that before language existed, the name of unknowing, of holy ignorance, as this would mark the end of our world. He is called Rudra, the one who makes people cry, who induces torrents of tears, swollen like rivers during the rainy season. He is destruction, but He is also the one who dispels pain (ru stands for ruk: disease, dra stands for for drāvi: melter, dissolver; Rudra is therefore the one who dissolves all the ills of life - samastarugdrāvi), He in whom effacement is supreme. The breath of Rudra is Agni. He has the nature of fire, the great cosmic sacrifice, the timeless oblation of life in death and of death in life. For he who remains hypnotised with fear before this spectacle, like a prey before his predator, Rudra offers the sweet oblivion of death.

"When beings are tired of action, of knowledge, of pain and pleasure, and seek the rest of dreamless sleep, they enter into Śiva the changeless state, the abode of joy, in whom the universe comes to rest and sleep."
Swāmi Karpātrī, Śrī Śivatattva Siddhānta II, 1941-42

For those who seek to go beyond appearances, He becomes the penetrating eye of investigation. Because He is Agni, He transmits the austerity of purification. This purification of the heart has the quality of Śiva's devastating fire that burns away illusion. All that can be added to us or taken from us is of no interest. Śiva then becomes the Lord of Yoga, internalising the cosmic sacrifice.

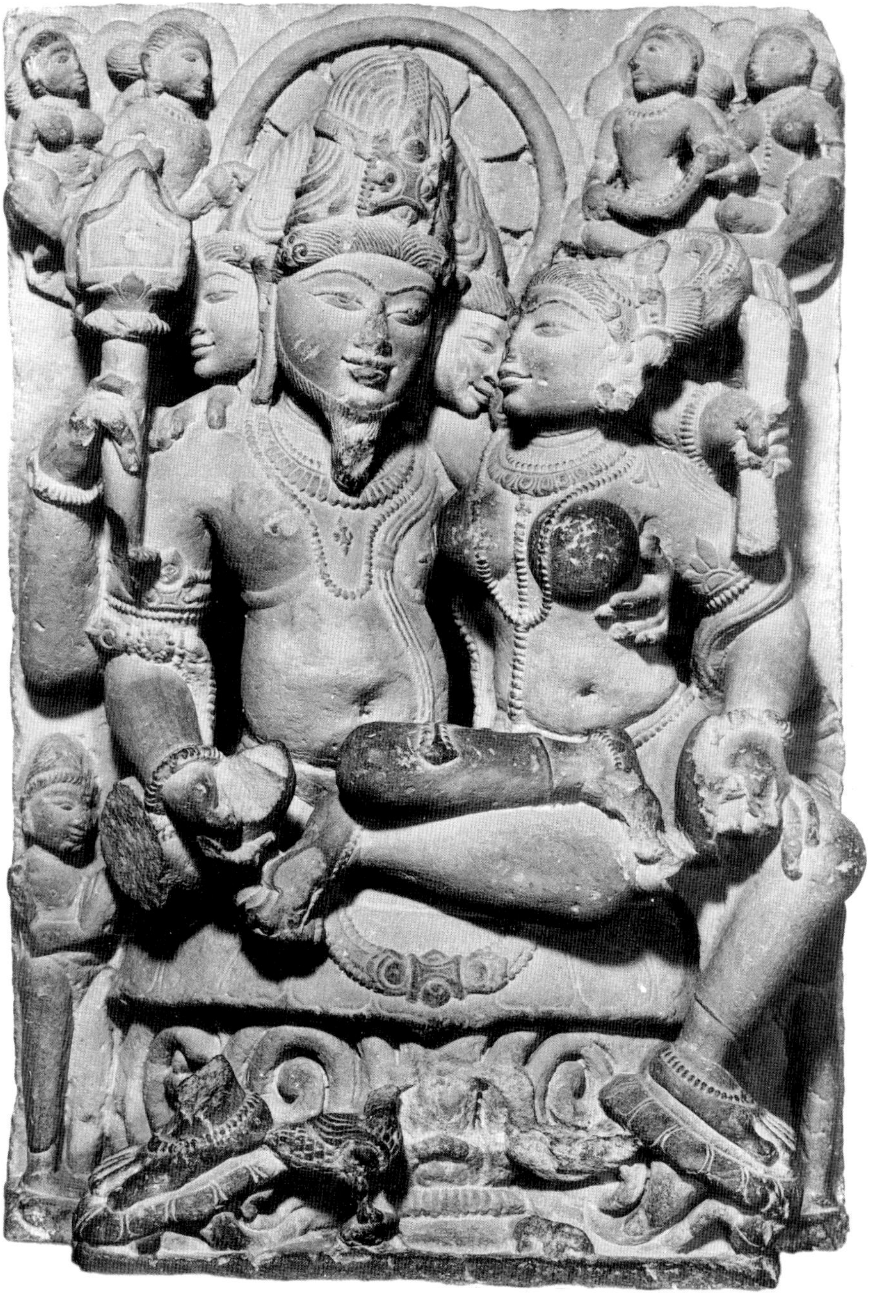

Brahmā and Sarasvatī
11th century
(Mathura District, New Delhi National Museum)

4

The Veils of Luminous Darkening

"Whatever is known as the composite form of Bhairava, that, O Goddess, is deceptive like magic, because it has no essence ...
This state of Bhairava is free from the limitations of space, time and form. It is not particularised by a specific place or designation. In reality, it is inexpressible, because it cannot be described."
VIJÑĀNA BHAIRAVA 8B-9A, 14

Once upon a time... there was a young prince who didn't believe in three things. He didn't believe in islands, princesses or God. His father the king had told him that these things did not exist. The prince believed him since he had never seen an island, a princess or any sign of God in his father's kingdom. Destiny then took him on a journey outside of the palace where he had always lived. When he reached the edge of the kingdom, to his great astonishment he saw a multitude of islands. At the water's edge there were boats waiting to take a group of strangely beautiful women, dressed in finery, to the islands.
A man dressed in a long tunic approached him.
"Are those islands?" asked the prince.
"Of course they are!" replied the stranger.
"And who are those creatures?"
"They are princesses."
"Well then," cried the young man, *"there must be a God!"*
"Of course there is a God. I am He."
Filled with excitement the prince returned as quickly as he could to his father.
"Father, I saw islands and princesses and I met God."
The king remained stoic. *"I told you, none of those exist."*
"But," protested the prince, *"I saw them as I see you now."*
"Tell me, how was your god dressed? Was he wearing a long tunic?"
"Yes."
"Were the sleeves of his tunic rolled up?"
"Yes."
The king smiled. *"You've been deceived. He was a magician and he tricked you."*
The prince raced back to the water's edge to find the stranger. And sure enough, he was there and seemed to be waiting for him. *"My father says you are a magician. This time you will not fool me. I know that these islands and these princesses are only illusions created by your magic."*
The man smiled. *"In your kingdom, there are also islands and princesses, but you cannot see them because you are under the spell of your father."*
The prince returned home again. *"Father, is it true that you are not really a king but a magician?"*
The king smiled and rolled up the sleeves of his long tunic. *"Yes, it is true."*
"So the man I met really was God?"
"No, he was another magician. We are all magicians creating the world as we wish to see it."
"I must find out the truth. The truth that lies behind the magic."

"There is nothing behind the magic", replied the king. The prince was overcome with terrible sadness.
"I will kill myself then."
The king made Death appear. Death ordered the prince to follow him. The prince shivered as he felt Death's icy breath penetrate him. Then he recalled the magnificent but unreal islands, and the unreal but seductive princesses.
"If everything is the result of my own magic," said the young man, *"then so too is Death. I can live with that."*
"You see, my son," said the king, *"you are starting to become a magician yourself."*

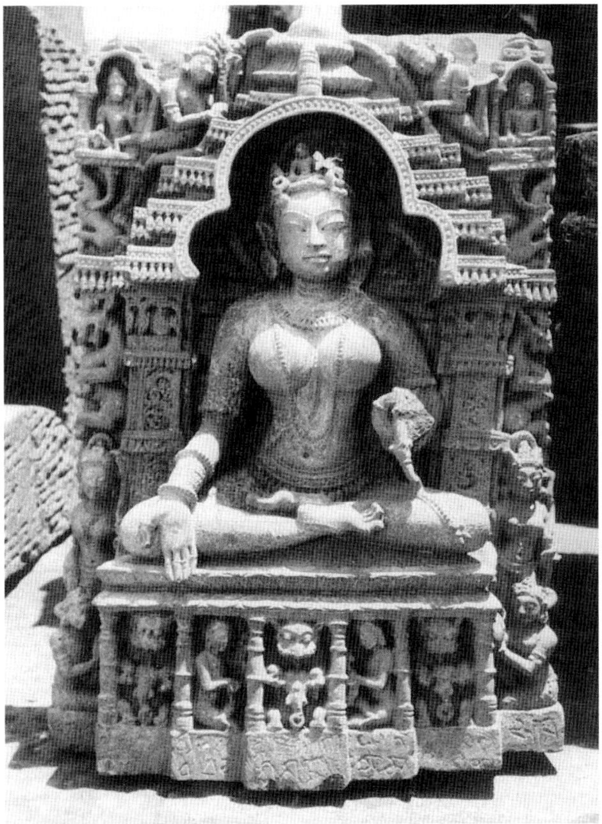

Devī *12th century*
(Viṣṇu Varāha Temple, Bilhari, Jabalpur, Madhya Pradesh)

Who has never stood in wonder at the marvelling gaze of a newborn child? Their eyes still staring into the great nothingness make us nostalgic for a wide-open space without limits. Our birth is a frontier beyond which we know nothing. The mystics speak of it as Terra Incognita or Holy Ignorance.
With our so-called birth begins the process of identification with what we call reality. Our representation of the world, which we take to be cast in stone, is merely a hoax. What we call reality is simply the result of different filters, tinted mirrors, reflections and phantoms. We are in a perpetual process of translation. *"Traduttore, tradittore"*, as the Italians say. Our life is nothing but ersatz.

The first filter is the nervous system. There are an infinite number of messages too subtle for us to perceive. Sound waves for instance less than 20 cycles per second, or greater than 20,000 cycles per second, cannot be detected by humans. The same goes for our eyes that are not capable of detecting certain waveforms. A bee's vision of the world or the olfactory experience of a predator must be very different from ours. This limitation of the nervous system creates a difference between what really happens and how we translate it. The brain itself is selective. That which is not useful for immediate survival is filtered out. Without this valve to reduce our perceptions, humanity, as we know it, would never have been able to survive. An individual would have non-conceptualised perception of space, but be unable to 'technify' it.

The second limitation is that of our social milieu, itself a product of the crystallisation of space through the first filter. It creates a model of representation conditioned by location, climate, culture and customs. Language is an expression of this. All our perceptions and sensations are labelled. The act of naming introduces the filter of conceptualisation. Words serve only to describe a system of conventions, a utilitarian reality. Outside of this reality,

words become a trap. The map is not the territory.
In Maidu, an Indian language of Northern California, there are only three words to describe the spectrum of colours: lak (red), tit (blue-green) and tulak (yellow, orange, brown). Whereas we would describe two objects of different colours - a yellow book and an orange book - using two different words, these same objects in Maidu would be described as 'two tulak books'. In the Inuit language, there are many ways to describe snow, its colour and consistency according to atmospheric conditions. In our language, we only have a few ways of describing the same type of situation.
In Sanskrit (from samskṛta, a past participle that means 'put together', 'elaborately constructed', 'perfect'), the language of the gods (gīrvāṇa bhāṣā), there are four levels of speech.
The first two levels, the grossest forms, are vaikharī and madhyamā. Vaikharī (corporal speech) is the empirical articulated sound that differentiates, and is the most opaque form of sound. Madhyamā (middle or intermediary speech between paśyantī and vaikharī) is the mental language that names, and comes before articulated sound. At this point, language is often only a reflection of our confusion, enclosing us in the even greater confusion of mistaking the description for what is being described. By nature it is dualistic, shrinking the field of perception to a subject-object polarity. The third level, paśyantī (the seer), is total perception without naming, and is in direct contact with the unbroken energy of the event.
The final level, parāvāk (the supreme word), is the source of all the other movements. Parāvāk is space itself, the screen onto which the other levels of speech are projected.

The third filter is that of individual limitations, the patterns and fixed representations we have of ourselves and of the world. These are generated by our personal history and by our experiences, both pleasant and unpleasant, which in turn lead to our conditioning.

These three filters, or knots (granthi), make up the three 'bites' of identification that forge the armour of separation. At no point however are these coagulations restrictive; they are only condensations filled by their own source and not separated from the space in which they appear.
In the next chapter we will look at this process of the emanation of diversity, like the swirl of a river that flows into itself.

Śiva Yantra

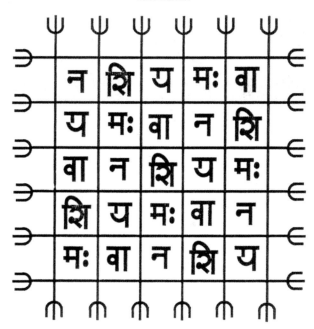

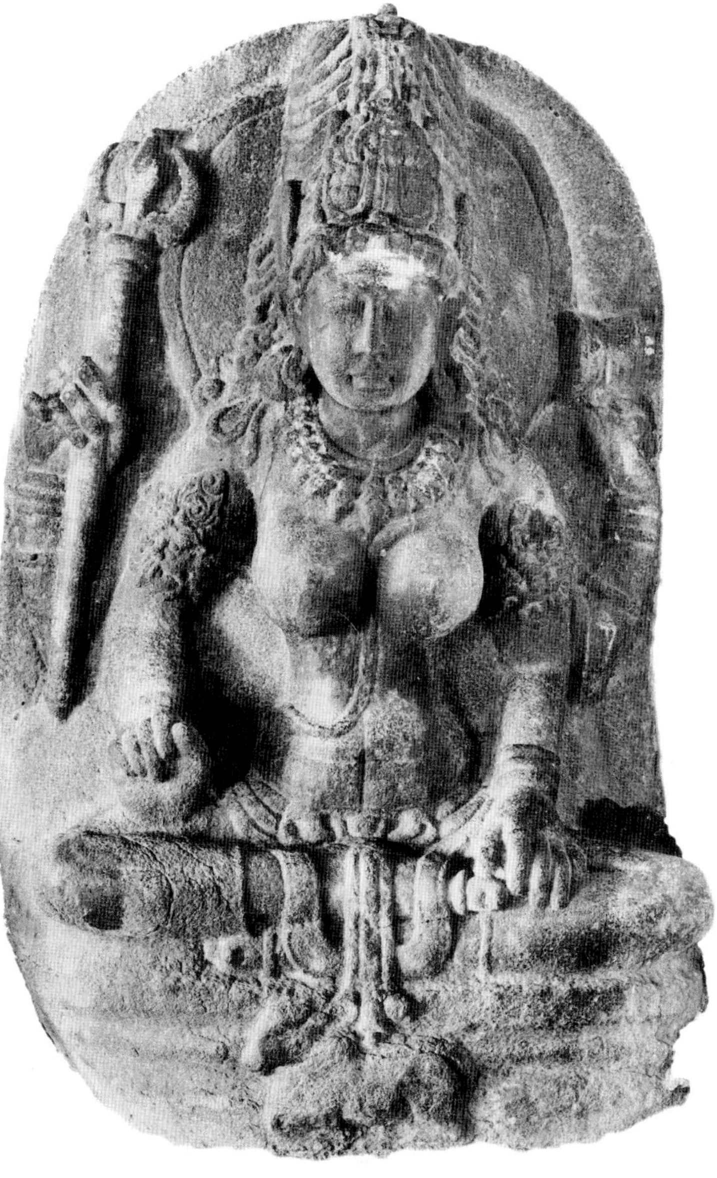

Maheśvarī *11th century*
(Rāmliṅgeśvara Temple, Narasamangala, Mysore Karnataka)

5

The Masks of God

Limiting Biographies (emanation), Identity (maintenance) and Sinking (resorption)

"Let Śiva who has taken the form of my individual being, offer salutation to His universal Being which is also Śiva, for the removal of obstacles which are indeed one with Śiva."
SOMĀNANDA, ŚIVADṚṢṬI I

"Since the seen in its totality is not different from the vision, and the vision itself is not different from the seer, the universe is itself the seer."
VĀMANADATTA, SAṂVITPRAKĀŚA

"The external manifestation of entities (objects) currently appearing in one's perception actually become possible just because they are already present internally as I."
UTPALADEVA, ĪŚVARAPRATYABHIJÑĀKĀRIKĀ I, 5.1

"Just as thin juice, thick juice, still thicker molasses, coarse sugar and refined sugar are all only the juice of sugar cane in different forms, so are all phenomena just different states of Lord Śiva."
"The flow of momentary Consciousness, the single self working in all minds, the power of animation, the universal soul shining as the whole phenomenon, the gross and subtle form, the generalities or species and lastly the individual being, all this consists of mere dialectical conception and does not at all exist in reality."
"No serpent exists in a rope, but the dread it causes could lead to death. Such immense power of delusion cannot be explained or discussed fully."
"In the same way, matters such as piety and sin, heaven and hell, birth and death, pleasure and pain, social castes and stages of life, and so on, never exist in reality, they only appear in the Self on account of the effect of delusion."
"The darkness of delusion is this; that all existing phenomena are taken as different from the Self, though these are non-different from it because of their becoming apparent only inside the light of Consciousness."
ABHINAVAGUPTA, PARAMĀRTHASĀRA 26-27-28-29-30

There is a certain heaviness in the gait of the ordinary man, who is not really that ordinary, having lost this original blessing for the singularity of separation he calls individuality.
There is therefore an uneasiness, a perpetual gnawing, whether we are at the head of an empire or whether we receive social benefits. It is as though each of our footsteps is hammered by anxiety, uncertainty, doubt and fatigue. Wherever we go and whatever we do, we wear our identifications like ramparts, which can of course bring us pleasure, but all too often expose our fear.
We are told we were born on such-and-such a date, in such-and-such a place. Since our earliest childhood, our peculiarities and shortcomings are engrained into us, throwing us to the lions of guilt. In all our actions, perceptions and emotions we wear the mask of separation that we have given

ourselves through the very farce of our individuality. The spontaneous flow of events is fixed, set in a story that begins by a so-called birth and ends with death. Between the two lies a long river of explanations aimed at proving our birth, since it did really happen to us and everything convinces us of it. We are convinced of our education, cultural heritage, successes, failures, choices, goals, and all that encloses us in perpetual contraction. The more we try to prove our birth, the more we want to escape the idea of our death.

And yet, in the depth of the night, in the silence of deep sleep, we return to our abode of peace, where all conflicts are resorbed into their source. We no longer need to brandish a membership flag, we have nothing left to prove as a man or a woman. We can only assume our functions through and by the presence of our own reflective awareness. Whether saint or psychopath, is it not ironic that whatever our motives, we act only by intuition, by the kiss of the source during deep sleep? In the early hours of the morning we can sense these faces that still carry the imprint of the ineffable, a shore of space and silence that pulses in the very heart of our most trivial activities. What then is this mysterious pulsation, so much ourself and so much more than ourself, that we have forgotten it?

"We offer our praise to Śaṅkara, the Lord of the glorious unfolding of the wheel of energies, to Him who in opening and closing his eyes makes the universe disappear and appear. To that in which all creation rests and from which it sprouts, to that where there is never any impediment anywhere; because of its essence nothing can hide it."
VASUGUPTA, SPANDAKĀRIKĀ 1

This great shiver of Consciousness manifests itself in a thousand and one forms and unfolds according to two aspects of exteriority and interiority. In essence, it is neither a question of exteriority nor interiority, but rather of the one and only Consciousness, indivisible and completely free (svātantrya), the radiating brightness (sphurattā) of the heart (hṛdaya), of all existence (mahāsatta). Kṣemarāja says the terms radiating brightness (sphurattā), wave (ūrmi), force (bala), essence (sāra) and heart (hṛdaya) are used in the Tantra as synonyms for spanda. Ghūrni is another term that is used, which, when referring to the eyes, literally means 'to roll in all directions', and denotes the state of inebriation. Ghūrni is therefore the ecstatic vibration of Consciousness whose infinite rapture makes one drunk.

Although these two concepts of exteriority and interiority refer to space-time and movement, spanda is neither of these, but is their source: interiority when the manifestation resorbs into its source, exteriority when there is emanation of 'this' and 'that'. Everything is a 'gushing forth', resonating (dhvani) with the 'initial vibration' (spandana) of the supreme subject (parampramātṛ). The declensions of this resonance propagate like waves, unfolding the totality of manifestations in the immediacy of reflective awareness (vimarśa), which shines unto itself and by itself (svaprakāśa). Spanda has various connotations: 'to beat' when referring to the heart, but also 'to shiver' or 'to tremble'. In the Tantra, this vital surge is called the goddess Kaulikī, who generates totality.

"In reality, Consciousness is spanda. Spanda is some kind of movement. If it were a progression from its own essence towards something else, this spanda would just be a simple movement, and we would not add 'some kind' (kiñcit); but on the other hand, if this progression were not a movement, it would not exist. Thus this surge of the essence in itself is called vibration (ucchalattā), without any progression and identical to wonder. The āgama describe it as a 'wave' (ūrmi) or the 'belly of the fish' (udara)." ABHINAVAGUPTA, PARĀTRĪŚIKĀVIVARAṆA, TRANSLATED BY RANIERO GNOLI, PAGE 132

These waves express different colourations of the absolute, like an actor playing different roles. They bear the names of supreme vibration (parāspanda), intermediate vibration (parāparāspanda) and lower vibration (aparāspanda). In parāspanda there is not yet a stage, and all the roles are contained in the supreme subject. Like the seed that contains the tree, this potentiality expresses the play of Consciousness in its immutable and dynamic aspects, unfolding its outer web.

It is this universal vibration (sāmānyaspanda) that is expressed as the particular (viśeśaspanda), in the same way the ocean is expressed as waves. Each of us experiences the particular in ordinary perception. The yogi listens to the vibration of differentiation in order to be immersed in the universal vibration. It is this universal vibration that gives the script and the roles, which change according to whether their direction is that of interiority or exteriority, and which move towards total subjectivity as well as towards the illusory separation of the object. It is this universal vibration that becomes the breath of life, acting at a grosser level as ordinary breath, giving power to the formulas (mantra) and making the wheel of divine energies turn.

The jolt of the cosmic drama can then be felt and the stage appears in the intermediate vibration (parāparāspanda). This is a wave of median contraction, between the total fusion of subject and object, and their energy of differentiation. The third wave (aparāspanda) unfolds the final contraction. This is the ultimate exteriorisation, which is expressed as the vibration of particularities (viśeśaspanda). It adorns the three guṇa, different armours and the cloaks of separation through the organs of the senses. It is here the Lord becomes masked, taking on the appearance of a limited personality, forgetful of His plenitude, seeing the universe as being separate from Himself. Since perception is veiled by incompleteness, we each tell ourselves the tragicomedy of our separation: tragic because it bears the mark of suffering, comic because there has never been any separation.

"Even though different, this vibration (spanda) unfolds itself in different states like waking, dreaming, etc., which are never distinct from Him. It never departs from its own nature as the perceiving subject." VASUGUPTA, SPANDAKĀRIKĀ 3

"According to Spanda teaching, the reflexive attention (svavimarśa) of the heart from which all things emanate, present at the start and end of the act of perceiving, is known as the universal vibration (sāmānyaspanda). It is the pouring out of Consciousness inside one's own nature. This vibration is a subtle movement (kimciccalana), totally independent, a pulse radiating with the reflexive and luminous attention of Consciousness that shines in everything. It is the wave (ūrmi) in the ocean of Consciousness that is never without waves. At times, it is natural for the ocean to be calm, without waves, and at other times agitated and full of waves. This reflexive attention is the essence (sāra) of everything, Consciousness being the essence of the universe, which is inert (jada) because its true nature depends on Consciousness itself. And the essence of all this is the Heart."

ABHINAVAGUPTA, TANTRĀLOKA IV, 182B-186A

However, even the densest darkness caused by the painful difference of being a separate entity, only exists by and in the shining brilliance of the supreme. Somānanda in his Śivadṛṣṭi, without using the term vibration (spanda), preferring the terms radiating brightness (sphurattā) and that which flows (prasāra), speaks of this recognition which can surge spontaneously during everyday activities, whenever strong emotions are felt, instantly stopping the flow of becoming.

"It can be discovered in the region of the heart at the moment of remembering an urgent task, when one is told exciting news, at the precise instant of a dreadful vision, at the sight of something unexpected, at the beginning of the seminal flow; or when reading rapidly or fleeing for one's life. In these occasions there is a shivering (vilolatā) of all the energies." SOMĀNANDA, ŚIVADṚṢṬI I, 9-11A

Spanda is the chant of Consciousness, which is beyond becoming. Although immutable, this pulsation is both static and dynamic.

"Of this spanda principle, two states are spoken about: of the doer or subject, and of the deed or object. Of these two,

the deed or object is perishable but the subject is imperishable." VASUGUPTA, SPANDAKĀRIKĀ 14

Bhaṭṭa Kallaṭa inverses the terms opening (unmeṣa) and closing (nimeṣa) of Śaṅkara's eyes to describe the expansion and resorption of the universe. When Śiva opens his eyes to subjectivity, the universe disappears; and when he closes his eyes to subjectivity, the universe appears.

"To Him who by opening and closing His eyes makes the universe appear and disappear." VASUGUPTA, SPANDAKĀRIKĀ 1

Śiva shrouds himself in five swirling energies, like the magician's swirling actions to fool us with the tricks up his sleeve. These energies reveal five functions (pañcakṛtya): emanation (sṛṣṭi), maintenance (sthiti), resorption (saṃhāra), dissimulation (tirodhāna) and revelation of His nature through his grace (anugraha). The comparison with a mirror is often used: even though a mirror reflects thousands of objects, it is not transformed by those objects. The comparison stops there since it cannot convey the subtlety of this intuition of the reflection of the universe (pratibimbavāda) by Consciousness. A mirror reflects objects external to it. But here, nothing is external. In the ocean of the absolute, waves appear. These waves can be considered during a moment of amnesia as differentiation, as 'this' and 'that', but even this outer expression is the ocean itself.

"As we have said, the supreme blazing that is Bhairava is nothing but light. For now, we are examining its aspect of pure freedom. The nature of this light is to illuminate all things. The universe is not separate to it, and if it were, it would not be manifest. Thus, Parameśvara, with His total freedom, manifests all the different aspects of cosmic emissions and resorptions in the firmament of His own Self. In the same way earth, water, etc. are reflected in a mirror without being confused, all expressions of all things shine from the supreme Lord, who is nothing other than pure Consciousness." ABHINAVAGUPTA, TANTRĀLOKA III, 1-4

An āgama says: *"O beloved! One, who learns from the books or the master's mouth the nature of water and ice, has no more duty to perform. This present birth will be the last."*

All by-products of milk are already present in the milk. Similarly, nothing is separate from Consciousness, and although it seems to take ever more contracted forms, passing from pure subjectivity (śakti) to diversity in unity (vidyā), where one can feel the germination of phenomenon, through to the final contraction in objectivity (māyā), these are merely reflective manifestations (ābhāsa) of itself. Its total freedom (svātantrya) gives birth to this game of reflections, resulting in the belief of enslavement.

"To the following objection, how in reality can the pure subject, fully conscious, become an object, and in the process, unconscious? It is answered that in reality Consciousness stays essentially the same. Nothing can be added to or taken away from it; but because of its own and total freedom which makes the impossible happen, this Lord is very skilful in hiding his own self."
ABHINAVAGUPTA, TANTRĀLOKA IV, 8-10

One day, a king with no heirs who felt death approaching had a dream. The next king will be the first creature encountered at the palace gates at dawn. He informed his ministers and they were dismayed. Despite their protests, the king wouldn't change his mind. They did as they were told. At the gates at first light was a dozing beggar. He was taken to the palace where preparations for the crowning ceremony were begun. After the ceremony, the new king sat on his throne in his magnificent new clothes, a sceptre in his hand, surrounded by the whole court. He asked the time. When he was told, he said in an anxious voice: *"I must go now. People will soon be leaving the temple and it's the best time to beg!"* Forgetful of our heroic and royal nature we become beggars of duality, when, in the thick of identification, we tell ourselves the story of our lives. We take our different psychophysical clothes for our total reality. They are like

Balzac's 'magic skin' that shrinks every time we identify ourselves with them, and they are never to our satisfaction. We feel imperfect (incompletness, āṇavamala), we have a certain appearance and certain characteristics (illusion of contraction, māyīyamala), and we have a certain function (contraction of the action through the actor, kārmamala). Nevertheless, *"the gross state is merely the blossoming of the essence, and subtlety is merely the bud of the gross state."* (ANONYMOUS)

At the end of the day, when we are through with our daily occupations and we feel the silence of night shrouding us, we all know the pleasure of getting rid of our clothes and functions. When the body abandons itself, just before the kiss of sleep, the flow of exhalation points the way to the resorption of our various sheaths, from the grossest to the subtlest. These sheaths are known under the name of categories or principles (tattva).

"The tattva comprising the twenty-five of Sāṃkya and additional eleven are no realities per se, but the pervasive general principles underlying all existent entities."
ABHINAVAGUPTA'S HERMENEUTICS OF THE ABSOLUTE, B. BÄUMER, PAGE 143

According to the Sarvajñānottara (34), *"The tattva are imperceptible and pervasive in the whole world."*

In his Īśvarapratyabhijñāvimarśinī (III, 1.2), Abhinavagupta defines tattva (the essential nature of that) as *"one that shines undivided in the various groups of things, with distinctive features, and so serves as the cause to justify their being represented as belonging to one class."*

Traditionally, these tattva are described either in a 'descending' order towards the densest principle or in an 'ascending' order towards the subtlest. The terms 'ascending' and 'descending' should not be taken literally, for they are simply an allusion of transcendence in immanence and immanence in transcendence. These principles are merely a reflection (ābhāsa) of pure and undivided Consciousness. The mouth of becoming only opens phenomenally; in the absolute, nothing happens. In the dream state, entire universes may loom up and we can feel the whole gamut of emotions. But even if we wake up in a sweat, our body trembling from a nightmare, from the point of view of the dream it was all very real, but from the point of view of the waking state nothing happened.

"Like a King, master of the entire earth, in the joyous exaltation of his power, can, just for fun, do the duties of a simple soldier. Thus the All-Potent in his exuberant joy, enjoys himself as the multiple forms of this universe."
SOMĀNANDA, ŚIVADṚṢṬI I, 37B-38

The absolute exhaled (visarga: emission) thirty-six breaths, or mists, in which he shrouded himself.

"Sometimes God in his unfolding appears through the energy of His will as the sole energy (Śaktitattva), sometimes through the excess of his cognitive energy he appears as the eternal Śiva (Sadāśiva), or through the extension of his energy of activity he appears as the sovereign state (Īśvara). Sometimes He assumes the state of pure science (Śuddhavidyā) or sometimes He likes to hide Himself and shows Himself as illusion (Māyā). Thus He puts on the aspects of the thirty-six levels of reality, successively embracing the different stages up to the gross manifestation of the earth, unconscious, dense and resistant." SOMĀNANDA, ŚIVADṚṢṬI I, 29B-33

The first two tattva are called Śivatattva and Śaktitattva. They are only named tattva for pedagogical reasons, in order to describe the immutable aspect of Śiva and his dynamic aspect, Śakti. Śiva represents the transcendental unity of 'I' (ahaṃ), and Śakti the felicity of 'I am' (ahaṃ asmi). Śiva is never separate from Śakti and vice versa. They are one with the source Paramaśiva and are not part of creation.

"The divine action, vibrating inwardly as well as outwardly

in accordance with time sequence, belongs to none other that the infinite Subject of knowing. Therefore infinite knowledge and action are mutually inseparable."
UTPALADEVA, ĪŚVARAPRATYABHIJÑĀKĀRIKĀ III, 1.1

These two tattva still remain in the realm of perfect subjectivity. The total subjectivity of 'I' is filtered by a very subtle objectivity in realising 'I am this', which corresponds to the unfolding of objectivity as 'this' (idam). This fine mist is called Sadāśivatattva. There is then a subtle differentiation with the opening (unmeṣa) of the eyes, symbolising extroversion of the universe, of 'this' and 'that'. The feeling 'I am this' becomes 'this I am' in Īśvaratattva, which corresponds to the closing (nimeṣa) of subjectivity as 'I' (ahaṃ). In Śuddhavidyātattva there is a grosser subjectivity which differentiates, but which does not yet separate the 'I' (ahaṃ) and the universe (idam). Both are balanced. Śuddhavidyātattva is the final tattva of pure subjectivity.

"Īśvara is the extroversive aspect of the absolute and Sadāśiva is the introversive aspect, the former being known in the āgama as unmeṣa and the latter as nimeṣa."
UTPALADEVA, ĪŚVARAPRATYABHIJÑĀKĀRIKĀ III, 1.3

Exteriority expresses itself in six armours (ṣaṭkañcuka, which will be looked at in more detail in a later chapter) that are the next tattva. In māyātattva, objectivity breathes through various limitations and contractions. These contractions plunge us into amnesia of our primordial nature, making us believe we are its limitations and giving us the impression of being separate; the illusion of individuality. All that we perceive is different, foreign. Kalātattva limits creativity. Vidyātattva limits knowledge. Rāgatattva limits our actions. Niyatitattva limits space. Kālatattva limits time. Paramaśiva is now disguised in finitude and becomes Puruṣatattva, also called jīva, aṇu, paśu, terms that denote limitation, restriction.

"Bound by the energy of limitations, he is named Paśu."
ABHINAVAGUPTA, ĪŚVARAPRATYABHIJÑĀVIMARŚINĪ ĀGAMĀDHIKĀRA II, 3

Forgetting subjectivity favours a reality of objects that seem to have a separate existence, and which unfolds the next tattva, the root substance (prakṛtitattva, mūlaprakṛti) or principle substance (pradhānatattva). Prakṛtitattva unfolds the other twenty-three principles. The internal organ (antaḥkaraṇatattva), comprising intellect (buddhi), mind (manas) and ego (ahaṃkāra), cements the fortress of personality and allows, as in a play, the entrance of characters so the play of Consciousness can unfold. The ego principle (ahaṃkāratattva) is the actor's mask that appropriates action. What we did and shouldn't have, what we didn't do and should have, what we did that fills us with pride or with shame. Ahaṃkāratattva fixes us in a role that is itself narrowed by the intellect principle (buddhitattva). It is all the considerations relating to the validity of an action. Must it be done or not? Is it good or bad? These considerations vary according to place, culture, climate, and only have circumstantial value.

"Good and bad are part of the artificial, of the evanescent, of what is not your real nature and from which we part easily. If we take the prescribed and the forbidden for the criteria of truth, ultimately the sole criteria will be Parameśvara Himself, the omnipresent who transcends all and can make the prescribed forbidden and the forbidden prescribed."
MAHEŚVARĀNANDA, SAṂVIDULLĀSA

The actual mental process is the realm of the mind principle (manastattva), which is defined as saṃkalpasādhana or creation of affirmations (saṃkalpa) and thoughts, whatever they may be. The ten other tattva participate in grasping the universe through the five organs of perception (pañcajñānendriya) and the five organs of action (pañcakarmendriya). The organ of hearing creates sounds and grasps them with the ear (śrotratattva). The

organ of touch creates tactile sensations and grasps them with the skin (tvaktattva). The organ of sight creates forms and grasps them with the eye (cakṣutattva). The organ of taste creates flavours and grasps them with the tongue (rasanatattva). The organ of smell creates odours and grasps them with the nose (ghrāṇatattva). According to the Spanda School, the five organs of perception are expressions of the blazing of Consciousness. The idea they are gross elements is rejected and it is claimed their source is in the ego (ahaṃkāra) as the luminous principle (sattva) of Consciousness. At the heart of each perception, I feel, I see, I taste, etc., resides 'I-ness'. The organs of perception (jñānendriya) are externalised in the five organs of action (pañcakarmendriya). The organ of communication creates sound and is expressed with speech (vāktattva). The organ of prehension manifests taking or giving and is expressed through the hand (pāṇitattva). The organ of locomotion manifests movement in space and is expressed through the foot (pādatattva). The functions of elimination are expressed through the organ of excretion (pāyutattva). The functions of reproduction and urination are expressed through the sexual organ (upasthatattva).
For the person who believes himself to be limited, the organs of perception and action are used only to grasp and fragment the world. They only reinforce the tyranny of separation. For the hero, the organs of perception and action, as Abhinavagupta says, are *"Śiva, free, and of transparent essence, who ceaselessly vibrates. His supreme energy rises up to the extreme point of the sensorial organs. He then is just bliss and this universe appears too, as vibrating."* (Quoted in Maheśvarānanda's Mahārthamañjarī, translated by Lilian Silburn, page 90)

We will see in another chapter how, especially in the exploration of āsana, sensation itself is the sinking of separation. The solidification of reality, at its grossest level, acts in the next ten tattva: the five subtle elements (pañcatanmātra) and the five gross elements (pañcamahābhūta). The pañcatanmātra are the subtle forms of pañcamahābhūta. The element of sound (śabdatanmātra) is expressed in the element of ether (ākāśatattva). The element of touch (sparśatanmātra) is expressed in the element of air (vāyutattva). The element of form (rūpatanmātra), or rather the localisation of the sensation of the object, is expressed in the element of fire (tejastattva). The element or sensation of taste (rasatanmātra) is expressed in the element of water (jalatattva). The element where the sensation of odour arises (gandhatanmātra) is expressed in the element of earth (pṛthivītattva).

The spell of this incredible magician unfolds an infinite play of mirrors to make us believe in our finitude, like in tales where we find stories within stories, one after the other until we forget the start of the story. The final touches of make-up have been made. We will now witness the most incredible of performances, where unity will take on the face of diversity. Each of us has a script and we will be such good actors that we will forget ourselves in our roles. O, mysterious dance of Śiva (tāṇḍava)! This amnesia too is fake since it shines with the resonance (dhvani) of the supreme essence.

"The ruler of the gods binds himself and frees himself. He is himself the subject who experiences pleasure and pain. He is himself the knowing subject. Therefore let him investigate himself too."
Sāraśāstra

As in theatre, the three blows are heard, making the stage vibrate and freeing the round of guṇa. Let the party begin!

"The actor of the cosmic drama, Śambhu, pure Consciousness, becomes an individual soul whose amazing state is to assume all roles."
Maheśvarānanda, Mahārthamañjarī 19

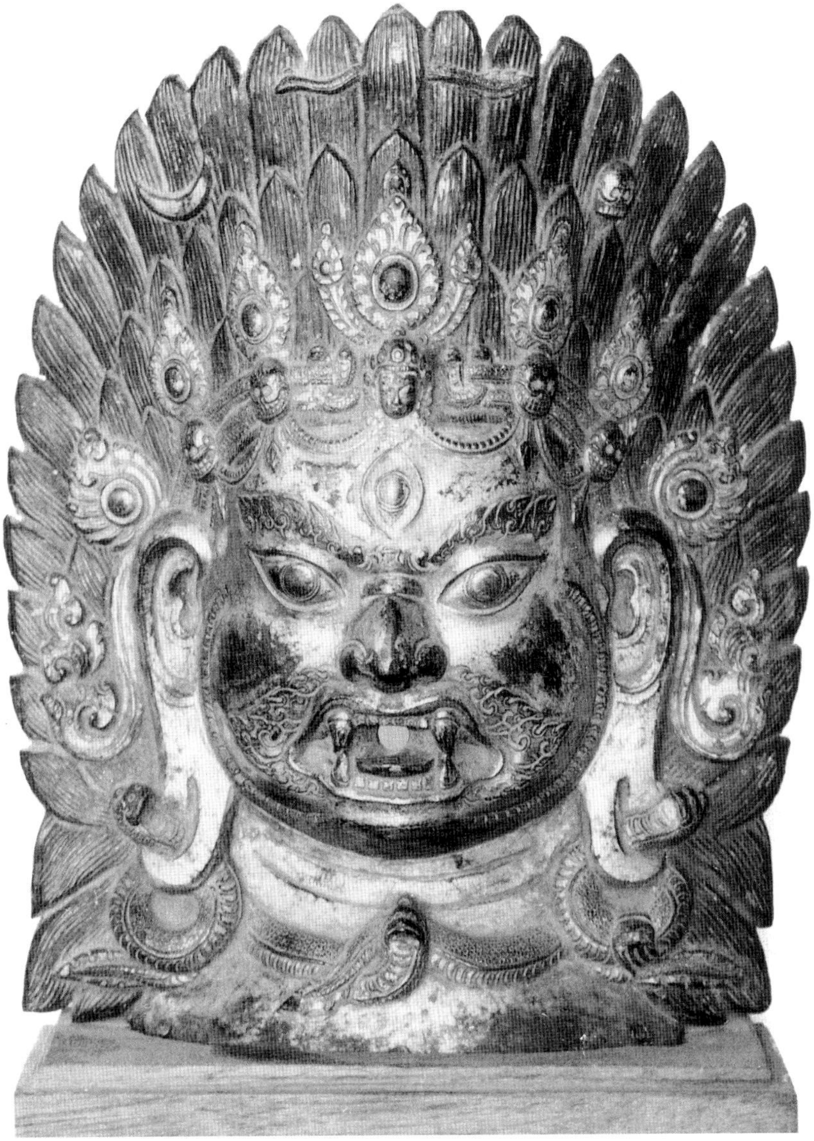

Mahākāla *19th century*
(Bharat Kala Bhawan, Vārāṇasī)

6

The Armours of Amnesia

"In the ultimate Reality, there is neither appearance nor disappearance. Only the supreme and vibrant energy exists, which, although beyond temporal sequence, is revealed as space-time. It is merely pure metaphor to say it 'appears and disappears'."
Somānanda, Śivadṛṣṭi I, 29b-33

"He takes delight in hiding his own self and to appear as illusion."
Kṣemarāja, Spandanirnaya I, 21

"When the milk comes out of the cow's udder, it goes through some transformation but it does not mean that it is not milk anymore."
Somānanda, Śivadṛṣṭi I, 18-20a

In the Mahābhārata there is a story of a game of dice that leads to a fratricide war. Knowing Yudhiṣṭhira's passion for the game, the Kaurava challenge him. Yudhiṣṭhira cannot refuse, but he is a very poor gambler and is challenged by a professional for whom the dice hold no secret. Yudhiṣṭhira has no chance.
We know that after this game the Pāṇḍava lose everything, even themselves! They are saved from slavery by a technicality. Yudhiṣṭhira gambles Draupadī after having lost himself. By a stroke of luck, Draupadī wins back their freedom, but they must spend twelve years in exile. The thirteenth year must then be spent in total secrecy and if they are discovered, they will be exiled for a further twelve years. During this thirteenth year the Pāṇḍava have functions that are completely opposed to the dharma of their caste. Knowing what is going to happen, Bhīṣma asks Kṛṣṇa if he should intervene: *"Is it not better to avoid the worst?"*
"What is the worst?" asks Kṛṣṇa.
"The loss of dharma", replies Bhīṣma.
"And if it must come to the worst in order dharma is preserved? This is why I ask that no matter what happens do not intervene. Let each of them play to their limit."
Kṛṣṇa reminds us of the song of the absolute. Let everyone reach their limits, those of the body-mind, whether it be in pleasure or suffering. Let everyone reach the limits of their identification. This total vulnerability has the stability of a rock. All limits collapse into non-limit.
The power of illusion and contraction (māyāśakti) is nothing other than the power of liberty, of totality (svātantrya), of the absolute in its darkening phase. Māyāśakti injects three venoms (mala: impurity) into objectivation, referred to as gross impurity (sthūla), subtle impurity (sūkṣma) and supreme impurity (parā).
The flow of universal, spontaneous energy of action (kriyāśakti) is obscured into partial and conditioned

actions, ending with the play of the organs of action in carrying out mundane activities (kārmamala: impurity of action), and deeds deemed to be 'good' or 'bad'. The flow of intuitive knowledge (jñānaśakti) is obscured into partial knowledge, by the extension of the internal organ (antaḥkaraṇa) and the senses, ending in the impurity of differentiated perception (māyīyamala), tainted with ignorance. The flow of the energy of will of the absolute (icchāśakti) is obscured into the incompleteness of the limited being (aṇu), ending in a feeling of finitude, individuation (āṇavamala) and a sense of lacking, as if we were not complete (āpūrṇa).

"Omnipotent, omniscient, perfect, eternal and non limited, the Lord through the unfolding of his five energies appears as an individual with the opposite qualities."
MAHEŚVARĀNANDA, MAHĀRTHAMAÑJARĪ 18

This kiss of māyā, which gives us the taste of individuality, leads us into a whirling oblivion. It is a bit like deep sleep for Puruṣa, where the activity of Consciousness is reduced to a minimum. Māyā cloaks Puruṣa with five armours (kañcuka) to stimulate us, but in a limited and conditioned way. These five armours change the qualities of the absolute into a series of contractions. It is just a different point of view, two sides of the same coin.
Omniscience contracts and appears as spatial localisation (niyatitattva): 'I live in England, I am English'.
Eternity contracts and appears as temporal localisation (kālatattva): 'I have a certain age, at a certain time.'
Plenitude contracts and appears as lacking, incompleteness (rāgatattva), giving us the insatiable desire to fill the void.
Intuitive knowledge contracts and appears as limited knowledge (vidyātattva) that is always lacking because always insufficient.
Spontaneous effusion contracts and appears as creativity that is always partial, limited by the energy of fragmentation (kalātattva).

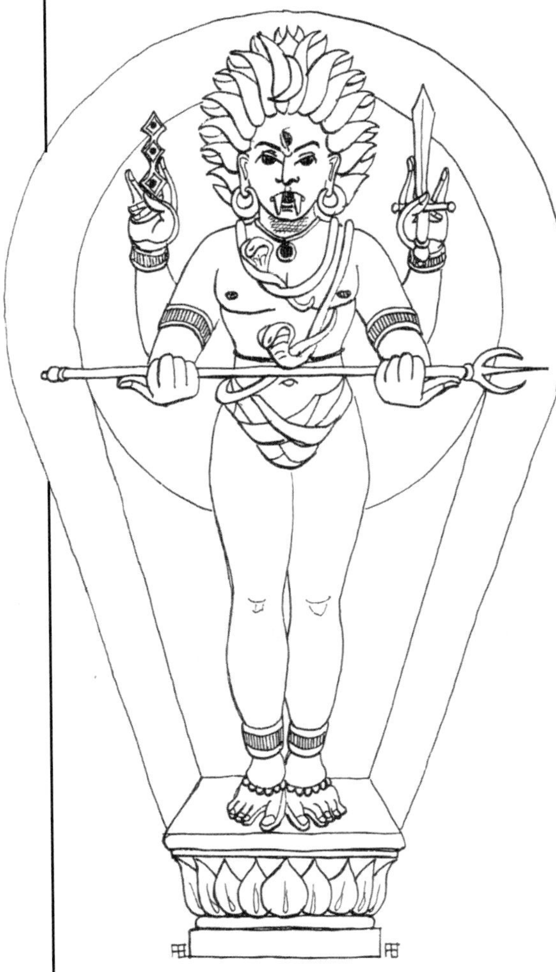

RAUDRAPAŚUPATAMŪRTI

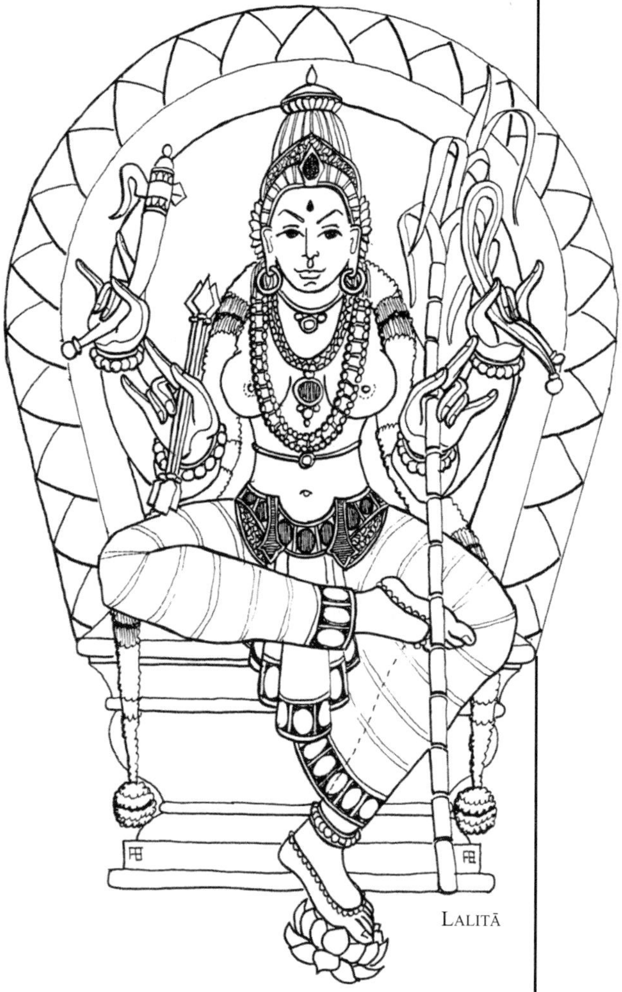

Lalitā

Who has never looked with astonishment at their passport photo, thinking 'am I really like that'? The records of our experiences, that we've accumulated in order to try to define and situate ourselves, all wear out with time and provide only a lame defence against the assault of the unexpected.

We believe we belong to a country, a culture. We bear our age with the burden of memory. Although we have everything we need, we are starving for experience. We chase after a myriad of trinkets, as though they are miraculous destinations, in the hope they will calm our burning. If we are alone, we want to meet someone. If we are with someone, we tell ourselves we would be better off alone. We have an ill-fitting, second-hand knowledge that cannot quieten our fear of the unknown. Even if we are an expert, we feel helpless against the daily humdrum. In certain moments of grace, without warning, we are touched by the ever-incomprehensible intuition that all this is only a game. We are our own divinity, wearing the mask of separation.

"Here the divinity is Consciousness, as our own Self, questioning itself and being on the verge of revealing itself."
Abhinavagupta, Parātrīśikālaghuvṛtti, Introductory Stanza

"In this supreme state of Bhairava which is not a state, happiness and pain, shackles and freedom, Consciousness and unConsciousness, are just denominations. They are just pointing to the same and sole reality, like the words 'pitcher' and 'pot' apply to the same object."
Abhinavagupta, Tantrāloka II, 19

"The Śaivite reality remains the same, at the heart of all things. Only those with erroneous convictions separate upper and lower. This reality (Śivatattva) is eternal and infinite. It is the essence of differentiation since the true nature of the Lord is to take on multiple forms."
Somānanda, Śivadṛṣṭi I, 48-49

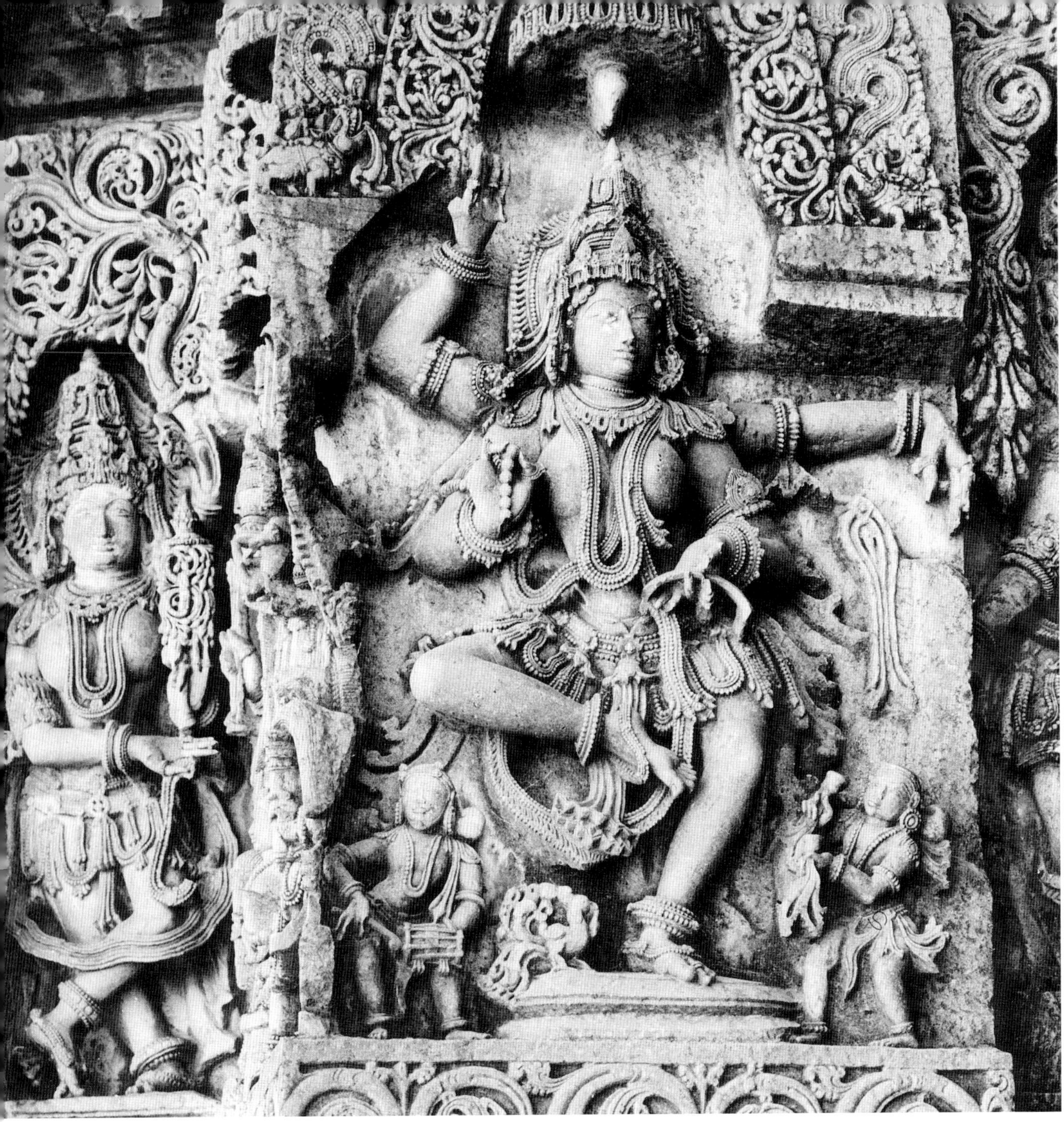

Sarasvatī *12th century*
(Hoyśleśvara Temple, Halebad, Mysore)

7

The Five Gaping Mouths of Consciousness

"From one sole and unique energy comes emanation and resorption.

On one hand, awakening and emanation of the universe,
with the apparition of different elements from Śiva to the earth:
emission with an infinite variety which engulfs the essence of the undifferentiated.

On the other hand, this same energy resorbs all exteriority
when there is emergence of the essence which erases all differentiations."

BHAṬṬA KALLAṬA, COMMENTARY ON SPANDAKĀRIKĀ 1

Consciousness manifests the actors (Śiva, Mantramaheśvarā, Mantreśvarā, Mantra, Vijñānākala, Pralayākala, Śakala) and the various roles they must play. According to their level of subjectivity and spheres of objectivity, they unfold one or resorb the other, thereby showing that appearance and disappearance are only an insinuation of that by which and in which they are manifested.
These beings incarnate either the divinity, like the Mantramaheśvarā, or become completely limited under the grip of impurities (mala) and the five armours (pañcakañcuka), like the Śakala, which literally means 'those who are divided, caught in the flow of time'.

"A person who sees objects as his own form is called a master (pati), while one lying under the effects of delusion and seeing objects as different from him is called a bound being (paśu)."
UTPALADEVA, ĪŚVARAPRATYABHIJÑĀKĀRIKĀ III, 2.3

These actors unfold according to a hierarchy in which the superior actors perceive themselves as the source of objectivity, and those who are lower perceive themselves as subordinate.This reality reflects the five main energies of the absolute:
• The energy of Consciousness, one and indivisible (citśakti);
• The energy of plenitude (ānandaśakti);
• The energy of will (icchāśakti);
• The energy of intuition (jñānaśakti);
• The energy of spontaneous action (kriyāśakti).

Iconographically, they are depicted as the five forms (pañcamukha) of the manifestation of Śiva Svacchandanātha:

Īśāna, Tatpuruṣa, Sadyojāta, Vāmadeva and Aghora. Pañca comes from the root PAÑC meaning 'to spread'. These five forms are merely a metaphor for the extraordinary diversity of the one thousand and one emanations of he who is faceless, formless, beginningless and timeless (niśkālaśiva). They represent the five directions, the five elements, the five races, the fives senses, etc. The epithet associated with Śiva represents his position, as well as his energetic colouration. Īśāna, the governor, looks up towards the sky and symbolises absolute knowledge. Tatpuruṣa, the Supreme Being, faces east. He is affiliated to the priest caste (brāhmaṇa) and symbolises knowledge in beatitude. Sadyojāta, he who is born suddenly, faces north and is the embodiment of the mind and sexual organs. He is affiliated to the servant caste (śūdra). Vāmadeva faces west. He is the embodiment of ahaṃkāra and the organs of action. He is affiliated to the merchant caste (vaiśya). Aghora, he who is ignorant of fear, faces south. He is the embodiment of death and the end of discriminative knowledge. He is affiliated to the warrior caste (kṣatriya). These faces chant the hymn of reality according to five different savours, thereby expressing the tantra. The term tantra is used here in the sense of intuitive revelation (āgama), of expansion, transmission, long extension (tanu viśtare), rather than referring to the actual texts, although traditionally we talk about the revelation of the ten dualistic tantra (bheda), eighteen dualistic/non-dualistic tantra (bhedābheda) and the sixty-four non-dualistic tantra (abheda).

Our perception of reality depends on our reading of it. We may have a dual reading (dvaita), where all perception comes from a sense of separation between

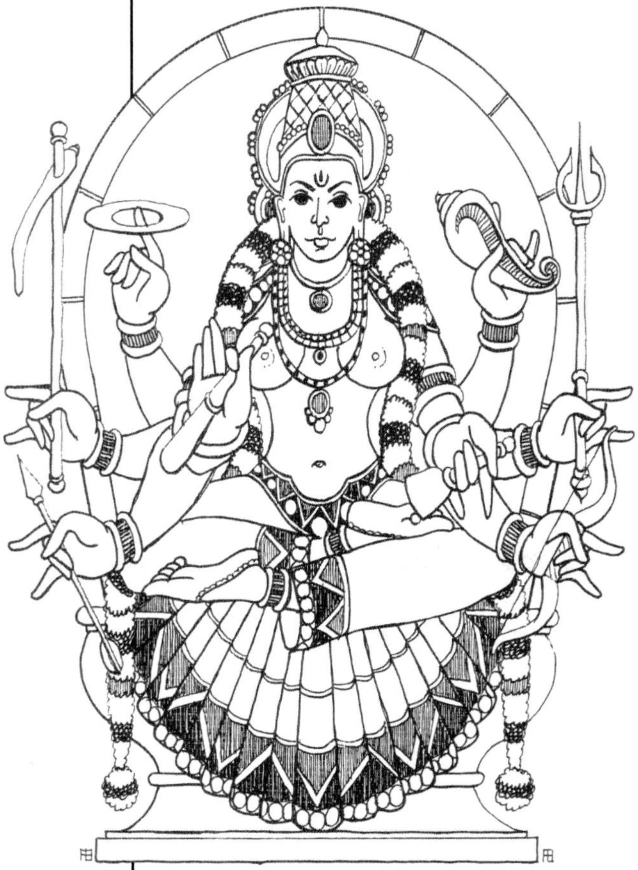

Mahāsarasvatī

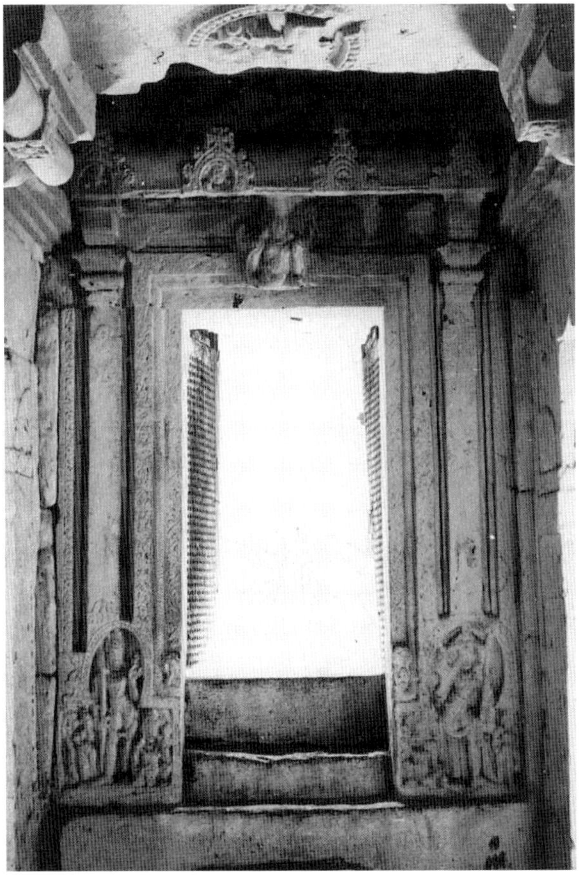

Bijapur
7th century
(Badami, Karnataka)

ourselves and others. Here, everything exists in separation. To describe this state of mind the image of two battleships confronting one another can be used. Each is exclusive of the other. The notion of territory is preponderant and all that we meet seems strange, potentially dangerous. When our reading becomes more refined, we are more inclined to sense diversity in unity (viśiṣṭādvaita). We don't now insist so much on the exclusivity of the two battleships, but instead we begin to open up to the inclusiveness of the ocean. And yet there remains a boundary between unity and diversity, as in the theory of internal differences (svāgatabheda) of viśiṣṭādvaitins, where there is a clear demarcation between creator and creation, even though they are intimately connected like the body and soul. These two melodies, dvaita and dvaitādvaita, then melt into the song of non-duality (parādvaita), where only the inclusiveness of the ocean remains.

In this intuition, all phenomena are mere reflections, manifestations unseparated from the absolute. Here, everything is perceived as being the source of itself. Nothing is foreign, all things are merely one's self. Even the concepts of diversity and unity are included in what is their source.

"Genuine non-dualism is the vision which sees unity in the diversity of these points of view: this is diversity, this is unity and it is also both, diversity and unity at the same time."
ABHINAVAGUPTA, MĀLINĪVIJAYAVĀRTIKA I, 626

"In the same way one teaches a pupil not yet familiar with certain synonyms that a jar is also a pot, thus it is said that the Lord is all manifest phenomena."
ABHINAVAGUPTA, MĀLINĪVIJAYAVĀRTIKA I, 929

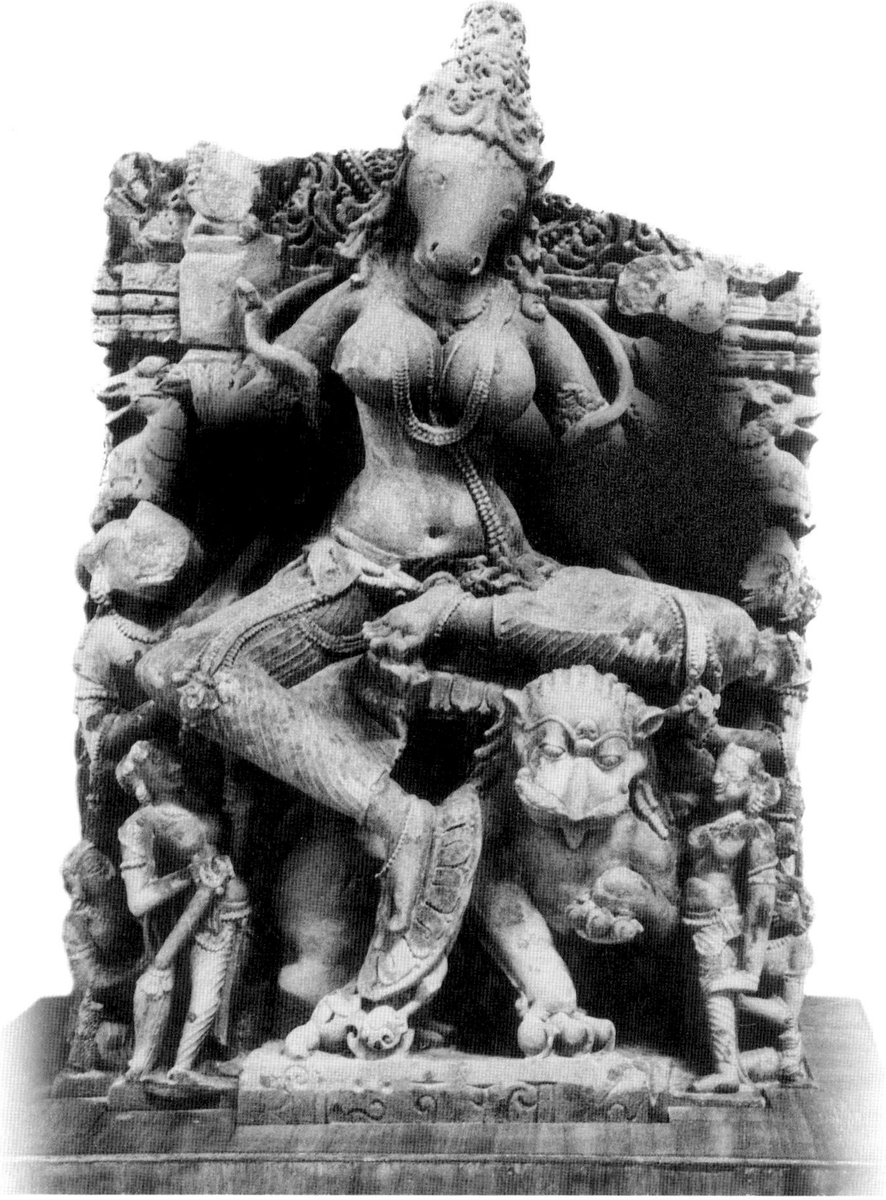

Itarala *11th century*
(Gurgi, Madhya Pradesh)

8

The Texture of Reality: Faces and Expressions of Space-Time

"All this is nothing but the phantom for frightening children,
or a sweet given by the mother to attract the child.
These descriptions are only meant for the spiritual advancement
of the unenlightened."

VIJÑĀNA BHAIRAVA 13

The path of objectivity is a path which only comes to an end in its source: Consciousness, Śiva. This path is metaphorically depicted as being the corridor of the worlds (bhuvanādhva). We speak of one hundred and eighteen worlds to describe the continual and futile cycle of trying to find anything in objects, in the gross (sthūla) corridor of the external world. The external worlds (bhuvana) are the grossest manifestation of space as a stage and crystallisation of the body-mind. Gross perception focuses on the scintillation of the tens of thousands of objects in these worlds created by our desires. The corridor of the worlds is a vast supermarket in which we rush from one aisle to another, fascinated by the display of all that is on offer to meet our fantasies for worldly, emotional and spiritual security.

When we become tired of this constant investment in objects, we can sense that this scintillation is nothing more than the reflexive light (vimarśa, prakāśa) of Consciousness. The object itself only exists by and because of this scintillation. It is merely a reflection that could not be perceived if this reflexive light of Consciousness did not exist.

The corridor of the worlds (bhuvana) then becomes the corridor of principles (tattvādhva). This world is merely the gross, objective crystallisation of more subtle elements. The objective world is merely a shadow. We open up to the possibility of what is behind the scenes of perception, once freed from grasping. The thirty-six tattva are themselves the scintillation of the five energies, which are the essence of these principles. The restrictive emanation of these energies is referred to as kalādhva, made up of five expansions. These five expansions unfold the thirty-six principles, declaiming the gamut of subjectivity and objectivity.

In its gross aspect, reality is constantly narrowed by concepts, by names (mantra). At an intermediate level, names become syllabic (pada), and in its subtle aspect, reality becomes the expression of phonematic energies (varṇa). What we call reality is only a fabric of changing points of view, different contents, constantly shifting. We experience reality through three states: the waking state (jāgratavasthā), the dream state (svapnāvasthā) and the deep sleep state (suṣuptavasthā). When an object is grasped by the organs of perception, this is called the waking state. If no object is recalled by thoughts, this is called the dream state. When there is neither object nor memory, this is the deep sleep state. When only pure Consciousness prevails, this is the fourth state (turya).

For the yogi, the ever-changing nature of the waking state (jāgratavasthā), which for us represents the ultimate reality, is only identification with the world from the point of view of exteriority and separation. What we call 'waking state' is the hypnotic belief in a reality that is separate and exists by itself. This waking state is itself however coloured by our incessant projections, thus giving it a particular tone. If we are in love, the whole world seems to be in love; if we are depressed, the whole world seems depressed. This waking state disappears in the dream state (svapnāvasthā). Although objectively we favour the waking state, the dream state resonates more with subjectivity. The waking state is cramped by social convention. In dreams our mask disappears, and we are touched by more intense emotions and may often have reactions contradictory to our social image. The realisation that dreams are merely an emanation of ourself is more obvious than realising the same is true of the waking state. This is why, even if it only happens intermittently, the dream state is described as being filled by itself, by the subject. When all impressions of objectivity in the waking state and impressions of fluctuating subjectivity in the dream state, due to the sensation of being a body-mind, are drowned in deep sleep (suṣuptavasthā), this state becomes the state of great pervasion (mahāvyāpti), of establishment in the original form (svarūpastha), of peace (śantībhāva). Whatever these states, they can only exist through and in the reflexive light of Consciousness.

"All the states of Consciousness, impressions of happiness and pain, exist only because of the knowing subject which is their background. Without the permanent support of the knowing subject, these experiences could not exist."
Utpalācārya, Spandapradīpikā 4.4

"On the single thread of Self-Awareness the yogi strings the sequent states of waking, sleep, dreamless slumber and undifferenced awareness, as though he were stringing a necklace of many-coloured gems."
Maheśvarānanda, Mahārthamañjarī 61

Thus perception may become an opportunity to taste the essence of sensations, contemplating their Heart as undifferentiated Consciousness. The sinking of exteriority and interiority in deep sleep is characterised by absence. But even this absence can only be known through presence. It's a bit like being in a dark room and saying 'I can't see anything'. When this absence is resorbed into presence, this state is called turyāvasthā. It is described as the fourth state or statelessness beyond form (rūpātita), in which all differentiation is devoured.

"That which is night for all beings, in that the wise one is awake. That in which all beings are awake is night for the sage who sees." Bhagavad Gītā II, 71

"The word night means māyā, which is the cause of the delusion of ordinary people...
The conditions of life in which ordinary people are awake, i.e., engaged in performing activities, these conditions are night for the yogin. This is because a yogin is not awake for worldly activities.
We can say that māyā imposes its influence on ordinary people by applying two different means. First, it gives names and forms to various objects. Second it gives a false

experience of pleasure that is derived from the experience of various objects. It is because ordinary people fail to recognise the real nature of the objects which possess various names and forms, that they continue to live under the spell of experience based on pleasure and pain..."
ABHINAVAGUPTA, GĪTĀRTHASAṂGRAHA
(COMMENTARY ON THE BHAGAVAD GĪTĀ)

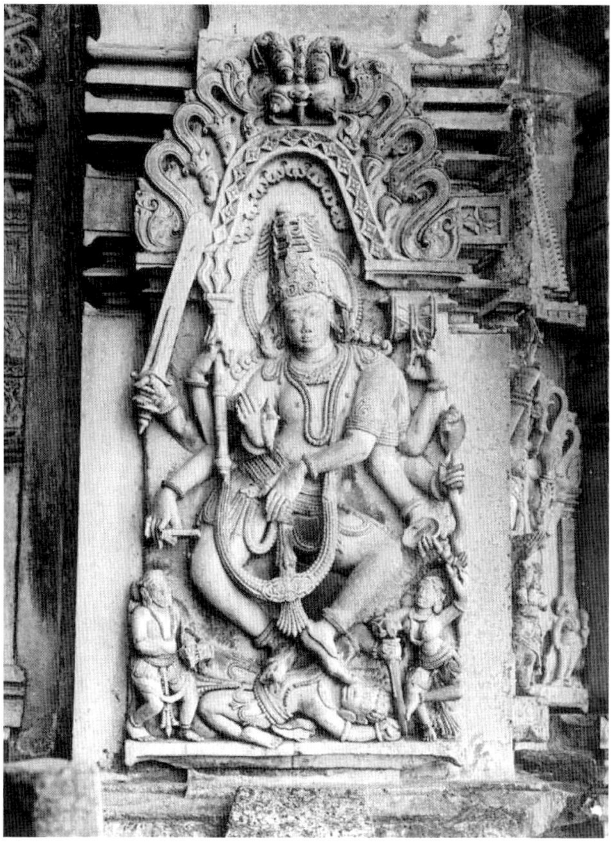

Śiva Naṭeśa
12th century
(Keśava Temple, Belur, Karnataka)

We speak of these different flows as states (avasthā). They have a beginning and an end, but they are only states and therefore only objects of experience. Hence they have the relative nature of all experience. These three states emerge from and submerge into their source, which cannot be defined as a state. In Her bosom, presence and absence no longer have meaning. Every way, every path, every goal and every form of experimentation by any kind of activity is impossible. Any hope of acquiring a new state or of losing an established condition is just a joke the Lord plays on himself, like a child who likes to scare himself. It is here the yogi experiences the spontaneous activity of divine Consciousness and the futility of doing anything in particular.

"He who sees all the diversity of the manifested universe as a reflection in Consciousness is truly the universal Sovereign. Thus, this intuition, which rises spontaneously and ceaselessly without any differentiation whatsoever, characterises the divine way (Śāmbhavopāya). All other things, religious conventions, purifications, vows, recital of mystic formulas are of no use whatsoever to Him."
ABHINAVAGUPTA, TANTRĀLOKA III, 268-270

Yet even the subtlety of this fourth state (turya) only shines by and in the eternal Presence, Śiva, who is not a state.

"Concepts are too pale to describe Him and thus He is sung in the hymns as surging from a spontaneous shiver. He is praised as beyond the states (turīyātīta) and ceaseless (satatoditam)."
ABHINAVAGUPTA, TANTRĀLOKA X, 283

"This supreme state which is not a state is neither being nor non-being, nor the two together. It is neither the absence of being nor non-being. Its indescribable transcendence makes it difficult to conceive."
ABHINAVAGUPTA, TANTRĀLOKA II, 28

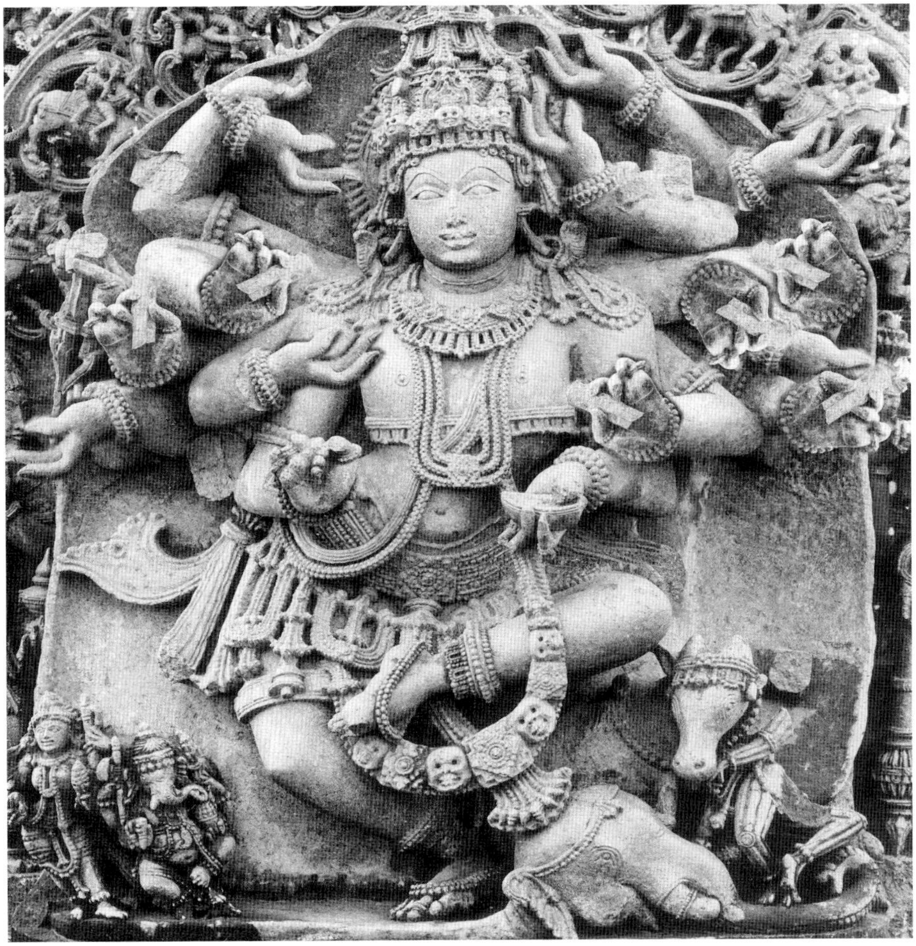

Śivagajāsurasaṃhāramūrti *12th century*
(Amritpur, Mysore)

9

Actors, Fairground Entertainers and Bargain Dealers Ranting on the Subject

"Behold my forms, O Pārtha, a hundred-fold, a thousand-fold, various in kind, divine, variously coloured and shaped."

"Behold the Āditya, the Vāsu, the Rudra, the two Aśvin and also the Marut. Behold O Pāṇḍava many wonderful beings never seen before."

"Behold, O Guḍākeśa, here and now, the whole universe, moving and unmoving, and whatever else you might want to see; that all exists in My body."

BHAGAVAD GĪTĀ XI, 5-6-7

When Vedavyāsa chants the Mahābhārata, the epic poem that encompasses all other stories, he unveils the meanderings of the fable Consciousness recites to itself in order to become a separate entity, forgetful of its origins. In these tales of recognition, roles only exist to illustrate the subject. Like a sheet of music unfolds scales of notes to reveal the music of silence, characters and situations are merely reminders.

Thus Arjuna cannot be Arjuna without Karṇa, and the wisdom of Yudhiṣṭhira is revealed by the madness of Duryodhana. The multitude of characters reveal different savours of the subject according to their depth and point of view, putting the accent either on the subject (pramātṛ), the process of perception (pramāṇa) or on the object of perception (prameya). Symbolically, each of us unfolds these different facets, reciting the text adapted to our situation, where little by little we divide the subject into ever more contradicting polarities, between subject, perception and object of perception.

Thus the first declensions of the subject are not declensions. They belong to akala (Śivatattva and Śaktitattva) and are only the actors of pure subject. They are known as akala because they are unseparated, free from division (kalā). They are neither limited by the object (prameya) nor by perception itself (pramāṇa).

The premise of a story's beginning then emerges, with the role of Mantramaheśvara who expresses the perception 'I am this' (ahaṃ idam). The plot thickens with the role of Mantreśvara who expresses 'this I am' (idam ahaṃ), where the accent is more on 'this' (idam) than on 'I' (ahaṃ). Placing the accent on the object, which is still connected to the subject, is part of the role of the Vidyeśvara, where diversity in unity is more prevalent. Even though the savour of unity is still predominant, the premise of diversity arises. And although admittedly we are still immersed in the ocean of our own nature, a fluctuation arises between the realisation that exteriority is the expansion of our own nature (ahaṃ ahaṃ) and the feeling that this exteriority is separate from the 'I' (idam idam).

"The multiplicity of beings rests in the One, and from that One alone multiplicity spreads out."
Bhagavad Gītā XIII, 31

The Vidyeśvara give way to the kingdom of māyā. With the kiss of māyā and its five suits of armour, everything is in place so that the epic poem we are going to act out may unfold. With the Vijñānākala, the mist of incompleteness (āṇavamala) settles in. This incompleteness takes the polarity of attention without action or of action without attention. A dichotomy is established between them.
When the Pralayākala enter the scene, they recite the peace and quiet of the abyss. Here there is still only silence. It is state of negation where exteriority disappears, as in deep sleep. But this void is not aware of itself. It is a state of absence. In this absence there is the seed of differentiated and dualistic perception (māyīyamala) and the illusion of being the doer (kārmamala). These two polarities are as yet still latent. Who would go to the theatre to look at an empty stage, or to contemplate the curtain that hides the stage? Who would go to the cinema to stare at a blank screen? We want to see drama, empires and lives collapse; we want to feel the tingle of love, the tears of separation and the kiss of death.

In the Mālinīvijaya Tantra it is said that the Lord, though not made of parts, objectifies Himself in diversity. The Śakala (those who are divided, made up of parts) are the last declension of the subject, the grossest since they are centred only on the object (prameya). The Śakala recite from the three limitations of incompleteness (āṇavamala), differentiated perception (māyīyamala) and action (kārmamala).

Here is where all roles and functions take shape, where all passions are unleashed in heaven and hell. Here is where we believe we are a president or a prostitute. Here is where we dream of other more exciting, less mediocre lives, forgetting that these roles are only a function of circumstance since:

"All actions are performed by the guṇa, each following their own individual role. He whose mind is confused by the sense of separation thinks he is the doer."
Bhagavad Gītā III, 27

Here is where we long for situations and experiences, because we believe the answer can be found in the object.

"Bound by hundreds of hopes, overwhelmed by desire..."
Bhagavad Gītā XVI, 12

"They were exhausted by the multiplicity of their ways, never saying 'let's rest'." The Bible, Isaiah 57-10

Yet although the theatre of our existence is limited and conditioned, it spontaneously resonates with the vibration of the inexpressible (anuttara).

"O Lord, the threefold path existing in this universe directs Your devotees to God Consciousness. It may be joy, it may be sadness or it may be sluggishness, it all directs Thy devotees to God Consciousness."
Utpaladeva, Śivastotrāvalī I, 10

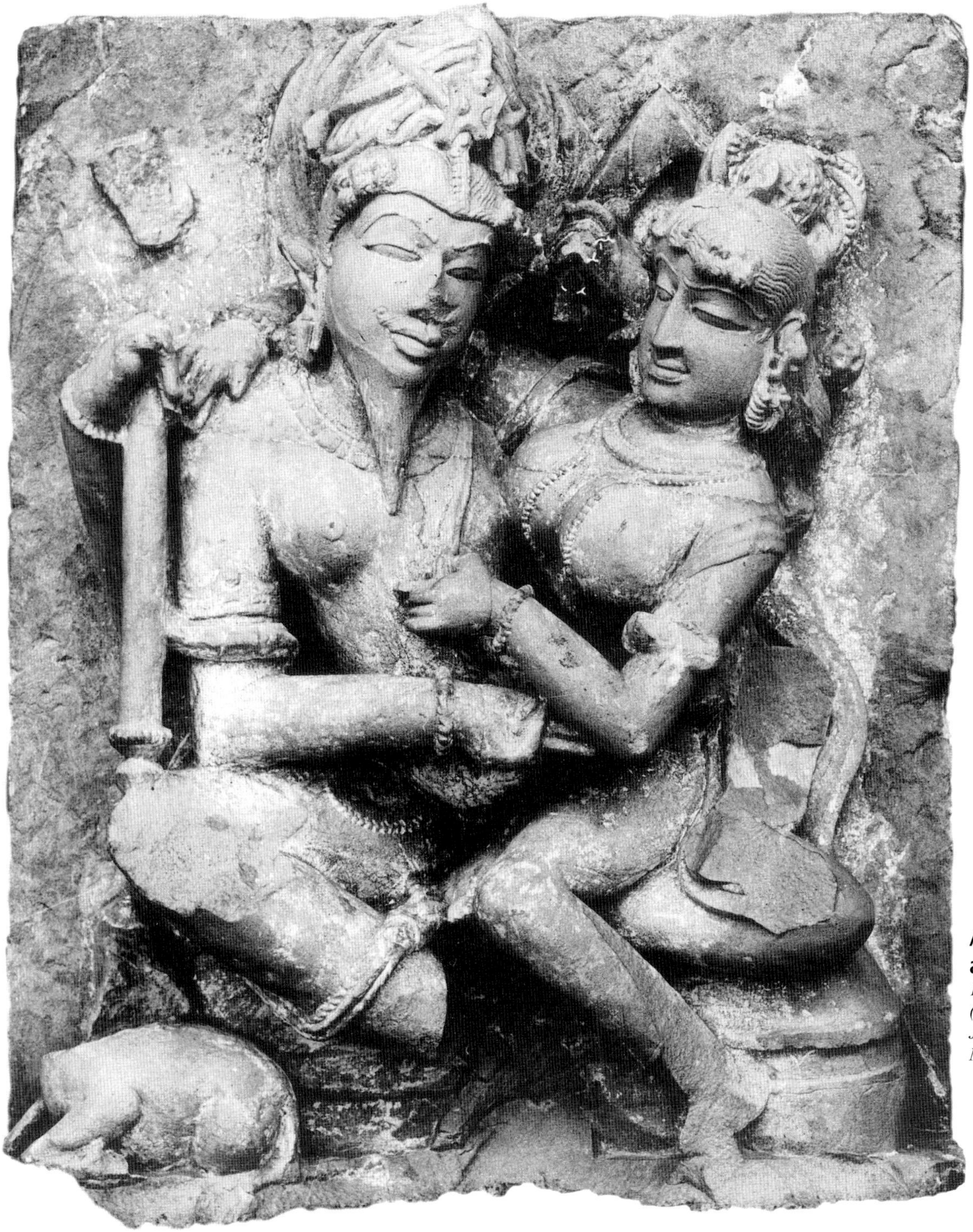

Agni and Svāhā
11th century. (Karitalai, Jabalpur District, Madhya Pradesh)

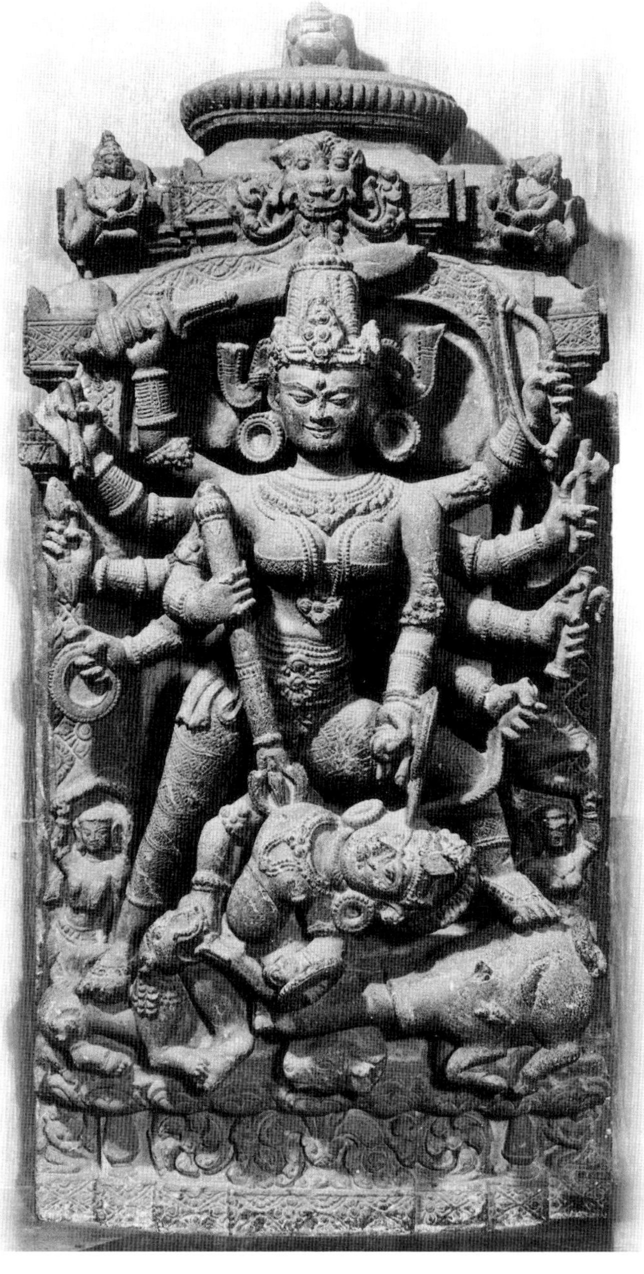

Mahiṣāsuramardinī
10th century
(Mahaliṅgeśvara Temple,
Indian Museum, Calcutta)

10

Means, Techniques and Other Desperate Endeavours

"The aim of all exercise is to create an idea within the body,
and eliminate its opposite. In the ultimate Reality, there is nothing to remove.
Duality itself does not exist separated from Consciousness.
It is simply the absence of intuition of its true nature."
ABHINAVAGUPTA, TANTRASĀRA IV

"Ritual and yogic practice cannot serve as a means because Consciousness is not born out of activity;
it is the reverse, activity proceeds from Consciousness."
ABHINAVAGUPTA, TANTRĀLOKA II, 8

"A path cannot reveal His essence because He is eternal,
it cannot make Him known because He is self-shining,
nor take away the veil which darkens Him since no veil can cover Him;
since nothing is separate from Him, nothing could penetrate Him."
ABHINAVAGUPTA, TANTRASĀRA II

"This is the ultimate Truth. There is no control of mind;
it does not rise at all; there is none bound;
no spiritual practitioner, no seeker of liberation and there is no realised soul."
AMṚTABINDŪPANIṢAD 10

It is told there was a young fish that heard about a vast expanse of water, with no limits as far as the eye could see. His parents told him that it was only a myth for dreamers. In his search, he meets other fish that tell him he must travel very far, that this expanse of water is to be found elsewhere. He travels as far as he can, but finds nothing. One day, exhausted, he meets a fish that tells him: *"This vast expanse of water is within you and there is a path to reach it; but first you must find those who can help you get there"*. He goes from one master to another, from one technique to another, but nothing works. He is just as far from his goal as he was when he started out. One day, however, he meets a fish who simply tells him: *"You are already there. You are already swimming in this vast expanse of water, and you always have been"*. Kabīr says: *"I laugh when I hear that the fish in the water is thirsty."*

Consciousness (saṃvit) is beyond all means (anupāya), all paths, all techniques and all practices, because you cannot become what you already are. It is described as gatopāya, where all means disappear. It is neither conditioned by time nor space; no language can define it, and it cannot be realised by any means of knowledge. Since it is the substratum of all activities, there is no activity able to reveal it. This spontaneous, free radiating light of Consciousness, which is our own nature, and in which the universe is reflected, is what characterises the absence of means (anupāya).

"As for those who wish to directly discriminate this essence in some way, they are nothing more than fools that try to use fireflies or glow-worms to apprehend the sun."
ABHINAVAGUPTA, TANTRĀLOKA II, 14

"O Lord, the reality of your presence is spontaneously obvious and omnipresent, thus those who seek You using means, are certain not to discover You."
JAYARATHA, TANTRĀLOKAVIVEKA II, 14

We have never been different, or near, or distant to what we are. This intuition is beyond all effort, all becoming, all process and all objectivation by some experience or other. There is nothing to gain, nothing to renounce. Fantasies of attaining some state or other, or of being in a state different to that of the sky of Consciousness, are a far too tiring venture. Let the realised and illuminated tell their cock-and-bull stories of enlightenment to those willing to listen.
"From the viewpoint of absolute reality there is no shackle, and in the absence of shackles there is no deliverance, as both are forged by dualising thought."
VĀMANADATTA, SAṂVITPRAKĀŚA

Here, the master-disciple relationship is merely a mind construction, or only takes the form of a function. There can be no relationship since all relationship is based on separation. Since Consciousness is the essence of all things, *"who other than the Self could teach it and to whom?"* (MAHEŚVARĀNANDA, MAHĀRTHAMAÑJARĪ 64)

Consciousness is joy (ānanda) that eludes all means, but contains them all. The upāya describe how the fragrance of the inexpressible is realised in the different levels of subjectivity, perception and objectivity. When one is identified with the body-mind, they can be considered as a classification of techniques, but fundamentally they are allusions from the absolute when we are touched by grace. Hence we talk more of immersion, absorption or interpenetration (samāveśa) rather than of means. There are three types of immersion according to how we experience reality, how we understand reality, and the dominant interpretation we have of reality. The means of Śambhu (śāmbhavopāya) becomes established in the spontaneous efficiency (icchā) of the 'I'. Śāktopāya tells of the emergence of intuition (jñāna), of the non-fragmented energy of Consciousness. Āṇavopāya utilises the contemplation of action (kriyā) through the body, breath, mind and intellect so as to be immersed in their source.

In śāmbhavopāya, the intuition that all appears in the sky of Consciousness and that nothing is beyond the heart of Consciousness predominates. There is nothing to do, nowhere to go, no psychological destination.

"He who perceives non-action in action, and action in non-action is wise among men. He is established in yoga and is the performer of all actions." Bhagavad Gītā IV, 18

In śāmbhavopāya, the immersion referred to is that of Mātṛka Yoga. In its purely technical aspect, mātṛka yoga is the esoteric study of grammar. In essence, it is the contemplation of the syntax of subjectivity. Everything is perceived as emanation, a reflection of vowels taking on the aspect of consonants from Ka to Kṣa, which are the vibratory aspect of all phenomena (tattva). The first sound in the Maheśvara Sūtra is the vowel A. It is said:

"Let the sound A be the nature of ultimate reality, without qualities and the essence of all things. The sound A generates the other sounds. It is this that illuminates..." (Nandikeśvarakāśikā 3)

The last sound is 'Ha' that ends by the anusvāra (m) or nasalisation. The phonetic emanation, which is that of the universe, can thus only be expressed by 'I' (ahaṃ).

At the end of his dance, Śiva strikes his ḍamaru fourteen times, thus making the Śivapratyāhāra or Maheśvarasūtra vibrate, which unfolds the emanation of phonemics into fourteen groups. The resonance of the ḍamaru is merely the spanda of pure subject (paramaśiva). All we perceive is merely a reflection of the subject itself. We can only encounter the supreme subject, which is nothing other than ourself.

The Kulayukti says: *"That which brings us down is also that which lifts us up."* Śāmbhavopāya contemplations focus on all that arises, a mirror of the heart of Consciousness.

"The complexity of all manifestations of existence is merely a reflection in the sky of Consciousness."
Abhinavagupta, Tantrasāra III

Śāmbhavopāya is instilled with non-dual feeling, which generates contemplations full of this intuition. The means of Śambhu (śāmbhavopāya) is established in undifferentiated Consciousness (anupāya) through subjectivity.

Whenever the feeling of diversity in unity predominates (bhedābheda), the different energies are contemplated to take us back to the radiant and reflexive light of Consciousness. Śāktopāya is fundamentally the purification of the mind process, which here does not refer to the control or stilling of thoughts as described in Patañjali's Yoga.

For the tantric yogi, thoughts, whatever they may be, are mantra (*cittaṃ mantraḥ - The mind is mantra,* Śivasūtra II, 1) because they stem from the vibratory and energy emanation of the phonemes, which are merely the radiant reflection of Consciousness. Doubts that generate dualistic perception are therefore severed at the root.

"The way of energy (śāktopāya) is one with that of knowledge (jñāna). The yogi must therefore purify dualistic thought (vikalpa), leaving way for intuitive reason (sattarka), which is beyond mundane thought and open to reality." Abhinavagupta, Tantrāloka IV, I-32

This contemplation of energies as being undifferentiated Consciousness is done during interstitial gaps (saṃdhyā), between two thoughts, two breaths, two actions, between waking and dreaming, when the ebb and flow of emanation and resorption are at rest.

"Meditating on the knowledge of two things or states, one should rest in the middle. By abandoning both simultaneously, the Reality shines forth in the centre."
Vijñāna Bhairava 61

Dualistic thought arises from the distinction between pure and impure, good and bad, attraction and repulsion, and all other opposites (bhedābheda).

The undifferentiated energy of Consciousness creates opposites, but also burns them. Śāktopāya is therefore the contemplation of these opposites, which are first of all experienced separately, and then reunited as a single and unique energy. These energies are the dance of the absolute in its forms of unity (abheda), diversity in unity (bhedābheda), diversity (bheda), and omnipresence of the subject in these three states. They are described as the twelve Kālī with their metaphorical forms of goddesses. Contemplation of the wheel of energies and their qualities *"always eager to hide their own essence"* (SPANDAKĀRIKĀ 20), takes the symbolic form of Vāmeśvarī, who spews out the universe.
These qualities, spewed out by the Supreme, can trigger either recognition or subjugation.
Thus **Khecarī**, the śakti who moves in the space of Consciousness is, in her appeased form, the recognition of the savour (rasa) of plenitude; but in her agitated form, is the painful kiss of armours and limitations.
Gocarī, the śakti who moves as the internal organ (antaḥkaraṇa) is, in her appeased form, the recognition of the rasa of undifferentiated unity; but in her agitated form, is the painful kiss of difference.
Dikcarī, the śakti who moves in the ten spatial and sensorial directions is, in her appeased form, the recognition of spatiality; but in her agitated form, is the painful kiss of grasping.
Bhūcarī, the śakti who wanders the Earth with specific qualities of objectivation (smell, taste, form, touch, sound) is, in her appeased form, the recognition of the body of the inexpressible; but in her agitated form, is the painful kiss of bodily identification with the experience of birth and death.

In śāktopāya we mustn't lose sight of the fact that these energies are merely different cloaks with the same weave. In its 'caricatured' or strategic version, śāktopāya becomes merely an attempt to manipulate energies, either to control or sublimate them. In śāktopāya we become immersed in the contemplation of diversity in unity. These different energies are shadows of the absolute. A tree's shadow leads us to the tree. Symbolically, śāktopāya takes the form of a sacrifice where the one who performs the sacrifice, the sacrifice and the object of sacrifice are one.

"Consciousness takes on the faces of the worshipper, worshipping and the worshipped. Only Consciousness exists. And this is spontaneous worship."
VIJÑĀNA BHAIRAVA 153

As Abhinavagupta says in his Īśvarapratyabhijñāvimarśinī (III, 17): *"Nothing new is obtained, nor what was really non-manifest is made manifest. Only wrong ideas about that which is shining, as not shining, is removed."*

The means of energy (śāktopāya) is to become established in undifferentiated Consciousness (anupāya) through perception. In śāmbhavopāya the emphasis is placed on subjectivity. In śāktopāya it is placed on perception in the act of self-awareness. When the rasa of diversity (bheda) predominates, objectivity is used as a reminder of the subject. Diversity is the gateway in āṇavopāya. Āṇava is the term used for beings limited by notions of individuality, but it also describes the objective nature of contemplation. Identification to the body is so powerful that it is used as an object of immersion in the subject. This immersion is considered to be subtle or gross depending on the contemplations used and the inclination of each individual. If the predominant belief is that of being uniquely and only this body, contemplation of its different parts, whether anatomical or physiological, will reveal the fragrance of spatiality of a non-gripped body. There is therefore no limitation or graduation attached to these contemplations since they are not a process. They are simply suggestions according to one's personal inclinations. Hence immersion into the body can open into śāktopāya, leaving the energetic aspect predominate, and quieten into śāmbhavopāya where the body is sensed as a reflection in Consciousness.

"If one contemplates in a thoughtfree way on any point in the body as mere void even for a moment, then, being free from thoughts one attains the nature of the Thoughtfree."
VIJÑĀNA BHAIRAVA 46

When the body again becomes the seat of all sensations, of all savours (rasa), the organs of the senses (karaṇa) trigger the immersion. The body is recognised as a savour whose source is Consciousness. In the immersion known as 'meditation on prāṇa' (uccāra), the breath is the object of contemplation. Here we explore the modalities and different colourations of the breath (pañcavāyu: apāna, prāṇa, samāna, udāna, vyāna). We contemplate the sound and resonance (dhvani) of the breath. Contemplation of the source of inhalation and exhalation, and of the interval between the two, becomes the point of immersion.

"O Bhairavī, contemplate the junction point at the confluence of inhalation and exhalation. In these two voids, let the Presence shine forth."
VIJÑĀNA BHAIRAVA 25

These different savours are the contemplation (dhyāna) with form of different bodily activities, which are nothing more than the coagulated mind (buddhi). The space-time aspect of the world can be internalised in the body, which becomes the cosmic body and an object of contemplation.

"If one meditates on the subtle and subtlest elements in one's own body or of the world as if they are merging one after another, then in the end the Supreme Goddess is revealed." VIJÑĀNA BHAIRAVA 54

When misunderstood, the way of the individual (āṇavopāya) may appear to be based on the idea of a seeker and a process that leads somewhere. The motor behind the so-called seeker's strategy is the fear of death, because he wants to continue existing, no matter what. It is here we find the kingdom of spiritual remedies, enlightenment and mystical experiences, all bought at a steep price, and of yoga methods boasting salutary techniques and vindicating perfect body-mind, all of which accentuate the illusion of separation. The way of the limited individual (āṇavopāya) is to become established in undifferentiated Consciousness through objectivity.

"When you throw your frail barque on the ocean of God, happy are you when it sinks." ANGELUS SILESIUS

For Abhinavagupta, all the upāya have the quality of subjectivity and interiority (antara), apart from the subdivisions of the last upāya, which he defines as being external injunction (bāyavidhi), and concerns religious duties.
The upāya are permeable. There is no separation between them since they bathe continually in the three energies of will (icchā), knowledge (jñāna) and action (kriyā). At each moment, we all unfold these three energies simultaneously. There is the intention (icchā) that knows (jñāna) itself in the action (kriyā). In all the upāya we merely rehearse and ritualise our own death. In śāmbhavopāya we learn to die in subjectivity; in śāktopāya, in the act of perceiving; and in āṇavopāya, in objectivity. In the way of the individual, we become completely ordinary and embrace our limitations. We realise that the limitations of individual Consciousness are anchored in divine Consciousness. In their essence, the immersions (samāveśa) leave a lingering fragrance of the absence of differentiated knowledge, ungraspable, forever incomprehensible.

"There is neither bondage nor liberation for me, they are just like bogies for the fearful. This world is like a reflection in the mind, just as the sun is reflected in water."
VIJÑĀNA BHAIRAVA 135

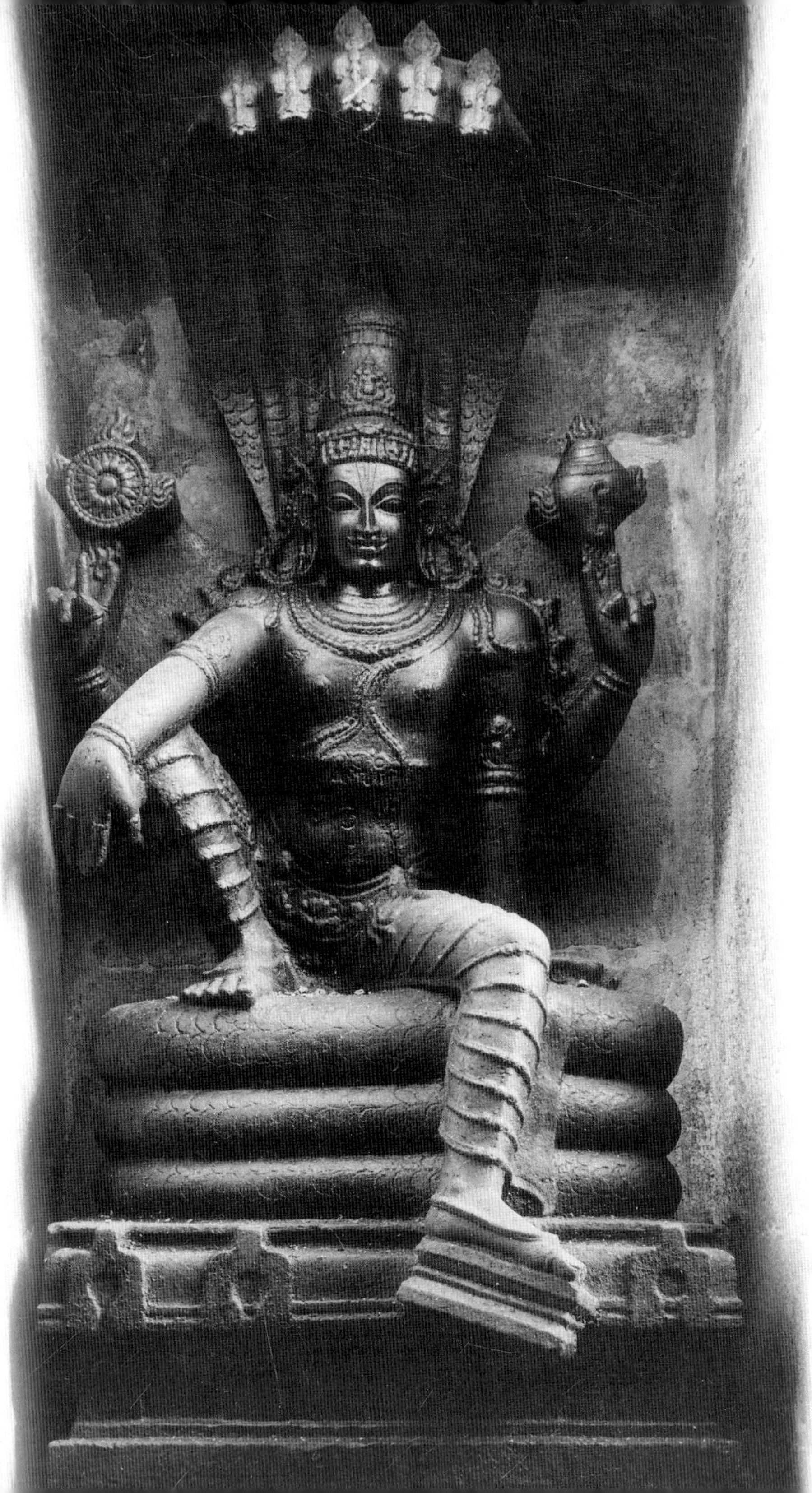

Keśava *17th century*
(Bhaktavatsala Temple, Perumal, Tamil Nadu)

11

The Field of the Lord

"The Lord said: This body, O son of Kuntī, is called the field,
and he who knows this field, the learned call the knower of the field."
"Know me as the knower of the field in all the fields, O Bhārata; the knowledge of the field and its knower,
and know that through this knowledge alone I can be realised."
"Hear briefly from Me what the field is, what is its nature, what are its modifications,
from where these modifications come, and who the knower is, and what is his nature."
"The five elements, the sense of I, the intellect and also Prakṛti,
the ten senses and the mind and the five objects of the senses, desire and aversion,
pleasure and pain, the body Consciousness and the upholder of prāṇa,
these are briefly described as the field along with its modifications."
BHAGAVAD GĪTĀ XIII, 2-3-4-6/7

"This entire universe is born from Me, it is reflected in Me and it is never separate from Me."
ABHINAVAGUPTA, TANTRĀLOKA III, 280

Yājñavalkya said to Bṛhaspati: *"This Kurukṣetra is for all the gods the abode of the divine sacrifice and which is for all beings the abode of realisation of Brahman, wherever you go, it is there that you have to recognise Him. This abode itself, where everyone is this body, where one is incarnated, is the Kurukṣetra, the divine abode of the sacrifice for the gods and the spiritual centre for all beings. Furthermore, it is Avimukta (that which we cannot leave) which is Kurukṣetra, the divine abode of the sacrifice for the gods and the place of realisation of the absolute for all living beings. It is there that Rudra gives the initiation into the ultimate reality. Thus one should ceaselessly be in touch with Avimukta, and not leave for a single instant the place of the One who is neither free nor bound."*
JĀBĀLOPANIṢAD I, 3-4-5

We associate the body with a solid and compact form, cemented by the image we have of it and which we project. This projection is filled with insecurity and fear, identifying us with an incessant spinning wheel of clichés gleaned from magazines. We are tempted to believe in the myth of the perfect body, a body that will always be different from our own and which sees anything that puts our identification into question as dangerous. A body that is like a fortress, which fears being slightly overweight, having grey hair or wrinkles, being sick, and which most of all fears its end, its death. A body of a Hollywood hero who, even in the most dire of situations, doesn't lose his presentable image, or that of 'big-screen' yogis on the covers of glossy yoga magazines, selling a body and politically correct wisdom that reeks of performance. Yet even this grossest of identifications is also a blessing because it contains its own sabotage and causes disidentification with a body that doesn't actually exist. Which is the body we can claim as our own: the body of the waking state, the dreaming state, or of its total absence in deep sleep? Which body defines us? Which body represents us? The body of our childhood, our adolescence, that which we have when we wake up in the morning, or that after a good meal when our stomach is full?

"When one is filled with joy arising from the pleasure of eating and drinking, one should meditate on the state of fullness. Then the great bliss will arise." Vijñāna Bhairava 72

Whilst lying on grass, the body welcomes its touch and takes on its quality. When in water, it becomes fluid; when caressed by the breeze, it becomes like the wind. Who can put limits on such a body? Who can trace a border if it were not for references to an image? The body is only sensations. Are we the body of pleasure during the embrace of love, when it dissolves into the infinite? Are we the body of pain in its contraction? Or are we the space in which sensations and the body itself appear?
Kṣetra (field) comes from the root KṢI or KṢAY, meaning 'to live', 'to reside'. The different levels of meaning of this term flow down like waterfalls. In the Vedic period, it denoted the country, the region, the house one lived in, earth and the soil one toils. Kṣetrapati means the lord of the soil, he who possesses the earth. The earth itself becomes the place of dharma, of accomplishment (dharmakṣetra), an auspicious place (subhakṣetra). It is also spoken of as a place (sthāna) and as a geographical location (deśa), auguring notions of sacred places (tīrtha) and their geometric representations (maṇḍala). The Vāstusūtra Upaniṣad thus describes a perfect geometric form that encompasses cosmic representation (rūpakṣetra). It can also become a womb, like in the Śarīrasthāna (II, 3) where it means uterus. In certain Purāṇa, the earth, the position of the stars and the universe itself become kṣetra. Certain places can participate in the consecration of the universe, and are places (tīrtha) to remind us of the sacred, of the expansion of the radiant and reflexive power of Consciousness.

"The entire universe is a form of Śakti." Śaktidarśana

These places are sung of in the Mahābhārata and the Purāṇa. Kāśī, Kāmarūpa, Bhāskara, Puruṣottama, Nārāyaṇa, Gayā and Prayagā are all places of supreme accomplishment (siddhakṣetra). Kurukṣetra, Kedāra, Varāhamūla, Gajakṣetra and Puṇḍarīkṣetra are all places of meritorious acts (puṇyakṣetra). Each tīrtha is the privileged site of certain deities. Thus, Kurukṣetra, where the Pāṇḍava and Kaurava slaughter each other, is also known as Brahmākṣetra, the sacred field of Brahmā, of all dharma.

"Dhṛtarāṣṭra said: When my army and the army of the Pāṇḍava assembled on the field of dharma, on the field of the Kuru, the meeting place of all kṣatriya, what did these two armies do, O Sañjaya?"
"Field (kṣetra) is that which enables sense organs to operate. That word kṣetra in the expression dharmakṣetra refers to a field in which both worldly dharma and supreme dharma come into existence. If the word kṣetra is derived from the root kṣad, meaning 'to attack', 'to confront', then the body is the meeting place (samāgama) of mutually contradicting feelings, such as passion and dispassion, anger and tolerance, etc."
Abhinavagupta, Gītārthasaṃgraha I, 1

Purī is sacred for Viṣṇu (Viṣṇukṣetra), Bhuvaneśvara is sacred for Śiva (Śivakṣetra) and Jajpur is sacred for Pārvatī (Śaktikṣetra). According to the Purāṇa, Kāśī is the ultimate abode of all tīrtha. Kāśī (Vārāṇasī or Benares), which means light, personifies Śiva.

"In Kāśī the light shines.
That light illuminates everything.
Whoever knows that light, truly reaches Kāśī.
I am that Kāśī whose essence is self-knowledge."
Śaṅkarācārya

There is a legend that tells the story of Brahmā, Viṣṇu and Śiva debating their respective supremacy. Śiva transforms into a pillar of light that pierces the earth and sky. Viṣṇu changes into a wild boar and digs into the Earth. Brahmā becomes a bird and flies up into the sky. It is said they looked for the end of this light for thousands of years, but couldn't find it. Upon his return, Viṣṇu admits defeat but Brahmā refuses to do so and lies, saying he saw the end of the light. Śiva takes the form of Bhairava and cuts off the fifth head of Brahmā! Having become the murderer of a brāhmaṇa, he must now wander around carrying the skull of his victim. It is said that Śiva ends his expiation in Kāśī. This is why Kāśī is called that which we can't abandon (avimukta), and also the forest of bliss of Śiva (ānandavana), his garden of joy (ānandakānana), and the abode of Rudra (rudravāsa). It is also known as the great crematorium (mahāśmaśāna).

Kāśīkṣetra, the field of perpetual light, is delimited by a circle (bṛhat pañcakrośi yātrā) with a diameter of 11 miles, or 5 krośa. Another meaning for this term is envelope, sheath (kośa). Kāśī, like the human being, is made up of five sheaths, and becomes the cauraśikrośi yātrā, thereby covering a circuit of 168 miles. It is divided into eight directions (aṣṭadik), each with a protective śakti, representing the zodiac and the months, and which symbolises the different cycles and tides of time. The pilgrim reactivates in himself the one hundred and eight sacred sites of the pañcakrośi yātrā, which is a clockwise circumambulation that is smaller (laghu) than the cauraśikrośi yātrā, and which must be accomplished within five days. The yātrā accomplished by the pilgrim symbolises the different energies of Śiva, which watch over and sanctify the cardinal directions: piṅgaleśvara (east), kāyāvarohaṇeśvara (south), dardureśvara (north), bilveśvara (west). The internal consecration of these one hundred and eight places of worship participates in the cosmic sacrifice of the different elements (earth, water, fire, air, ether, etc.) within the body of the pilgrim.

The pañcakrośi yātrā represents all the tīrtha, all the gods and all the planets, thus becoming the ultimate tantric maṇḍala. According to the Kāśīrahasya, this maṇḍala was revealed in different forms. In the Kṛta Yuga, Kāśīkṣetra had the form of Śiva's trident (triśūla), in the Tretā Yuga it was a circle symbolising the cakra of Viṣṇu. In the Dvāpara Yuga it had the form of a chariot representing the sun, and in the Kālī Yuga it is a conch, which represents Śiva's body, the womb of the universe, the cosmic egg (hiraṇyagarbha).

Kāśīkṣetra is situated on Śiva's triśūla, beyond space and time, for which He is also their source. Śiva's trident represents the three energies: energy of will or vital surge (icchāśakti) and its function of subject (pramātā); cognitive energy (jñānaśakti) and its function of knowing (pramāṇa); energy of action (kriyāśakti) and its function of known object (prameya).

The five subtle elements (tanmātra) from which the universe is woven are also represented. The five textures of reality or sheaths (annamayakośa, prāṇamayakośa, manomayakośa, vijñānamayakośa, ānandamayakośa) are found in these five sacred circles. The first marks the entrance to the cosmic maṇḍala, for which Gaṇeśa is the guardian. The second circle is that of the pañcakrośi yātrā. The third is the holy city (Nagarī Pradakṣiṇa). The fourth is Śiva's inner sanctum (avimukta, that which cannot be abandoned). Antargṛha is the fifth circle, the saint of saints (Viṣveśvara, Madhyameśvara), becomes the bindu, the place of emanation and resorption. The three segments define the three worlds (triloka) of earth, atmosphere and heaven. The exteriority of these tīrtha is merely the expression of a primal emotion, where the boundary between external and internal fades.

"Empty inside, empty outside,
like an empty jar in the space.
Full inside, full outside,
like a jar immersed in the ocean."
HAṬHAYOGAPRADĪPIKĀ IV, 56

In the tantric approach, the body is seen as a maṇḍala. One of the interpretations of maṇḍala according to Abhinavagupta is a circle in which there is a deity (devatācakram), representing the universe. The two are merely the reflection (ābhāsa) of Consciousness (saṃvid).

"The yogi should contemplate simultaneously on the whole world or his own body as filled with the bliss of the self, then by his own blissful nectar he becomes united with the supreme bliss." VIJÑĀNA BHAIRAVA 65

In his Tantrāloka, Abhinavagupta describes the mystical kṣetra in the body.

"To the knower of kṣetra located inside the body, the kṣetra are eight. They are the eight petals of the heart lotus. The names of the kṣetra are Prayāga, Varaṇā, Aṭṭahāsa, Jayantī, Vārāṇasī, Kaliṅga, Kulūtā and Lāhulā."
ABHINAVAGUPTA, TANTRĀLOKA XV, 89-90AB

The Lalitā Sahasranāma describes the body of the goddess as having the nature of the field and as encompassing all manifestation.

"Kṣetra, Kāmarūpa and other abodes, and the thirty-six categories from earth to Śiva, these form her body. The Liṅga Purāṇa says: Devī, the wife of the destroyer of the three cities, becomes kṣetra (matter). The divine and eternal Lord becomes the knower of the fields (body)."
LALITĀ SAHASRANĀMA 127A

The variations of kṣetra are infinite, as if it wanted to encompass the infinity of forms of Consciousness, suggesting geometric and geographic spaces, the body and its different sheaths.

"The truth of Consciousness (Cit) itself is the truth of the universe; this Existence itself is the body of Consciousness."
YOGAVASIṢṬHA

Fields of sensation and perception, where the body becomes the place of all geometries, all geographies, of all spaces taking the form of constellations, planets, oceans, rivers, lands. The body is a mirror of the universe; it sings of its mineral, vegetal, animal, human, demonic (asura) and divine (deva) structures, expressing all attitudes (bhāva) and emotions (rasa). It thus expresses the semantic articulation of the radiant and reflexive vibration of Consciousness. It becomes an echo of the tantric principle: *"Everything is the essence of everything (sarvam sarvātmakāma)"*, and you can hear the body itself singing Śaṅkarācārya's Hymn of Kāśī:

"The body is the sacred field of Kāśī.
If all this dwells within my body,
What other place of pilgrimage can there be?"

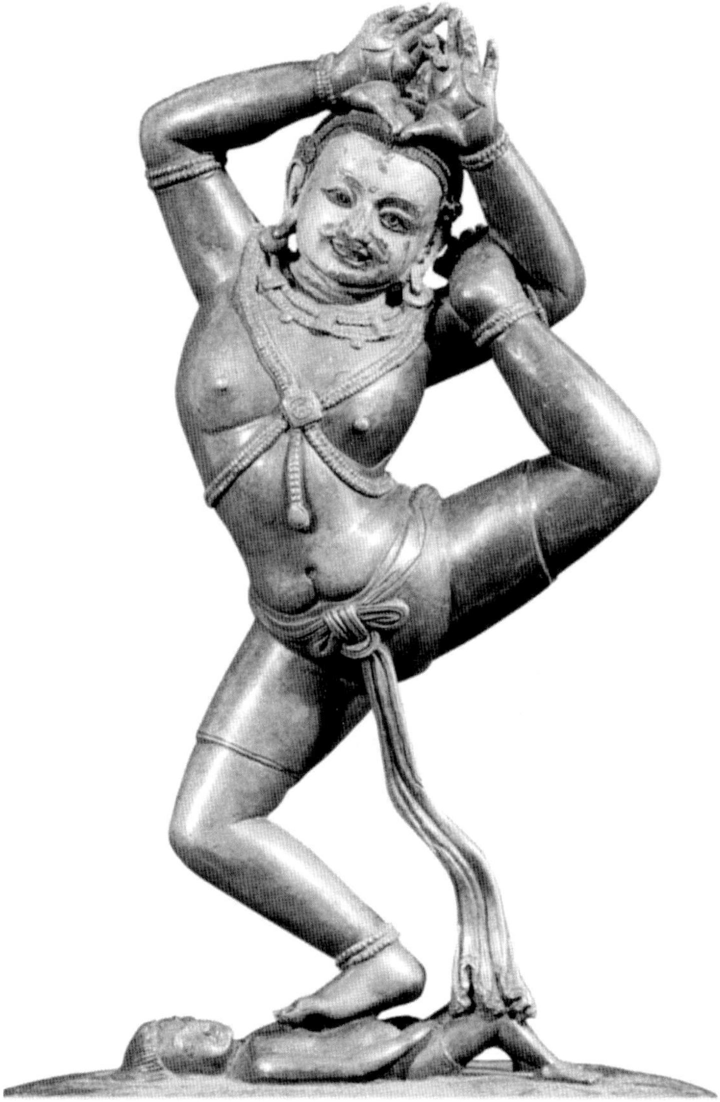

Hevajra

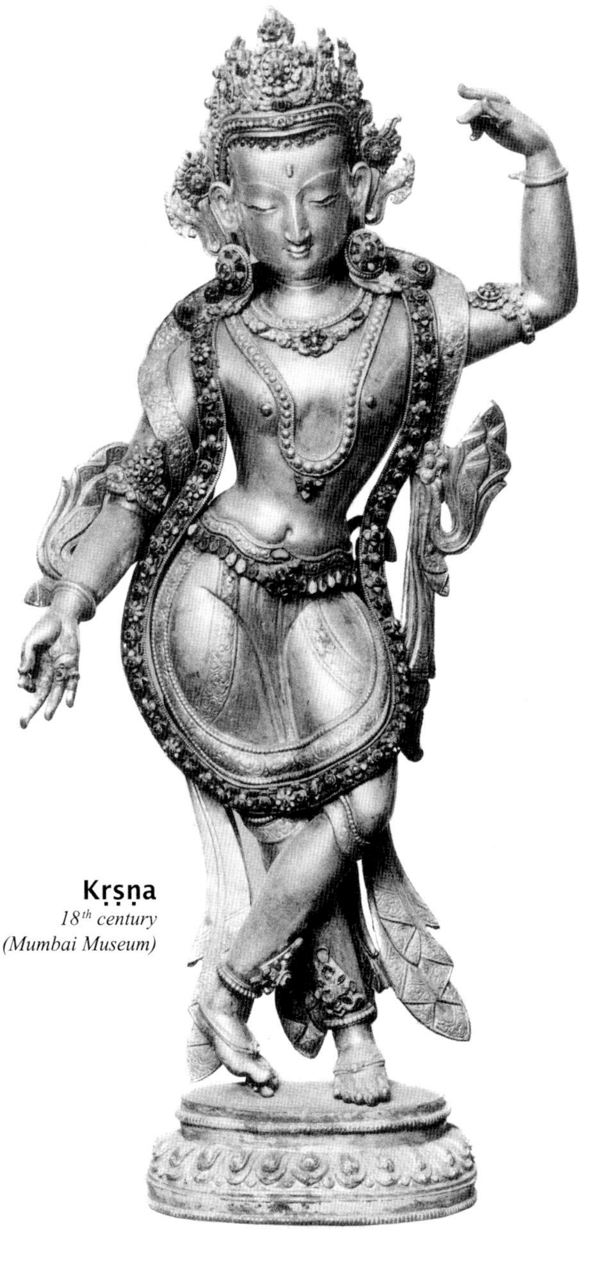

Kṛṣṇa
18th century
(Mumbai Museum)

12

Consecration of Embodiment and Rituals of Fullness

"The ignorant man does not observe the magnitude of the delightful enjoyment of the most precious wealth lying in the body, prāṇa, etc. and feels overwhelming depression in his heart. If the Supreme goddess who feels particular relish in bringing into being the entire universe enters his heart, then oh! she sportively functions as the full and final oblation in reducing to ashes the depression that has been plaguing him."
ABHINAVAGUPTA, PARĀTRĪŚIKĀVIVARAṆA, JAIDEVA SINGH, PAGE 95

"The body is the oblation." VASUGUPTA, ŚIVASŪTRA II, 8

"I praise the wheel of deities within the body, eternally arisen, trembling, the essence of experience, end of everything and constantly present." ABHINAVAGUPTA, DEHASTHADEVATĀCAKRASTOTRA 15

"Thus the body should be seen as full of all the paths, filled with the varied operations of time, and seat of all the movements of time and space. The body seen in this way is in itself composed of all the divinities, and thus must be an object of contemplation, of adorations and of rites of fulfilment. He who penetrates in the body achieves liberation."
ABHINAVAGUPTA, TANTRĀLOKA XII, 6-7

At the height of identification, the body serves as proof of separation, like a dyke of fear to stop the tidal wave of existence. Without referring to memory, we cannot know what the body of separation is. The image of the body allows us to get a grasp of ourselves, to define ourselves as a man or a woman, with certain characteristics, pleasant or unpleasant, reducing space into a simple contraction. We know nothing of this body other than the story we continually tell ourselves: a particular age, a particular shape, in a particular place, carrying out particular tasks. Although this story has an aftertaste of lacking, we are very attached to it. As a matter of fact, we take great care to protect this wardrobe full of beliefs, prejudices and preferences, which create and fix us in a form, a structure that we call our body.

"How did pleasure (sukha) and suffering (duḥkha) appear? Whence did they come? In truth, none of the material objects in this world are either favourable (anukūla) or unfavourable (pratikūla). For the practitioner of Yoga, the change in prakṛti will not result in sukha or duḥkha. He will be like that ākāśa that is unaffected by anything. Beneficial or harmful, all is in the mind."
NĀTHAMUNI, YOGARAHASYA, KĀLĀDHYĀYAH 2-3-4

What a marvellous mystery it is to see the fear of space give itself a name and a shape! What a marvellous mystery it is to see this open space dress itself and forget itself in a structure, a scaffold, a setting that becomes the sole and unique reality! Is it really me that I see in the mirror of my projections, seeking to plug the breach of reality? Am I my twenty year-old self or my seventy year-old self, the youth of my body or its old age and pain? We still have within ourselves, like a murmur, the light-heartedness of the carefree child's body, full of effervescence, with fluid movements that unfold spontaneous mudrā, sacred gestures, both in joy and in tears. We still bear the ever-present light-hearted celebration of our childhood dances, intoxicated by our own fullness.

"Once upon a time in your tavern my friend I took a little wine. I threw off this earthly robe. I saw, thanks to the tavern, that the world is all harmony, built up or broken down; it is for this reason that I spin this way."
JALĀL AD-DĪN MUḤAMMAD RŪMĪ, RUBĀ'IYĀT, INTOXICATION V

All our sensations cry out for the sinking of separation, so we may glimpse the body as a breath, a morning mist foretelling the nascent light of day, a divine veil.

"This entire world is the shadow of His essential parts.
And those who exist through the veil of His life,
Are not just part of him, they are His very Self."
JALĀL AD-DĪN MUḤAMMAD RŪMĪ, RUBĀ'IYĀT, THE QUEST III

He is called śarīra, kṣetra, piṇḍa, rūpa, purpura-puri, aṅga, mūrti, deha, all of which describe the body as being no more than a pointer, the signifier of the breath, the caress of the absolute. The body's ephemeral nature is beyond all doubt. As the Īśa Upaniṣad says, *"the body has its end in ashes."* Yet even with its ephemeral nature, the body is the city of gods (Ayodhyā).

The body (śarīra) is explained in these terms:

"That which decays and gets destroyed is śarīra."
KṢĪRASVĀMĪ, COMMENTARY ON THE AMARA KOŚA II, 6.70

As for the Garbhopaniṣad, it uses the following definition: *"Why is he (embryo) called the body? Because in it lie close fires, namely the fire of knowledge, the fire of seeing and the gastric fire."* (5)

The body (śarīra) refers to different condensations and coagulations. Contemplation of the total evanescence, of the non-substance of this body, is the ultimate oblation.

"The existence of the body from where pleasure and pain proceed, that is the inexpressible attitude (mudrā). The spontaneous flow of breath, that is the prodigious yoga."
ABHINAVAGUPTA, ANUBHĀVANIVEDANA 3

The body is the vibrating place of tides, called sheaths (kośa), which are different waves (ūrmi) of crystallisation and conditionings. The exploration of the process of coagulation of Śiva's seed (Śiva bīja: spandaśarīra, śaktaśarīra, puryaṣṭakaśarīra, prāṇaśarīra, sthūlaśarīra), from subjectivity to objectivity, in the so-called gross body, becomes the ritual of consecration of the body, upon which the accent is no longer placed. According to Yājñavalkya, the sun performs the function of oblation. From this oblation comes the rain which fertilises the earth and transforms it into vegetal life. This food (annarasa) is transformed into seed (śukra) and other constituents (dhātu), which in this context means 'to hold together'. From the seed comes the process of transforming food, called phlegm (śleṣman), which generates the humours (rasa), blood (rakta), flesh (māṃsa), fat (meda), bones (asthi) and marrow (majja), which in turn reproduce the seed (śukra).

"When the intentness of worldly objects is shed and limitation is discarded, what remains as the body is nothing other than Śiva's bliss. The body itself is completely full

with the blissful essence of Śiva and is the very abode of the thirty-six principles. One should behold it in this way day and night and worship it as such."
Abhinavagupta, Tantrāloka XV, 284cd-286ab

The ritual of consecration is the actualisation of fullness in the limited and conditioned body. As we saw in the chapter on the upāya, the means can never achieve anupāya, which is beyond all activity and is the source of all activity.

"All means, external and internal, are dependent on that Consciousness (Saṃvid Śakti). How can these means reveal it?"
Abhinavagupta, Tantrāloka II, 11

What will be described in these rituals must not be taken in the literal sense of mundane liturgy where one accomplishes certain actions to achieve certain goals. The savour (rasa), the primal emotion (bhāva), which is the upsurge at the heart of these rituals, is that of fullness.

"That is whole; this is whole; from the whole, the whole becomes manifest. From the whole when the whole is negated, what remains is again the whole."
Īśāvasya Upaniṣad, Opening Verse

Downstream, this upsurge adopts the gross forms of fragmentary activities that we impose on our body. The mundane ritual, born out of a sense of lacking, attempts to obtain a body-mind more in line with its desires, and we thus become slaves to the 'more or less' syndrome. We set ourselves into a practice of reform, change and intentions. Whether it is a movement of accumulation or renunciation, both manifest the farce of separation. It is unavoidable that this very movement, even in its grossest expression of hegemonic and colonialist practices, recognises itself (pratyabhijñām) upstream as being the upsurge from the heart.

"Bhairava is upsurge." Vasugupta, Śivasūtra I, 5

There is no seeker, only seeking that tires itself out. There is no practitioner, only a practice of offering, like drawing patterns in water that become lost in its depths.

"Neither renounce nor possess anything. Enjoy yourself freely, resting in your self, just as you are!"
Abhinavagupta, Anuttarāṣṭikā 2

The śarīra and its different sheaths become the vantage ground for the exploration of the states of Consciousness. This process is known as karaṇa, where the body and its attributes are used as means of contemplation, so it may be revealed, free from superimposition and grasping.

"The varieties of karaṇa are meant to subordinate and ultimately assimilate all objective phenomena to the Consciousness of the essential Self."
Jayaratha, Tantrālokaviveka V, 129

There is always a certain contraction due to the image we have of the body, to its definition that bogs us down. The purpose of karaṇa is to resorb our grasping of the body.

"O gazelle-eyed Goddess, if one contemplates on all the elements constituting the body as pervaded by void, then this evocation will become permanent." Vijñāna Bhairava 47

The observation of bodily processes lets its structure rest in its natural conditioning.

"There are two categories of conditioning: the necessary and the unnecessary. The unnecessary has it roots in ignorance and a sense of separation. When this is relinquished, the necessary conditionings only hold up the body. It is purely biological."
Yogavasiṣṭha, Nirvāṇa Prakaraṇam

The Postural Field (Kṣetrāsana)

Like an ancient epic poem recounting the deeds of heroes, āsana are a celebration of the Absolute, in all its forms and savours. The various groups of āsana bear witness to a circumambulation (parikrama) that follows a rhythm, whether practising or teaching.
For Kṣemarāja, āsana is not a psychophysical posture (here the term posture is used for want of a better word), but the power of the supreme Śakti as conscious light, unlimited by space and time or by bodily activities.

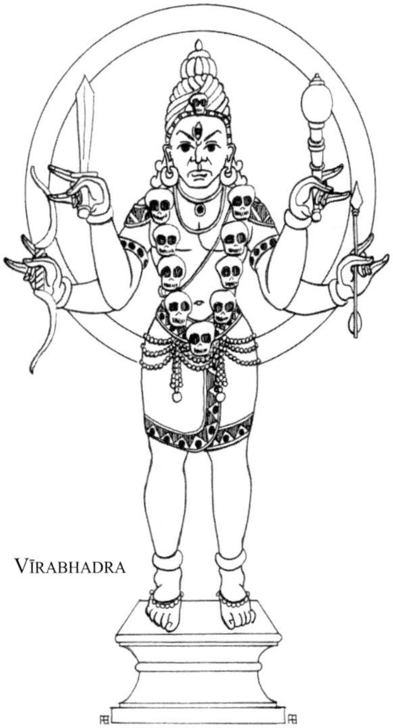

VĪRABHADRA

*"That on which
the yogi seats
with a sense
of full identification
with the divine
is āsana or seat.
The seat in this context
is the power
of the highest Śakti."*

KṢEMARĀJA,
ŚIVASŪTRAVIMARŚINĪ
III, 16

Standing Āsana (Utthiṣṭha Sthiti): The Epic of the Auspicious Hero (Vīrabhadra)

"O Vīrabhadra, best of Gaṇa, destroy the sacrifice of Dakṣa with all the auxiliary adjuncts and then return to my abode quickly. Even if there be deva, gandharva, yakṣa or others, reduce them also to ashes quickly."
ŚIVAPURĀṆA, RUDRASAṂHITĀ II, 32

Consecration of the body starts with standing āsana. The entrance is Samasthiti (also called Tāḍāsana). Sama means equilibrium, evenness. This word has many declensions rich in meaning:

• Samavāya indicates reunion, meeting, contact, the relationship between the parts and the whole. *"Samavāya is the perpetual reunion of the earth and the other elements, and of their qualities..."* (CARAKASAṂHITĀ I, 150)
• Samabuddhi or samacittatva (mental evenness), samadarśana (unified vision), samadhāna or samādhi. According to the Yogasūtra of Patañjali, *"That meditation having the manifestation of Truth, as if devoid of its own form, is called Samādhi."* (III, 3)
• Samādhi, for which the Nirukta gives this definition: *"When the mind is established in the understanding of the Self, that understanding is called Samādhi."*
• Samāna, referred to as 'even breath', is one of the five breaths (vāyu) and participates in the union of apānavāyu and prāṇavāyu.
• Samarasa is the unique essence of all things.
• Samasaṃsthāna is the state of equanimity of psycho-physical fluctuations. In Vācaspati Miśra's Yoga Bhāṣya (II.46), it is described physically as being Baddhakoṇāsana.

Sthiti comes from the root STHĀ, which means 'to be standing'. One of the literal meanings of this term is the action of standing in a steady and stable manner. It is also used to denote the continuum of existence. In cosmology, it comes after the emanation phase (sṛṣṭi). Whatever has

the quality of stability is called sthiti, like the Earth. According to the Vaijayanti Kośa, sthiti means continuation (maryādā) and maintenance (dhāraṇā), but also installation (niveśa) and disposition (racanā).
All these nuances are found in the term Samasthiti, which is the art of verticality, wherein all notions of differentiation are lost in the feeling of unity. It is therefore not merely the act of standing, which would be an activity, but being or being held in and by the cosmic dharma (brahmadaṇḍa).
Sensorially, this savour (rasa) of unity is actualised in the diversity of standing āsana. The first stage therefore is to make contact with the various parts of the body, moving away from the shackled image of a 'thought' body to a 'felt' body. We get to know the body's limbs through their vivisection, and when we bind and hold them during movement. The different areas and constellations of the feet, legs, hands, arms, trunk, hips, abdomen, chest, neck and head are all explored.

"To work on a part of the body you have to work on the whole. So also in order to work the whole you have to work each and every part individually as well as collectively."

Sparks of Divinity, Yogācārya Śrī B.K.S. Iyengar
Noelle Perez-Christiaens, Page 263

The action of cutting the body into its various parts is called khaṇḍa. It has the effect of banishing inertia and lethargy from the body, but also introduces spinal or vertebral extensions, be they vertical, horizontal, lateral, forward, backward or twisting. All these extensions are deepened in the other groups of āsana, which is why standing āsana are the śakti (power, energy) that initiates all other āsana (except in certain instances where they are therapeutically contra-indicated).
This vivisection is done with unified perception of the essence (sāra) of the body itself, which at first takes the form of redistributing weight and balance to give muscular freedom and synchronised mobility of the joints. The effervescence initiated by standing āsana help to awaken the impulses of the nervous system and vitalise its spreading, culminating in a widespread, even and clear awareness of the breath (cittaprasādanam). Standing āsana are therefore the initiators of all other āsana.
Khaṇḍasāra yoga or vivisection within the essence not only aims to free the trunk, arms and legs, a kind of esoteric amputation, in order to access the various breaths (pañcavāyu) in the three diaphragms (pelvic: mūlabhanda, thoracic: uḍḍiyānabandha, vocal: jālandharabandha), but also to destroy the mental image of the body.

Sitting Āsana (Upaviṣṭha Sthiti): Establishing the Throne

"He suddenly takes his seat in the fourth state; the one who by the grace of this mudrā in which are fused moon, sun and fire, takes possession internally of the process of emission and resorption."

Abhinavagupta, Tantrāloka, Kulayāga 153-154

"That which is well-known as the origin of all beings, and the support of the whole universe, which is immutable and in which the enlightened are completely merged, that alone is known as Siddhāsana."

Śaṅkarācārya, Aparokṣānubhūti 113

Sitting āsana are an intermediary between standing āsana and forward extensions. Firstly, they relieve tiredness in the legs from standing āsana, as well as providing some rest. To understand sitting from its root, certain parts of the body must be free and unblocked (toes, feet, ankles, knees, hips, groins). The extension of the spine in sitting āsana comes from the freedom of the coxofemoral region, sacroiliac, glutei and hamstrings. The freeing of these areas, already initiated in standing āsana, continues with sitting āsana and culminates in forward extensions.

Sitting āsana not only serve as an intermediary stage, but also as a study of the various prāṇic flows in the pelvis, allowing us to observe how the pelvis resonates when the legs are 'amputated' from it in Daṇḍāsana, Vīrāsana, Svastikāsana, Padmāsana, Baddha Koṇāsana, Mūlabandhāsana and Kandāsana, as well as in their supine phase (supta) variations.

Forward Extension Āsana
(Paśцimā Pratana Sthiti): The Western Gate (Paścimādvāra)

"Stretch out both legs and keep them apart; firmly take hold the head by the hands and place them on the knees. This is called Ugrāsana, the terrible posture. It excites the motion of the air, destroys the dullness and uneasiness of the body, and is also called Paścimottānāsana. That wise man who daily practices this noble posture can certainly induce the flow of the air along the posterior channel (suṣumṇā nāḍī)."
ŚIVASAṂHITĀ III, 92

The posterior channel illustrates the peaceful quality of the mood in forward extensions, which above all pacify the nervous system. Standing āsana stimulate and develop endurance, while forward extensions quieten and teach us how to immerse ourselves in the silence of this energy. Here we begin to understand the movement of introversion, where we establish ourselves in the silence of the nascent nightfall, and which culminates in inverted āsana and Śavāsana.

"And when, like the tortoise withdrawing its limbs from all sides, the yogi withdraws his senses from sense-objects, his knowledge stands established."
BHAGAVAD GĪTĀ II, 60

In order to feel the posterior channel, the anterior spine has to find its full length. This is what we learn in forward extensions. To paraphrase Yogācārya Śrī B.K.S. Iyengar, one places the absolute in the ground.

Lateral Extension Āsana
(Parivṛtta Sthiti): The Gesture of Matsyendranātha

"To twist the torso in such a way that the abdomen seems to have become the back and to maintain that attitude with energy... this āsana is called the one of Mastyendra."
GHERAṆḌASAṂHITĀ II, 23-24

This group of āsana cleanse any residual blockages in the back, shoulders, neck and hips, and prepare the spine and back muscles for the deeper work of backward extensions. After forward or backward extensions, they return the spine to a certain neutrality. By rinsing out the abdominal and pelvic cavity, they purify the apānavāyu and its excretory function, as well as stimulating the digestive fire (jaṭhara agni).

Abdominal Toning Āsana
(Udara Ākuncana Sthiti): Preparing to Take Flight

"The Bandha that I am going to explain is called uḍḍiyānabandha, because by means of it the great birds (the vital breaths) take wing ceaselessly."
HAṬHAYOGAPRADĪPIKĀ III, 56

These are the āsana that tone the abdominal girdle. They help to dispel gas (Pavanmuktāsana), distension and abdominal wind. They are preparation for the powerful suction that is indispensable in Uḍḍiyānabandha and Mūlabhanda.

Balancing Āsana (Baka Mudrā): The Gesture of the Crane

"He who remains the same in pain, pleasure and in sleep; who looks upon a clod, a stone, a piece of gold as of equal worth; who remains the same amid pleasant and unpleasant experiences; who possesses firm intellect; who regards blame and praise of himself as one, he who is the same in grace and disgrace, impartial to friends and foes and who has given up all initiative of action, he is said to have transcended the guṇa." BHAGAVAD GĪTĀ XIV, 24-25

At first, in balancing āsana, the weight of the body and the action of gravity are experienced. When these are mastered, complete weightlessness of the body is experienced. Paradoxically, gravity can become an ascending force. This becomes possible when the body's centre of gravity is positioned in such a way that it escapes the pull of gravity. The contractions applied to the abdominal organs in balancing āsana strengthen them, particularly during the Bakāsana cycle from Śīrṣāsana. In balancing āsana, the outer spine is trained which gives it strength and resistance.

Binding Āsana (Granthana Sthiti): The Art of Knotting the Body

"This worship should be done by a penetration from Consciousness which flashes as it cuts through the twelve knots right to the ultimate exhalation (visarga) so as to be nothing more than energy."
YOGINĪHṚDAYA, PŪJĀSAṂKETA, ŚRĪCAKRAPŪJĀ 135

In these āsana (Eka Pāda Śīrṣāsana and its variations, amongst others), the body is knotted in order to release it from certain grips and to gain access to important prāṇic junctions. Here the abdomen is subjected to different kinds of contractions.

Backward Extension Āsana (Pūrva Pratana Sthiti): The Eastern Gate (Pūrvadvāra)

"This supreme energy which blossoms in felicity is like the cobra as it lifts itself..."
ABHINAVAGUPTA, TANTRĀLOKA XXIX, 248-251

Backward extensions are not introduced until the other peripheral movements of the spine have been integrated by practising the other groups of āsana. The scapular, dorsal, lumbar, sacral, coccygeal and gluteal regions must first have been freed from their initial rigidity. This is why standing āsana, forward extensions and lateral extensions are introduced beforehand as they are essential in understanding backward extensions.
Backward extensions provoke a deep churning. When the gods and the demons churned the cosmic ocean, the first thing to come out was a poison so terrible that it was capable of destroying the universe! In these āsana, pain, discouragement and frustration may accompany the traveller. Yet even here, effortlessness should be the starting point for all effort. These āsana train the nervous system to open up to greater intensity, like when the power of an electrical circuit is increased. In backward extensions, the adrenal glands are strongly stimulated. It is therefore important they are then pacified by an appropriate sequence of āsana.

Inverted Āsana (Viparīta Karaṇī Mudrā): The Seal of the Great Resorption

"The sun (Sūrya) dwells at the root of the navel and the moon (Candra) at the root of the palate. Man succumbs to death because Sūrya swallows up the ambrosia.
That process by which the Sūrya is raised up and the Candra is carried lower down is called Viparīta Karaṇī

Mudrā, which is kept secret in all the Tantra.
With the head on the ground and the legs lifted while using both hands as a support, remain stable in this inverted position.
By constantly practising this mudrā, decrepitude and death will be conquered. The power it bestows ensures the consequences of the dissolution of the universes are not endured."
GHERAṆḌASAṂHITĀ III, 29-30-31-32

Inverted āsana, even Śīrṣāsana, which is a stimulating āsana, teach the art of resorption. It is in these āsana that the withdrawal of all the energies into their source culminates.
In Śīrṣāsana, the pelvic and thoracic diaphragms are explored through Mūlabhanda and Uḍḍiyānabandha. The fulcrum of Śīrṣāsana is the crown of the head, which is in contact with the element of earth, while the feet are in contact with the element of space. Hence there is an 'inversion' of the sensation of elements within the body. In Sarvāṅgāsana and Halāsana the vocal diaphragm is explored. The whole area of the shoulders, neck, throat and back of the head are released, which teaches Jālandharabandha. In Setu Bandha Sarvāṅgāsana we learn to unfold the three bandha.
In these āsana, we move from a frontal brain or verbal perception that categorises the world, to a more holistic perception of the primitive brain. They therefore participate in cerebral integration where a harmony of perception exists between the two hemispheres and the so-called internal and external realities. The khaṇḍasāra in inverted āsana is the beheading!

"One should contemplate the entire sky which is the nature of Bhairava as if it is pervading one's head.
Then one experiences everything as the form of Bhairava and one enters into the glory of His nature."
VIJÑĀNA BHAIRAVA 85

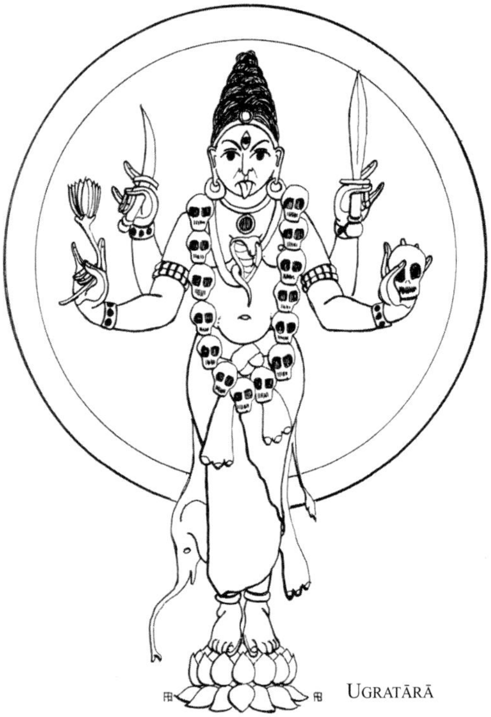

UGRATĀRĀ

Postural Contemplation
(Bhāvanāsana)

"One should know that the real āsana is the one in which the meditation of Brahman flows spontaneously and unceasingly, and not any other that destroys one's happiness." Śaṅkarācārya, Aparokṣānubhūti 112

One of the etymologies of the word āsana is 'to be seated'. The essence of being seated is establishing all sheaths of the śarīra in their source.

"Taking his seat in the middle breath (udāna) in between the passages of inhalation and exhalation, holding firmly on the cognitive energy (jñānaśakti), the stable posture that the yogi acquires is the real āsana."
Kṣemarāja, Commentary on the Śivasūtra (III.6)

What then is this āsana if it is not the pulse of spanda, which takes on a myriad of forms? Thus the āsana become a mirror of this pulse, of this sensation (sparśa), also called tingling (pipīlikā). This pulse is expressed in all forms, which is why the different groups of āsana recreate the infinity of all these structures, whether geometric, geographic, mineral, vegetal, animal, human, heroic, demonic or divine. Touch (sparśa) is the most radiant act of consecration in āsana.

"The organs of sight, hearing, taste and smell are to be found in a subtle way in the earth and the other elements, belonging to the lower level of reality, the highest not outstripping the level of illusion (māyātattva) while touch inhabits at the upper level of the energy as an inexpressible and subtle sensation to which the yogin ceaselessly aspires, for this contact is achieved in a Consciousness identical to the pure, brilliant firmament of its own luminosity."
Abhinavagupta, Tantrāloka XI, 29-33

1
Postural Rituals
(Kriyāvasthā)

"That which begets felicity and delights the heart, this is what is suited to this veneration."
Abhinavagupta, Tantrāloka XXIX, 106-107

All traditional arts demand an apprenticeship. Great musicians are able to improvise, forgetting technique, because they have been absorbing it over many years of intense practice.
In the Vāstu Sūtra Upaniṣad (the Upaniṣad of architects, sculptors and temple builders), it is said that there are six disciplines essential to this art. These can be applied equally to the art of āsana: knowledge of stone (śailam), which in our context is the body, composition of diagrams (āsana), the vital points (marman), stone cutting (śailabhedana), which in our context is the arranging of the body's limbs (aṅgaprayoga), the emotional attitude evoked by the composition (nyāsabhāvanā) and intuition of the unity underpinning the composition (saṃbandha prabodhana).
The first contact with the body reveals its inertia. At first, āsana will simply create movement and mobility. It is a return to sensation, to non-verbal perception, in which the body is no longer 'thought' or 'named'. The āsana become an opportunity to observe how the body is constantly agitated, restricted and contracted. This is why the first, very gross phase is called kriyā (here referring to the foremost etymology, which is action or ritual, and not the various cleansing processes known as ṣaṭkarman; these processes were only used as a last resort when the organism proved incapable of detoxifying itself, and because of their aggressive nature were never part of a regular practice). This stage is also called Cikitsā Krama or gradual purification.
The language of posture refers to three rhythms; these

are described as: emanation (sṛṣṭi), maintenance (sthiti) and resorption (saṃhāra). The Vaijayanti Kośa defines sṛṣṭi as the natural state (svabhāva), sthiti as the act of maintaining, of continuing (maryādā), and saṃhāra as that of ending, of dissolving (pralaya). The pulse of spanda is already implied when entering into an āsana, holding it and releasing it. Everything perceived, the universe itself, is regarded as the field of Consciousness. The universe, as yantra or maṇḍala, unfolds in eight directions: east (pūrvā), west (paścimā), south (dakṣiṇā), north (uttarā), north-east (īśa), south-east (āgneya), north-west (vāyavī) and south-west (nairṛta). When these directions are applied to the maṇḍala of the body, the anterior side is the east, and the posterior side the west, the north being the head and the south being the feet.

"According to the space-directions, the guardians of the quarters are worshipped (Āditya in the east, Yama in the south, Varuṇa in the west, Soma in the north and Agni in the centre)." Vāstu Sūtra Upaniṣad V, 23

The sense of direction in an āsana is the basis of alignment. By alignment, we are referring to the concept of equanimity (samatva).

"Absorption in the unity of Brahman should be known as the equipoise of the limbs and not the mere straightening of the body, like that of the dried-up tree."
Śaṅkarācārya, Aparokṣānubhūti 115

At first, external means of movement and action are used. Movement can be vertical, horizontal, spiral, lateral, expansion and contraction. These movements are applied to different parts of the body in the various āsana. The body thus becomes the object (grāhya) of dynamic concentration, taking support on the different parts (aṅga) of the organism. Mobility will become action, which is intelligence in motion, unfolding different and opposite senses of direction, some parts being stable and others mobile. Precision when adopting the āsana and the refinement of the shape itself reveal its external texture.

"The features of the character arise from the measured gestures of the body."
Vāstu Sūtra Upaniṣad IV, 7

The median line (brahmakila or brahmadaṇḍa), like the centre (bindu), is the support of all āsana. Alignment or median line is only another name for cosmic order (dharma or ṛta).

"All limbs have to be set along lines."
"The middle line is the support."
"The hole is the centre (marman) and is to be contemplated as Brahman." Vāstu Sūtra Upaniṣad II-8, IV-26, VI-8

Thus the source of āsana is the savour of tranquillity (śāntarasa). Samasthiti, the art of verticality, is merely the other side of the same coin. Samasthiti is therefore the even posture, where fluctuations of opposites are resorbed in the centre.

"The Bindu is like Brahman, Brahman is immovable."
"The Bindu obtained in the centre is the life-breath of the earth." Vāstu Sūtra Upaniṣad VI-11, II-14

Every āsana has its source in Samasthiti, which is the actualisation of śāntarasa. If Samasthiti is present, the wave of resorption (Śavāsana) is also present.

"There where day and night have been abolished, where the course of the sun and moon is interrupted, the vital breath ceases to circulate through Iḍā (left) and Piṅgalā (right) and surrenders into Suṣumṇā (centre), because Suṣumṇā consumes time." Haṭhayogapradīpikā IV, 17

The different attitudes (bhāva) give way to the taste of unity (samarasatva).

"O good-looking one, as bees make honey by collecting the essences of trees standing in different quarters, and reduce the juice into a homogenous whole; and as they do not have such distinctive ideas as, 'I am the juice of this tree', 'I am the juice of that tree', so also O good-looking one, all these creatures, after merging in Being, do not know this: 'we have merged in Being'."
CHĀNDOGYOPANIṢAD VI, 9-1, 9-2

2
Attention and Bodily Sensations
(Vijñānacarasa)

"Sacrifice is an appeasement that one celebrates as a blossoming."
ABHINAVAGUPTA, TANTRĀLOKA XXIX, 107

In the initial phase, dynamic concentration was fragmentary, dividing the body into parts, using movement and action (kriyā). It must now give way to attention (vijñāna) that is no longer focalised, but on the contrary, diffuses into a unifying whole, like warm oil spreading out. Here, sensation predominates and the body's texture in the flow of the āsana is observed. The phases of adjustment and action are minimised. Alignment in the kriyā phase placed the emphasis on the outer shape of the āsana and the aesthetics of the limbs in space, without being concerned by the final form.

"By a harmonious form a meditative mood is induced."
VĀSTU SŪTRA UPANIṢAD II, 23

In the vijñāna phase, this principle is obsolete. It remains present, rather like musicians who tune their instruments before playing, but who do not spend all their time just tuning them; or like gliding birds that use rising currents of air, occasionally moving just one feather, but who do not exert themselves by beating their wings incessantly. Here, āsana become mudrā, symbolic gestures of the three energies: energy of will (icchāśakti), energy of knowledge (jñānaśakti) and energy of activity (kriyāśakti), where a contemplative mood gains the upper hand. The external manifestation of an āsana is just a pretext to recognise that the object (grāhya) bathes in the light of the subject (grāhaka) without separation.

"From the formless arises form."
VĀSTU SŪTRA UPANIṢAD V, 22

Technically, we 'undo' more than we 'do'. This phase is also called śaktikrama, the succession of energies.

3
The Sky of Consciousness
(Cidākāśa)

Here, even attention dies and evaporates into the space of Consciousness (cidākāśa). The āsana becomes a maṇḍala (from the root MAṆḌA, essence). All the dynamism of doing, of action, is extinguished and the āsana becomes a reflection of its source. The non-volitional aspect of the posture becomes a unifying obviousness. The āsana is merely the space of Consciousness. This non-doing completely burns up the object itself, so we may intuitively recognise what we are, through the discriminative emptying of what we are not.
This reminds us of the three aims (lakṣyatraya or trilakṣya) of Gorakṣanātha: the external aim (bahirlakṣya), the internal aim (antarlakṣya) and the median aim (madhyalakṣya). Lakṣya literally means 'that which deserves particular attention'.
In the external aim, any object whatsoever can be used: the blue of the sky, a sound, the sun, the moon, the flowing water of a river, etc. The external aim brings the

diversity of phenomena (vikalpa) towards undifferentiated perception. In āsana practice, the external aim uses the various parts of the body, their interaction and their unity. The internal aim uses the body's various internal geography, both organic and subtle. The organic aim will open into bridges of space (ādhāra), places of contemplation that unfold the five firmaments (pañcavyoman). Here, we become aware of the various flows of breath in these spaces, the pañcavāyu (apāna, samāna, prāṇa, udāna, vyāna). The internal aim thus creates intimacy with the marrow of life and reveals how it is robed in different colourations and contractions to become the so-called compact mass of the body. When these two aims reach maturity, they die into the median aim (madhyalakṣya), where all notion of body-mind disappears.

"Who am I when neither my will nor my knowledge has arisen? I am this in reality! Having become that, one should be merged in that and one's mind should be identified with that."
VIJÑĀNA BHAIRAVA 97

This stage is called adhyātmikakrama or plunging into the Self.

4
Incantation, Clarification and Resonance, or the Rhythms of Silence
(Vinyāsakramadhvani)

"The spontaneous outpouring that is expressed in the energy of phonemics, the expression of the non-manifest, of unarticulated sound, is called resonance (dhvani)."
ABHINAVAGUPTA, TANTRĀLOKA V, 131B-132A

The ritual of consecrating the body is expressed through nyāsa. This term, which is at the heart of vinyāsa, signifies impregnation, placing, establishing or mental welcoming of deities and their energies, accompanied by mantra and mudrā in various parts of the body. Hence the invocation: *"O Lord make your dwelling here (Om Pratitiṣtha Parameśvara)"*. In traditional nyāsa, the fingertips and the palm of the hand are used to consecrate different parts of the body. It is interesting to note the etymology of the Sanskrit word for hand (hasta):

"That which blossoms outwards (hasati vikasati)."
ĀGAMA KOŚA, VOL. 8, PAGE 81

The base of the thumbs (aṅguṣṭha) become the dwelling place for the waters of Brahmā, symbolising the creative force, the hypnotic power of the mind, which, like a coloured lens, projects our own expectations onto reality. *"When a pickpocket meets a wise man, all he sees in him are his pockets."* (INDIAN PROVERB) The index finger (tarjanī) is used to warn and reprimand, but also to point out. It discriminates. The ring finger (anāmikā) doesn't have a name; it is un-nameable because Śiva used it to decapitate Brahmā! It signifies the non-conceptual, the non-mind. The little finger (kaniṣṭha), the smallest or weakest, represents the dual nature (vikalpa) of the mind.

The middle finger (madhyama) represents the unifying vibration of Consciousness, where the characteristics of the other fingers no longer exist. In postural rituals, āsana become the offering of space (ākāśa) in the different parts of the body. The limbs and the anatomical, physiological, respiratory and sensory functions all participate in the nyāsa of impregnation.

Thanks to postural nyāsa, the infinity of the worlds and their geography are rediscovered in the completeness of the body. Far beyond the exterior nyāsa, āsana seal into the body the consecration of the gross elements (pañcamahābhūta): earth, water, fire, air, ether; the five breaths (pañcavāyu); the cakra and their bīja mantra; the seven constituents (saptadhātu): skin (rasa), blood (rakta), flesh (māṃsa), fat (meda), bones (asthi), marrow (majja), sperm, ova or vital energy (śukra); the three humours (tridoṣa): wind (vāta), bile (pitta), phlegm (kapha); the three qualities (triguṇa): inertia (tamas), activity (rajas), luminosity (sattva). The nyāsa thus become the expression of the five mouths of Śiva Svachandanātha (Īśāna, Tatpuruṣa, Aghora, Vāmadeva, Sadyojāta), or of diversity in unity, as well as the expressions of Consciousness that represent joy (ānanda), will (icchā), knowledge (jñāna) and activity (kriyā).

According to the Dhātupāṭha (dictionary of root meanings), the root of krama is KRAM, which means *"to take a step (kramu pādavikṣepe)."* (Dhātupāṭha I, 502) The three worlds are circumscribed by the three steps of Viṣṇu Trivikrama (Trīṇi Padā Vicakrame: Ṛgveda I, 22, 18), like three mad strides of the energy that creates, measures, conquers and transcends both the visible and invisible. Māyā comes from the root MĀ, meaning 'to measure'. The crazy wager and function of Viṣṇu (from the root VIṢ vyāptau, to spread out, to pervade) is to measure the immeasurable, which becomes space-time.

"Viṣṇu is truly the sacrifice, by striding he obtains for the gods that all-pervading power which now belongs to them. By the first step he gained the same earth, the second the aerial expanse, and by his last step, the sky."
Śatapathabrāhmaṇa 1-9, 3-9

Krama indicates a sequence in time, a cycle, like the succession of day and night, months and years, the cycle of seasons and the course of the sun in the sky. This succession is not left to chance; it follows an order, gradually in an orderly fashion (kramāt, kramena, kramaṣaḥ).
Circumambulation (parikrama), transition (saṃkranti), the process of transformation (pariṇāmakrama), of emanation (sṛṣṭikrama) and of resorption (saṃhārakrama), all speak of the same notion, a vital thread (sūtra) which links all phenomena and events within immanence and transcendence.

"The power of freedom, the will to create sequence and the sequence of time itself are manifestations of the power of the Omnipresent. May these three goddesses reveal to me the Unsurpassable (anuttara)."
Abhinavagupta, Tantrāloka I, 5

The intuition of a rhythm (emanation, maintenance, resorption) in the relative sequence of events leads us to their silence, to their absolute transparency.

"The pure Consciousness remains abiding in all the subject-object and in the instrument of knowledge of the universe. She (saṃvit) verily is one and any sort of limitation of sequential order is not possible in Her. Despite the absence of sequence, neither is it simultaneous. The essence of Consciousness (saṃvit) is beyond sequence (krama) and simultaneity (akrama), for it is really pure."
Abhinavagupta, Tantrāloka IV, 179-180a

Vinyāsa in āsana practice is the codification of bodily attitudes, of groups of āsana and of the precise positioning of various parts of the body, which begin to interact to produce certain effects. Only a glimpse of this art will be given here, as it would require an entire book in itself for a full and proper explanation!

Vinyāsakrama encompasses a diversity of definitions:
• The starting position, the attitude for entering into, staying in and for coming out of an āsana, according to a rhythm synchronised with the breath.
• The gradual linking of āsana according to a sequence, in a flow synchronised with the breath.
• The gradual preparation of āsana not yet mastered, spread over several months.
• Precision in establishing and unfolding an āsana.
• Unfolding variations for intensifying āsana or making modifications to an āsana.
• The resorption phase and āsana that unfold a feeling of calm (viśrānta karaṇa āsana).

Vinyāsa is to yoga what syntax is to literature. It is in a series that āsana reveal their melody and reflect their different energetic colourations. A series is an invocation that generates clarification and intuitive resonance of the absolute. The texture and savour of an āsana are different according to its place in the sequence. This however has nothing to do with counter-posture because āsana are not postures! Āsana mirror totality and unfold quietude (śāntarasa) in the body, breath and mind. Each āsana is thus self-sufficient and has no need for a so-called 'opposite action'. It is more a question of equalising energy (pratikriyāsana or samaśaktikriyā) to avoid certain undesirable effects or to reinforce certain desirable ones. For instance, we would not end our practice with Śīrṣāsana or with a backward extension, even if it was followed by Śavāsana, unless we were a master in the art of resorption!

"From the sequence of forms comes the condition of the mind; this procedure is the best."
VĀSTU SŪTRA UPANIṢAD VI, 24

The attitude referred to here is that of acceptance of the energetic flow of an āsana and its anatomical, physiological, neurological, sensory and mental repercussions. There is an introductory vinyāsakrama, an initiation into āsana. Thus the introductory vinyāsakrama for inverted poses would be supported Setu Bandha Sarvāṅgāsana, supported Viparīta Karaṇī, Ardha Halāsana, Halāsana and then Sarvāṅgāsana. When these āsana have been introduced, having themselves been introduced by other āsana, then Śīrṣāsana may be undertaken. Once Śīrṣāsana has been introduced, the vinyāsakrama for correct energy flow would be: Śīrṣāsana, Sarvāṅgāsana, Halāsana, Setu Bandha Sarvāṅgāsana, Viparīta Karaṇī.

"The conception of the composition (nyāsādhāraṇa) is most essential."
VĀSTU SŪTRA UPANIṢAD VI, 1

The various energetic colourations of āsana, or groups of āsana, are fundamental in the art of sequencing. Certain āsana are warming, whereas others are cooling. Certain may be stimulating and enlivening, calming and relaxing, simple or complex. To this must be added the process referred to as 'contraction' (langhana), which includes eliminating, fasting and drying āsana, and the process of expansion (brimhana), which includes nourishing, moistening and restorative āsana.
In elementary vinyāsakrama, we begin with standing āsana (utthiṣṭha sthiti), sitting āsana (upaviṣṭha sthiti), forward extension āsana (paścima pratana sthiti), lateral extension āsana (parivṛtta sthiti) and inverted āsana (viparīta sthiti). When these groups of āsana have created a degree of mobility, backward extension āsana (pūrva pratana sthiti) are introduced, followed by abdominal

āsana (udara ākuncana sthiti). A taster of supine āsana (supta sthiti) is given at the very beginning of the learning process with Śavāsana. As regards the vinyāsa of energy, Śīrṣāsana, backward extensions or sun salutations are never performed after Sarvāṅgāsana. Sarvāṅgāsana is one of the āsana of resorption, and because of the use of Jālandharabandha, must be followed by āsana that continue to unfold this 'wave' of resorption.

Vinyāsa has an infinite number of aspects. One of the grossest is moving from one āsana to another in a continuous flow. The link between āsana is the sun salutation (sūrya namaskāra). Here the movement is peripheral, and because we do not become fully established in the āsana, the notions explained earlier concerning alignment and maturation that come with duration cannot be truly understood. If used in an extreme way, one of the dangers of this method, whereby we are simply obsessed by the final pose, is that we may become like the mad monkey, stung by a scorpion and locked in a room without windows. This method is ideal for teenagers and young people who need a vigorous and challenging practice, for experienced practitioners who have a tendency towards inertia or dullness, or during cold winter weather. But it is very exclusive and therefore not suitable for everyone.

In the same vein, there is:

• Viśamanyāsa, which is a sequence of āsana that seem to oppose each other and have no links.

• Viloma Viśamanyāsa, which is the practice of a group of āsana, linked by an āsana in an opposite direction (e.g. backward extensions interspersed with Paścimottānāsana).

"The sculptors (Śilpakāra) apply a softening mixture."
Vāstu Sūtra Upaniṣad III, 8

A sculptor does not begin to use his chisel until he has applied four substances to make the stone malleable. This quotation introduces one of the most interesting aspects of vinyāsa, which is that of intimacy (paricaya) or welcoming (svāgatam). This is known as vinyāsakrama. Here, performing the āsana in its final external form is of no importance. A gradual approach is used to welcome the essence and unfolding of the āsana through passive observation of the neurophysiological processes.

Vinyāsakrama svāgatam proceeds from the simplest and most accessible to the most complex. Increasing resistance is 'welcomed', thereby letting us flirt with the more accomplished aspect of the āsana. By 'accomplished' we mean the unfolded sensation and texture of the āsana, without however moving into the so-called final posture. For example, in Halāsana, the feet, instead of being on the ground could be raised up. There exists therefore a gradual approach for each āsana. This vinyāsakrama, called 'framing' (sampuṭana kriyā), unfolds two processes: vitalising and pacifying.

One could adopt preparatory vinyāsakrama, which lead to a certain degree of maturity in observing the desired āsana, whilst allowing parasitic movements of agitation, panic and fear to be abandoned, and which would otherwise hinder breathing or create pressure in the throat, eyes, ears and tongue.

Śīrṣāsana can be framed using the pacifying progression of Uttānāsana, Adho Mukha Śvānāsana, Prasārita Pādottānāsana, Jānu Śīrṣāsana, Paścimottānāsana, Adho Mukha Vīrāsana, Śīrṣāsana, and then from Śīrṣāsana the āsana are repeated in the opposite sequence. The same āsana could be framed by a more dynamic postural environment by first doing Adho Mukha Vṛkṣāsana and Piñca Mayūrāsana for example.

A sequence only acquires its true value when accompanied by a yoga practice adapted to the needs of the individual (viniyoga). It should be in harmony with the internal and external environments, and not simply imposed. The constitution (deha), place (deśa), gender (liṅga), time (kāla), age (vayas), abilities (śakti), aspirations (mārga) and occupations (vṛtti) of the practitioner must be taken into account, whilst respecting the different stages of life (āśrama) and each person's

inclinations, which alter according to circumstances. If, for example, a person suffers from high blood pressure or if a woman is experiencing menopausal hot flushes, the postural programme must be adjusted. During the menstrual cycle, certain āsana such as inverted postures must be avoided, and greater emphasis placed on other āsana. Seasons and changes between seasons also have their importance. It is not possible to practise the same way in winter as in the middle of a hot summer.
The various techniques are adapted to meet the needs of the practitioner's age. Sṛṣṭikrama, which is for youths, is a purely dynamic practice where the emphasis is placed on expansion, agility, rapidity, suppleness and strength. Sthitikrama, which is for adults, places the emphasis on organic and prāṇic action. Antyakrama, which is for older people, is aimed at maintaining the circulatory and respiratory systems in good condition, and places the emphasis on the natural movement of resorption present at this time.

Cinnamastākayantra

Practice can also be adapted according to the needs of the moment and the maturity of the practitioner. Cikitsākrama is a purifying practice intended to cleanse and detoxify the body. Śaktikrama is for those who use āsana to create churning and effervescence, through the practice of more advanced āsana for example. Adhyātmikakrama is the practice of offering and oblation, where āsana are the surrendering of the body (śarīra) and its various sheaths into their source.
Respecting individual structure lets us mirror the different facets of our potential, at a given moment; rather like a plant which doesn't have ideal conditions yet is at one with its environment and makes the best of it. The body is no longer stifled by a personal commentary that restricts it within an image. This unity with its own constitution lets the structure breathe freely.

"After long deliberations, the sages pronounced that yoga can be divided into three categories of practice: Sṛṣṭikrama, Sthitikrama and Antyakrama. The practice of Yoga must take into account that Sṛṣṭikrama is for the Brahmacārin (adolescent, young man), Sthitikrama is for the Gṛhastha (adult man or woman with an active life-style, family and professional obligations, whether married or unmarried), and Saṃhārakrama (also called Antyakrama) is for the Saṃnyāsin (retired person)."
Śrī Nāthamuni, Yogarahasya, Viniyogādhyāya II, 3

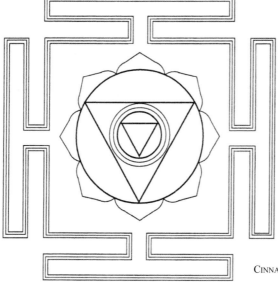

5
Supports for Contemplation, Junctions and Gateways to Space
(Ādhāra, Saṃdhi, Ākāśadvāra)

Ādhāra, from the root DHṚ, literally means that which retains, that which contains, but also supports; the word lakṣya, an object of contemplation, is also used. Gorakṣanātha describes sixteen ādhāra or supports for contemplation.

1. Pādāṅguṣṭhādhāra: the root of the big toes, and the space between the big toes and the second toes. These are of great importance in postural stability. The big toes must 'see'. It is said there exists a connection between the big toes and the optic nerves.

"The first support is that of the big toes. They should be contemplated like a bulb of light. Thus the gaze becomes stable." GORAKṢANĀTHA, SIDDHASIDDHĀNTAPADDHATI II, 10

2. Mūlādhāra: the perineum. This is the place of contemplation of the three paths (Iḍā, Piṅgalā, Suṣumṇā). It is from here the fire arises.

3. Gudādhāra: the rectum. This is the place of contemplation of apānavāyu. Numerous āsana help to vitalise apānavāyu, which, in this part of the body, regulates excretory functions. There are certain preferred āsana such as Samasthiti, Śīrṣāsana, Sarvāṅgāsana, Urdhva Dhanurāsana, Uṣṭrāsana and Paścimottānāsana that are used to learn expansion and contraction or to learn the upward suction of the rectum (vikāsa saṃkocana or aśvinī mudrā, also known as the horse's gesture because it is reminiscent of the stance of a horse when urinating). Apānavāyu becomes firm.

4. Medhrādhāra: the liṅga, situated at the root of the penis, though some say the penis itself. This is the place of contemplation of prāṇa, which rises with the syllable SVA, hence its alternative appellation of svādhiṣṭhāna, meaning pleasant. Here the life force (prāṇaśakti) becomes seed (bindu, vīrya, retas). Certain āsana induce a saturation of the body by the vital energy (bindu stambhana) and not its usual loss (bindu kṣaraṇa). Here, one rests in the secret cave of the bee, which unfolds Vajrolī.

5. Uḍḍiyānādhāra: situated above the navel. It controls the vitality of the digestive fire (jaṭhara agni), helping to cleanse the intestines, as well as the urinary and excretory systems.

6. Nābhyādhāra: situated at the root of the navel, also known as the bulb (kaṇḍasthāna), the root of the nāḍī network. It is in this place that sound is resorbed (nādalaya). *"In the lower region of Maṇipūra, turned towards the south and towards the north, is the area of the anus. At its centre, the bulb of the navel resembles the lotus flower and is said to be the receptacle of all the subtle channels (nāḍī)."*
GORAKṢANĀTHA, AMARAUGHAŚĀSANA

This ādhāra is the site where the praṇava (Om) becomes manifest in its subtle, still unified form. It is only in hṛdayādhāra that it becomes distinct, although still remaining continuous. It then bursts into an infinite number of sounds at the vocal cords.

7. Hṛdayādhāra: the heart. This is the place of contemplation of the union of prāṇa and apāna.

8. Kaṇṭhādhāra: the place of contemplation of the throat through Jālandharabandha, amongst others. It is here the fluctuations of the breath are stopped. Iḍā and Piṅgalā become stable in the centre.

9. Ghaṇṭikādhāra: situated at the root of the palate.

This is the place of contemplation of the nectar (amṛta kalā) that flows from the candramaṇḍala and pours into the sahasrāra.

10. Tālvādhāra: situated at the roof of the palate. This is the place of contemplation of the khecarīmudrā, representing unlimited Consciousness.

11. Jihvādhāra: situated at the root of the tongue. This is the place of contemplation of the emanation and resorption of corporeal speech (vaikharī).

12. Bhrūmadhyādhāra: situated between the eyebrows. This is the place of contemplation of the lunar disc. Here, one attains coolness and calm.

13. Nāsādhāra: situated at the tip of the nose. This is the place of contemplation of the gateways of breathing and of ākāśatattva.

14. Kapātādhāra: situated at the roof of the nose. This is the place of contemplation of the breath, and of its stability during inhalation. During exhalation, it is possible to observe the natural descent of the eyes and the roof of the nose, which tend to be pushed back upwards if the next inhalation is aggressive or unrhythmical. It is the place of contemplation of different lights.

15. Lalāṭādhāra: situated in the centre of the forehead. This is the place of contemplation and resorption of the frontal brain. Here, one becomes radiant.

16. Brahmarandhrādhāra: situated in the centre of the skull, but also in the area called 'the bee's cave' (bhramaraguhā) situated at the apex of the spine and in the lower parts of sahasrāra. This is the place of contemplation of space (ākāśa). Here, one worships the pair of lotus-feet of the revered guru.

In āsana practice, the notion of ādhāra is extended to the whole body and to all parts of the body. Different parts of the body thus become fulcrums for contemplation or absorption (samāveśa). These fulcrums are in fact a way of releasing the grips of the body, allowing the vital functions to spread out to their full organic extent and thus pour out their effervescence. This effervescence dissolves the boundaries of the body, spreading it out into the Universe. The ādhāra are the buds of life, and in their energetic aspect are recognised as divinities (devatā).

"The divinities of Consciousness, these masters of the sensory organs relish the universe transformed into nectar. Replete, they identify themselves with Bhairava, the firmament of Consciousness, God dwelling within the heart, He, the fullness."
Abhinavagupta. Tantrāloka III, 262-264

The practitioner contemplates how certain areas evolve in the āsana itself, but also how they are able to maintain their stability from one āsana to another. This junction is called saṃdhi. Saṃdhi is the meeting-point, the connection, the union. Saṃdhāna is a synonym of Saṃdhi that in Kashmir Śaivism signifies awareness and fundamental unity of Reality. The different moments of the day are known as trisaṃdhyā (dawn, midday, twilight), in which all the particular blend and melt into one another, leaving only the undifferentiated resonance of spanda. It is said that auspicious practices like prāṇāyāma or the worship of the Lord should take place at the saṃdhi.

"All acts of consecration should be done at the junction (sandhyā) where one is spontaneously united with the Lord." Abhinavagupta, Tantrāloka XXVI, 29b-33a

The demon Hiraṇyakaśipu was granted a boon from Brahmā protecting him from being killed 'by neither man, nor god, nor animal, nor during the day nor by night, neither inside nor outside a house'. In order to destroy

Hiraṇyakaśipu, Viṣṇu, in the form of Narasiṃha, the man-lion, used the saṃdhi of time (twilight) and that of space (threshold), representing the way in and out of the worlds. In grammar, saṃdhi are the junctions between vowels and consonants, which are transformed when they meet. It also refers to the coded or twilight language (sandhyābhāṣya) used in tantric texts to confuse neophytes! Saṃdhi also means the joints in the body, which, during āsana, become reservoirs of infinite space; or rather the synapses helping the diffusion of infinity between the limbs, thus avoiding compression. These reservoirs of space are not only the privilege of the joints, but also of the vital points (marman). According to this śloka, whose author is unknown, but quoted by Lakṣmīdhara in his commentary on the Saundaryalaharī:

"The point in which two lines meet is called saṃdhi and the point in which three lines meet is known as marman according to the view of those who have the knowledge of marman."

It also applies to the space that is the background between each breath.

"O Bhairavī, by focussing one's awareness on the two voids at the end of the internal and external breath, thereby the glorious form of Bhairava is revealed through Bhairavī."
VIJÑĀNA BHAIRAVA 25

Saṃdhi reveals the centre. Intuition and unfolding of saṃdhi are essential to āsana practice. There are gross saṃdhi that concern the outer conjunctions. For example, the position and opening of the armpits in Vīrabhadrāsana 2 helps the understanding of their positioning in Utthita Pārśvakoṇāsana. There are more subtle saṃdhi that correspond to the conjunctions of the organs of action and perception through the breath. Certain āsana educate the various diaphragms, which then become prāṇic junctions. The essence of all āsana is the contemplation of the incomprehensible, of the unknowable. This is what Śaṅkarācārya says of Mūlabandhāsana:

"That Brahman which is the root of all existence, and on which the restraint of the mind is based is called the restraining root (mūlabandha), which should always be adopted since it is fit for the Rāja Yogi."
ŚAṄKARĀCĀRYA, APAROKṢĀNUBHŪTI 114

These junctions, or doors of space, permit the practitioner to feel an āsana subjectively and to no longer objectivise it as exteriority. It is rather like two strangers who meet through a glance that intuitively reveals all, without the need for introduction.

6
Postural Emanation, Maintenance and Resorption
(Trikāla)

The intuition of 'what we are not' has no need of a process or progression in time. According to Abhinavagupta, it is instantaneous, like a flash of lightning. However its actualisation and diffusion, in order, as is said in the Śivasūtra, *"to implement the resorption of fragmentary activities within the body"*, takes time. This is why time (kāla) is an important element in āsana.
Duration does not matter to start with, but becomes dominant later on. When remaining in an āsana in a tactile manner, the body is no longer occupied verbally but is felt. What is felt is always new and leaves one free within the forever-renewed freshness of the sensation.
Two etymologies of the term kāla should be kept in mind: to list (kalyate iti kālaḥ), and to devour, to absorb (kal), which is associated with Śiva, Kālī and Mṛtyu, death or the great devourer. Kālī is known as the devourer of time (Kālasaṃkarṣiṇī).
Being established in an āsana means it can be evolved. Abhinavagupta speaks of two faces of energy: one fiery, effervescent (kṣobhita); and the other earthly, non-

effervescent (akṣobhita) (Tantrāloka III, 78-79). In its fiery aspect, the process of opening, of awakening (unmeṣa), of effervescence, of the unfolding of paths (adhvan), from the grossest to the subtlest, including all the tattva in the body itself, are incarnated; especially the five gross elements (pañcamahābhūta: earth, water, fire, air, ether), the five subtle elements (pañcatanmātra: smell, taste, form, touch, sound), the five organs of action (pañcakarmendriya: creation, excretion, foot, hand, speech) and the five organs of perception (pañcajñānendriya: nose, tongue, eyes, skin, ears). With duration, we can become immersed in a particular attitude, sparking a virile shudder of energy (vīrya) with a specific breath, and become impregnated with the savour and energetic colouration of an āsana and its resonance.

• Steadiness, heaviness, hardness, capacity to germinate, fragrance, strength, association, fixing and holding, are all qualities linked to earth (pṛthivī).

• Coolness, fluidity, dampness, oozing, flowing, lubrication, softness, salivation and bubbling, are all qualities linked to water (jala).

• Dreadfulness, brightness, burning, resplendency, redness, swiftness, intensity and what rises, are all qualities linked to fire (tejas).

• Uncontrollability, sense of touch, utterance of words, independence of movement, rapidity of movement, power, activity, agitation and subtle movements of the breath, are all qualities linked to air (vāyu).

• Sound, vastness, expanse, freedom, supportlessness, formlessness, indestructibility, inanimateness, immutability and mutability, are all qualities linked to space (ākāśa).

"When the seminal energy that has been lying within and identical with one's Self in a placid state is agitated, i.e. when it is in an active state, then the source of its pleasure is the Supreme I-consciousness full of creative pulsation, beyond the range of space and time, of the nature of perfect Bhairava-consciousness, the absolute sovereignty, full of the power of bliss."

ABHINAVAGUPTA, PARĀTRĪŚIKĀVIVARAṆA, JAIDEVA SINGH, PAGE 43

Then begins the process of involution, withdrawal (nimeṣa), which is described as the practice of fading, engulfing (Kālasaṃkarṣiṇī Kālī, the engulfer), linked to the earthly character of energy.

"In the cremation field where at night she dissolves the great elements and devours time and the divinities creating the circle of energies that fly through the sky across infinity. I pay homage to the unimaginable Kālī who blazes like a fire stirred by the wind."

ABHINAVAGUPTA, KRAMASTOTRA 11

All the different categories, from the grossest to the most subtle, are resorbed in their source. This process is also called purification of the elements: tattvaśuddhi or bhūtaśuddhi.

"Established in this attitude he dives easily into the lake of Consciousness." VASUGUPTA, ŚIVASŪTRA III, 16

"Absorbed in himself, the yogin rapidly becomes without colouration." ABHINAVAGUPTA, TANTRĀLOKA III, 103B-108

Implicit in the word purification, is the fading away of the objective world through dissolution of psychophysical references and grasps. Organically evoking the ritual of death in this way is at the heart of fundamental yoga practices.

"O Dear One, when the mind, the individual consciousness, the vital energy and the limited self, when these four have disappeared, then the nature of Bhairava appears."

VIJÑĀNA BHAIRAVA 138

Time in āsana allows the body to pause, so it can be surrendered in quietude (viśrānti).

"For those who succeed in taking their rest within this sacrifice, the hullabaloo of the world fades away like snow under the summer sun." ABHINAVAGUPTA, TANTRĀLOKA IV, 277

7
From Support to Supportlessness and the Caress of Spontaneity
(Saguṇāsana, Nirguṇāsana, Sahajāsana)

"Reject always whatever is assembled, whatever is conceptual, whatever is riddled with difficulties. Dedicate yourself to formlessness, to whatever is outside the realm of the mind, to whatever implies effortlessness."
Amanakṣa Yoga II, 27

The sensitivity of the body extends to the universe and encompasses it. Whatever is perceived becomes a direct extension of this intuition. Perhaps this is why āsana unfold archetypal energies which may at first seem strange to us, but which become us through unifying intuitive reasoning (sattarka): postures resembling a tree, a dog, a triangle, a half-moon, a warrior, the ferocious one, an eagle, a horse's head, a cow's head, a crocodile, a fish, a foetus, a cobra, a royal pigeon, a scorpion, a bow, an archer, a bridge, etc. Everything is support. Each situation becomes the support of the inexpressible, the indescribable, of a wonder prior to all knowledge or definition. The universe itself becomes an extension of this sensitivity.

"All comes from me, and all returns to me.
Split the log, I am within.
Pick up a stone, you will find me there."
Gospel According to Thomas, Verse 77

As regards āsana, introducing supports may help to awaken sensation, like an extension of awareness, or at least serve as a pointer. The support can point towards the 'marvellous form of the supreme firmament'.

This is how Śrī B.K.S. Iyengar describes the reason he introduced supports (props) into his own practice and teaching:
"Though I began Yoga in 1934 as a novice in the art of teaching, it was in 1937 that I got a chance through an invitation to teach yoga for 6 months in Pune. It was a challenge too as I was not only inexperienced but lacked the words to communicate or express myself. The responsibility of teaching was uppermost in my mind. Hence, I was preoccupied trying various ways to improve and perfect my own practice. I used to pick up stones and bricks lying on the roads and used them as 'supports' and 'weightbearers' to make progress in my mastery of āsana. Though these stones and bricks were rough and crude, they were helping me to some extent in getting the grip of the āsana. For example, take baddhakoṇāsana, where to place the stones and bricks exactly in this āsana, how to lessen the pricks and irritation, was a job. Often pieces from stone and bricks used to peel out, while I was keeping them and changing positions. By this way, realisation came to me that it is possible to learn many āsana with the help of 'supporters' the word prop came much later. I began to use whatever came handy like chairs, boxes, cots, cupboards, wooden pieces, rollers, grinding stones, and so forth. I learned from almost all household things including round drums to increase time in the āsana. Often these gave me tremendous backaches. Planks were cutting into my back (while trying backbends), but I would persevere by changing the position of the plank or the brick or whatever I was using. Methodical ways of using the props actually materialised after the Institute came into existence. As people began to approach me with their various problems and diseases, I realised the value of props. Though the members were getting relief with my occasional help, they were not able to sustain the pose independently and their problems used to recur fast. They were unable to retain the key points of action or adjust when the muscles and fibres went slack. Their genuine problems remained unsolved though they were sincerely trying to perform on their own.

I realised that raw students or patients could not derive maximum advantage. I thought that through 'indirect practice' (a passive state to stay with support) I could ignite interest in them to stay longer in each pose with props and without pain at the time of learning. By staying longer, their circulation improved, their respiratory system functioned better.

I engaged a carpenter to draw the shape of poses as I was performing and gave my thoughts to make them. Then I would test by doing the āsana on that unfinished material advising the carpenter to chop a bit here, to add there and so forth. Re-doing, re-shaping of each prop continued until the required final product was found out. Thus the birth of 'props' became a valuable gem of inspiration to do and stay longer and longer. The idea of Rope Śīrṣāsana was the inspiration of ancient yogis who were said to perform Śīrṣāsana hanging down from the branches of trees. This gave me the idea of fixing hooks to the roof and rope loops to the hooks. Thus the image of yogis performing Śīrṣāsana on trees came to my mind.

For angina of the heart and cardiac problems the idea of Arjuna making the bed of arrows for Bhīṣma struck me to support the top thoracic dorsal region where the cardiac nerves originate. So I arranged the bricks like arrows, which could support the thoracic dorsal spine vertebrae and muscle to protect the heart muscles to function with rhythm. Even Viparīta Daṇḍāsana, one of the most difficult backbends can be done by raw beginners with ease, without injury or harm. I had to break my head with the carpenter to prepare the design to perform this āsana. It is semicircular at the top, so that the back does not cut but the base is straight as the legs are taut and the feet get a foothold.

My Guru had a handwritten book on yoga called 'Yoga Kuruṇṭa' in Sanskrit language. In that book, there was a mention of wall ropes, like step ladders. Except for one or two āsana it was not as helpful as our 'loose' ropes which give more flexibility and scope for adjustment. My Guru was using two rings which restrict the movements of the body. The full range of action through lose ropes was my idea. All the props used now, like chairs, slanting planks, bricks are my own innovations, except the hanging ropes. By the by, Kuruṇṭi means puppet, a wooden doll. So 'Yoga Kuruṇṭa' is a method in which one learns to manipulate one's own body in various Yoga postures by means of a suspended rope, as if one were a puppet. Here the puppeteer and the puppet are one, performing their own puppet show.

First of all, Yoga is not an attractive subject. Nobody wants to take or bear pains. It is a mass psychology. Hence they are reluctant to take to Yoga as it involves extension, contraction and exertion. This means pain. Capacity to bear pain is limited. Will-power is limited, lacking in the present generation. In order to learn and perform āsana independently, certain limitations come in their ways. Some difficult āsana take years to understand or to make proper attempts. Often many are afraid even to attempt such poses. In Yoga, failures are inevitable. With props, fear complexes lessen and they build tremendous confidence in the doer. They check the overdoing and free the body from injury and damage. Props help to perform the āsana with ease. Pain factors are conquered through them. Even if the body pains, it becomes a bearable pain and helps the pupil to stay longer in any āsana. The student understands and learns āsana faster on props as the brain remains passive. Through this passive brain, one learns to be alert in body and mind. Props are guides to self-learning. They help accurately without mistakes. Normally, the practitioners do not use their inner body or inner organs as required evenly and properly while doing the āsana independently. For example take Sarvāṅgāsana. One doesn't know which elbow is in and which elbow is out. One cannot know which elbow is far away from shoulders and which is near. With the chair one fixes the arms in between the two legs of the chair or uses belts around the upper arm to keep the elbows in the correct position. So one cannot go wrong. This way props frame the body and mind to approach the āsana with retrospection. One can discriminate and judiciously adjust the body to the āsana dividing the body from the centre position evenly. By independent practice, one cannot study the alignment unless and until one develops that practical perception of seeing mistakes. In short, props become a real Guru in the absence of the living Guru.

Health is an everchanging state for a human being. Props are a great help in doing the āsana whether one is in a state of good health or in a state of bad health. Props oblige one to adjust to the condition of one's body, fitting accurately to the state of one's health, strength and endeavours. This will not be possible while doing the āsana independently. For example, one can do Śīrṣāsana on ropes with ease when there is stomach pain, but the same person will be reluctant to do so independently.

Now, talking of the pros and cons of using props, one of the criticisms levelled against the use of props is that one becomes habituated and lacks the will to attempt doing independently. Is it the fault of props? Certainly not! Props are used only as a guide, not to let in wrong practices. They are to feel the āsana. But I never say that they should be used on a permanent basis. Props give the sense of direction. When sense of direction sets in, I want my pupils to do the āsana independently sooner or later. As my pupils, don't you know that I often desist people from using props? The props are meant to give a sense of direction, alignment and understanding of the āsana. Once these points set in, one should do independently with retrospection and introspection comparing the feelings one gets with props. Simulating the same while doing independently is analysation. Movements of extension, expansion and circular actions which come from the props must be interpreted from the props toward independent performance. Compare the right movements with props to that of wrong movements when one does independently. Then one realises the importance of props and their utility. As a matter of fact, I do not use props at all. Even if I use them, is to educate myself and help others to get the same effects as I get.

But aged or diseased people perhaps may have to use the props permanently to do āsana. For example, a cardiac patient has to do Setu Bandha Sarvāṅgāsana on a bench. He needs the chair for Sarvāṅgāsana. A person with polio needs a trestler for standing for poses. They cannot do independently. The props show ways to discriminate and judge properly the accuracy of the āsana."

Yogācārya Śrī B.K.S. Iyengar
(70 Glorious Years of Yogācārya B.K.S. Iyengar, Page 391)

Props thus allow us to unfold the space of an āsana and acquaint us with certain āsana that may otherwise be too difficult to practise. Props create understanding of the correct gesture (mudrā) and attitude (bhāva) of āsana. Props let us stay longer in an āsana, thus permitting deeper penetration of unexplored bodily regions. It then becomes easier to incorporate certain breathing patterns and to see how the various colourations of breath (pañcavāyu: apāna, samāna, prāṇa, udāna, vyāna) move in different constellations of the body. Props can be regarded as an outer weave that points to the very essence of the āsana, in a purely subjective way. There will therefore always be some swaying between using an external prop and using the body itself as a prop. Ultimately, the body-mind is itself only an external prop.

"As for the Yoga depending on supports, the dependence on specific spheres, such as the hands, feet, etc. of the body is sālambayoga. As for the supportless Yoga, contemplation in which all names and forms are far distant and the Ātman is mere witness of all desires and other movements of the inner senses, free from dependence on them is nirālambayoga."

Tripadvibhūtimāhānārāyaṇopaniṣad, Adhyāya VII, 8

Perhaps it will become possible to intuit that when there is no longer focalisation on the gross and subtle bodies, and when they are resting in their source, the body itself is no more than a web of space.

"Either sitting on a seat or lying on a bed one should meditate on the body as being supportless. When the mind becomes empty and supportless, within a moment one is liberated from mental dispositions."

Vijñāna Bhairava 82

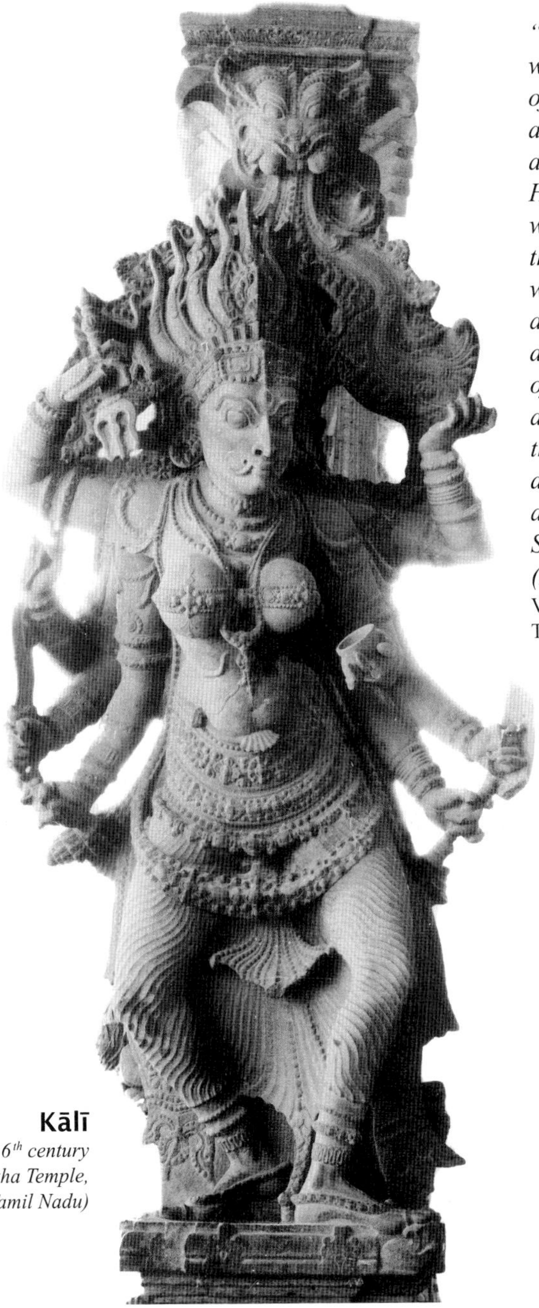

Kālī

16th century
(Kāśī Viśvanātha Temple,
Tenkasi, Tamil Nadu)

"Contemplate this funeral pyre
within your body, dazzling like the fire
of the final conflagration, where all subjects
are dissolved, where all categories
are consumed. In what would He not succeed,
He who penetrates into this body,
which is the abode of all divinities,
the place of cremation filled
with countless terrifying funeral pyres,
a desert frequented by Yoginī and Siddha
during their play. In this appalling field
of cremation, strewn with His own rays
and free of all differentiation,
the lineages of vanished darkness,
all individual bodies disappear
and only the kingdom of beatitude resides.
Such is for us the seal of death
(Karaṅkinī mudrā)."

VIRĀVALTĪTANTRA QUOTED BY ABHINAVAGUPTA,
TANTRĀLOKA XXIX, 182-186A

13

The Great Crematorium

Corporeal Worlds and Practices of Cremation

"Under the name of fire, He (God) consumes fortune and misfortune, happiness and sorrow:
all ways of being him are one. For he who has received the intimate touch of this fire,
nothing is too wide or too narrow.
The moment his flame burns within us, we are one with that which it devours:
being loved or hated, refusal, desire, loss or gain, at ease or troubled, in honour and in shame,
being with God in heavenly solace, or in the distress of hell, this fire makes no distinction.
It consumes everything it touches: damnation or benediction is no longer the question, I can assure you."

HADEWIJCH OF ANTWERP, MENGELDICHTEN XVI, XIX

"His temple is his own body, which bears the thirty-six categories and is perfectly endowed with windows
constituting its structure. It is there he resides, making immaculate offerings of the full Consciousness of the Self
to the auspicious divinity, the great Bhairava, the Supreme Self that accompanies his own energies.
As an offering, he throws the pile of great seeds, the differentiation of internal and external conceptual constructions,
into the blazing flame of his Consciousness. His oblation to the fire is made without effort.
His meditation has no respite, because the Lord creates wonderfully varied forms.
The fundamental reality shaped by the imagination, this is precisely his meditation.
His religious duty, which is very difficult to accomplish, but at the same time very easy,
consists of perceiving all things in unity and as representing Consciousness as resting
in the cemetery of the universe and bearing the emblem of the body's skeleton.
He drinks from the skull of a dead man, a fragment of the knowable object,
which he holds in his hand, and which is full of the liqueur of the essence of the universe."

ABHINAVAGUPTA, PARAMĀRTHASĀRA, 74-75-76-77-78-79-80

Kālīyantra

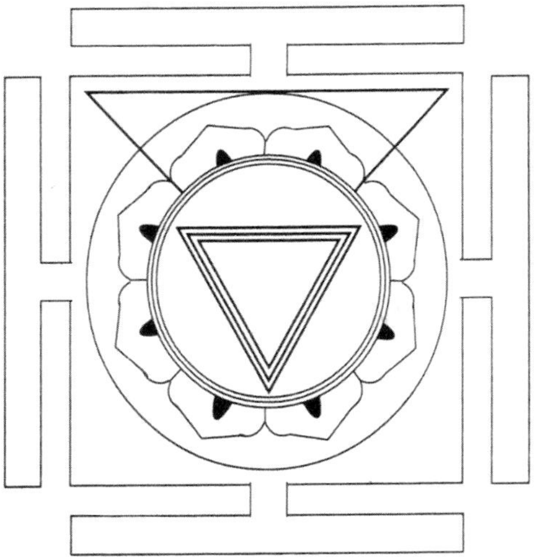

The texture of the body and that of reality are one and the same. They mirror the same fibre. The weave of the body shines with the constellations of infinite universes, the garments of deities exulting their energy. Worlds, whose peaks are unfathomably deep and whose abysses are heights of darkness, glitter in their eyes. One can taste oceanic depths and desert solitudes. Rivers of the sun and moon flow from inaccessible summits, abode of the immortal. Their winds tell tales of creation and destruction. One may encounter celestial vagabonds for whom these places are their playground. Their names murmur forgotten perfections. It is an eternal theatre where epics of feeling and passion take form.

"In this body, Mount Meru (the spine) is surrounded by seven islands; there are also rivers, oceans, mountains and the Lords of these lands. The seers and the sages reside there, as do all the stars and planets. Sacred places of pilgrimage, temples and the deities of these temples can be found there. The sun and the moon, as well as the creators and destructors can also be found there, as can ether, air, fire, water and earth. All living creatures that exist in the three worlds also exist in this body; devoting themselves to their respective functions around Mount Meru. But the common man does not know this. He who has glimpsed the universe of the body is a yogi. There can be no doubt about this".

Śivasaṃhitā II, 1-5

The pivot, the liṅga of light supporting these worlds, is embodied by Mount Meru, the axis mundi of creation. Allegorically, it is situated at the centre of the earth. In the purāṇa, it is described as a svastika with four arms radiating in four directions. Geographically, it is identified with the high land of Tartary, north of the Himalaya. It has various names: golden mountain (Hemādri), diamond peak (Ratnasānu), mountain of the gods (Devaparvata) and lotus mountain (Karnikacala). It is also compared to the pericarp of the earthly lotus, where the islands and continents are its petals.
In the body, this axis is the merudaṇḍa or brahmadaṇḍa: the spine along which different regions or worlds, the elements, the vāyu and the whirling energies of the cakra can be found.

"On the summit of Mount Meru is a hollow cavity, covered with snow. It is there, claims the sage, where reality lies. It is there where all streams have their source. It is from this void that Knowledge surges. From it flow the five streams."

Haṭhayogapradīpikā III, 52-53

The densest solidification of these five streams is found in the terrestrial region (bhūrloka), which comprises the earth and its seven continents, with Mount Meru in the centre encircled by the seven oceans and mountains, the seven lower regions and the seven underworlds. Below the base of Mount Meru (mūlādhāracakra) are found the intermediate regions and other hells. The corporeal worlds are magnificently described in the third chapter (On Understanding the Body – Piṇḍasaṃvitti) of Gorakṣanātha's Siddhasiddhāntapaddhati. Here follows an extract:

"The earthly world (Bhūr) is located in the region of the genital organs. The world of intermediary space (Bhūvar) is located in the region of the phallus and the heavenly world (Svar), in the umbilical region. Indra is the deity of these three worlds. Indra remains in the body as regulator of the organs of sense and action. He is truly powerful, like a king, having the powers of perception and action."
GORAKṢANĀTHA SIDDHASIDDHĀNTAPADDHATI III, 3

All these lands are merely emanations of mental states. They are only described as regions in a metaphorical, symbolic and poetic manner of speaking. We go through various environments, which, if not recognised as the colouration of the instant, can trap us in psychological states or bubbles; in worlds we project.
One feeling we can experience is that of intense claustrophobia, where everything seems closed, with no way out and with no air to breathe. This is hell in its original meaning of inferus, 'located beneath'. In this situation, we feel below ourselves. If we have realised the futility of our self-image, what situation or so-called entity could be lower than another?

As the poet Kabīr says:
"Heaven and hell are for the ignorant. I am no longer confused about sin and purity. Seekers, listen up, wherever you are, that is the entrance."

These worlds are sustained by the wrathful and dark aspects of earth, water, fire, air and space. One of the first worlds in this hell is avīci (static, unmoving). It gives the impression of extreme stagnation. Nothing moves, or wishes to do so, for here there is total apathy and inertia, like in a dream where we try to run but are paralysed. Here, we feel the weight of the second world, its stifling thickness, the abyss of time (mahākāla). Every second is like an abyss of boredom, waiting endlessly in a squalid station for a train that never comes. The sense of separation is intense. It becomes burning. Our thirst for change causes frantic agitation. There are not enough distractions. We live an endless rainy Sunday afternoon and have already watched all our videos, called all our friends, done all the workshops advertised in the new age supermarket, seen all the gurus and received all the initiations. There are not enough destinations, 'elsewheres' or miraculous aeroplanes to catch. We are always fleeing to escape the black hole of death. We need friction, the great burning of the third world, the frying pan (ambarīṣa). This constant over-stimulation makes us insensitive. We can no longer simply enjoy eating strawberries. We need an infinite quantity, and they are never big enough or red enough. So we create a whole new technology to produce bigger and redder strawberries. And then, because they aren't sweet enough, we drown them in an ocean of whipped Chantilly cream.
The hunt for sensations dominates us and we become extremely aggressive in our quest. We wander ghostlike searching for past and future pleasures. We stop at nothing to reach our goal. This state of mind characterises the world of raurava and mahāraurava (pertaining to a demon or asura). We feel cosmic hunger for inexistent stomachs, an ocean of thirst for sewn-up mouths. Then follows the desire for oblivion, for anaesthesia, which is preferable to feelings. This is the world of numbness, of any pill that can provide it. These worlds are known as the necklace of darkening (kālasūtra) and deep darkness (andhatāmiṣra).
The nether worlds (mahātala, rasātala, atala, sutala, vitala, talātala, pātāla) are not as limited as the hells, but remain purely mental and are more restricted than earthly manifestations. Pātāla comes from the Sanskrit root PAT, meaning 'to fall', 'to sink'. This is the playground of the asura, who take pleasure in the physical and material life force, and who oppose the gods (sura). Here, we also encounter heavenly musicians (gandharva); angel musicians (kinnara) who may have a head like a horse or feet like a bird;

demi-gods (kimpuruṣa) born of Brahmā's shadow, bearing swords and princely garb; yakṣa, the 'mysterious ones', gods of the forest and jungle; the malevolent (rākṣasa) who wander by night; Śiva's companion spirits (bhūta); terrifying phantoms (preta) roaming in search of a vehicle for their next reincarnation, companions of Śiva under the sway of Yama, the Lord of death; eaters of raw flesh (piśāca); dwarf demons (apasmara); female deities (apsara, which literally means 'those who move in water' or 'those who are of its essence', and which is derived from the word for water, ap); brahmarākṣasa, one of the sixty-four forms of Bhairava; kuṣmāṇḍa, a group of disease-carrying demons, servants of Śiva, able to take on any shape they please; and vināyaka, malevolent forms of Gaṇeśa that cause disaster and misfortune, the principal attendants of Śiva.

- The middle region (antarikṣaloka) is the intermediary space between the earth and the sun, populated by stars and planets, the playground of the siddha.
- The region of divinities (mahendraloka) is the abode of six groups of deities who have many powers and live for a whole kalpa (4.32 billion years).
- The region of prajāpatya (mahāprajāpatiloka) is the abode of four groups of deities who have mastered the elements and live for a thousand kalpa.
- The region of divine beings (janaloka) is the abode of four groups of deities who have mastered the elements and senses. They live twice as long as those in the preceding region.
- The region of austerities (taparloka) is the abode of three groups of deities who have mastered the elements, the senses and nature (prakṛti). They live twice as long as those in the preceding region.
- The region of certainty (satyaloka) is the abode of four groups of deities who live as long as creation itself.

Legend tells of sacred regions (pīṭha) that emanated from the corpse of Pārvatī as Śiva carried her over his shoulder. Viṣṇu's disc broke her corpse into pieces that then fell to earth. Through the ritual of nyāsa, all these worlds are in the body itself. Allegorically, they describe different states of Consciousness and the energetic vortices (cakra), apart from the last cakra which is beyond localisation. Through the consecration of the body, pīṭha becomes the expression of Consciousness (pratibhāvidyā) in its three energy forms: energy of will (icchāśakti), energy of intuition (jñānaśakti) and energy of activity (kriyāśakti); of the mantra sauḥ that is the seed of the universe; of kramamudrā, or the end of subject-object duality; and of the maṇḍala depicting the divine wheel of the energies. Symbolically, Śivaśakti are represented by the bindu, which has no objective reality, and no inner or outer localisation.

"It returns to supreme space,
the ultimate maṇḍala of extinction."
JAYARATHA, TANTRĀLOKAVIVEKA XXIX, 248D.A

Compared to the extreme situation of hell and the nether worlds, the other regions seem more pleasant. The expansions of Consciousness are no more than the luxurious suburbs of saṃsāra, where the gods live. Here, life seems to unfold without any upsets and all desires are fulfilled. There is the inebriation of power and we become intoxicated with self-importance and the arrogance of difference. This world however only sparkles with the artificial, and for the blessed ones whose stay can last thousands of years, they live in boredom. The idea of losing our territory provokes great fear, because with the boredom loiters the smell of death and decay. Whatever the experience, however divine it may be, it is still only objectivation, localised in space-time, conditioned in its expression.

"As long as one considers the bond with the body as being identical to Consciousness, one will continue to wander in the three-fold world. Thus adorned with the three energies,

the supreme Self remains the same, He, the mirror of absolute Consciousness, in which the universe is reflected."
GORAKṢANĀTHA, AMARAUGHAŚĀSANA

The Belly of the Fish

(Matsyodarī)

Abhinavagupta, at the beginning of his Tantrāloka, bows down to the mythical Macchanda, founder of the Kula lineage.
"Let Macchanda, the omnipresent, look upon me favourably; he who pushed back the vast and manifold glowing net of Māyā, made up of knots and holes, spread over all places."
ABHINAVAGUPTA, TANTRĀLOKA I, 7

For Jayaratha, commentator of Abhinavagupta, it is he who tears up the net of objectivity, red with passion (rāgāruṇa). Passion here is attachment to the manifest object as if it has its own light.
Jñāneśvar, in his work Jñāneśvarī, describes how this secret that has the power *"to calm and sooth all things"* was heard first by Matsyendranāth and handed down to his Guru Nivṛtti: *"This secret which, in immemorial times, the slayer of the demon Tripura whispered into the ear cavity of the goddess Pārvatī, exactly where we do not know, close to the sea of milk, this very secret was heard by Matsyendranāth, while abiding secretly in the belly of the fish."* (JÑĀNEŚVARĪ XVIII, 1729-1735)

He proclaims himself to be the son of Śiva and Pārvatī, having received the teachings of Adināth, the primordial, he without antecedent (Akula), family or relations.
Is 'the one without antecedents', who plays with identities, not the one who roams in India, Nepal and Tibet? All his names sing the same myth. Matsyendranāth, lord of the fishes, is revered as guardian deity of Katmandu, in the form of Śveta Matsyendranāth (Matsyendranāth the White), the representation of the Buddha of Compassion, Avalokiteśvāra. In the Kaulajñānanirnaya he is called Matsyaghna, killer of fishes, saying he is of the fisherman caste (kaivarta). Mīnanāth has the same connotations as Matsyendranāth, but here appears to make reference to the function of fisherman. He is also called Luipā, whose name is derived from Lohita, which describes the red colour of the waters of the Brahmaputra River in Assam. Having taught in Kāmarūpa, Matsyendranāth was known by the name of Lohipada (belonging to Lohita). Luipā could be an abridged form of Lohipada. The small cane used to catch fish is called a 'lui' in Bengal, hence the name Luipā (he who catches fish with a cane). The Tibetan translation of Luipā retains the meaning of 'one who eats fish guts', referring to the hero's ritual sacrifice. He is also given the names Macchaghnapāda, Macchendrapāda, Matsyendrapāda, Macchendra, Macchendapāda, Macchindranāthapāda, and Dzamling Karmo (the white lord of the world).
One tale relates that Mīna was a fisherman in the east of India. He spent most of his time in his boat, contemplating the line cast into the depths of the ocean. One day an enormous fish became caught on his hook. The fish was so big that Mīnanāth was dragged into the water and swallowed by the fish. At the same time, it is said that Śiva was to reveal the secret teachings concerning his true nature to his wife Umā. Although reluctant, he did so in the deepest part of the ocean, in total intimacy, where nobody could hear what was said. The leviathan that had swallowed Mīnanāth happened to be nearby whilst the Kula teaching was revealed, and which described the constant interpenetration of Śiva and Śakti, who are eternally inseparable. Perhaps this is why Śiva was so reluctant, since he was just repeating to himself (Śakti) what he already knew. In the belly of the fish, Mīnanāth was able to hear everything.
During the teaching, the goddess fell asleep! This is an

allusion to the utter freedom (svātantrya) of the ultimate reality, creating a forgetfulness that is no more than an optical illusion allowing the net of diversity to unfold. How could she forget herself or become unconscious? *"Are you listening to me?"* asked Śiva. *"Yes,"* replied Mīnanāth from inside the fish. Śiva saw that Umā had fallen asleep and the answer had come from another. Pleased with the fervour of Mīnanāth, Śiva decided to initiate him instead of Umā. It is said that Mīnanāth remained in the fish's belly for twelve more years to digest the teachings he had received. At the end of this term, he was freed when another fisherman gutted the fish.

In another version, knowing that Śiva was going to divulge his secrets to Gaurī, Mīnanāth followed the couple as they settled themselves on the banks of the Island of the Moon (Candradvīpa). Mīnanāth changed into a fish and was able to hear the ultimate secret of the tantra. Here again, Śiva's companion fell asleep. In some versions it is said that Mīnanāth made Gaurī fall asleep so she could not hear Śiva's teachings. Imitating Gaurī's voice, Mīnanāth muttered sounds at appropriate moments to make Śiva think she was listening. When Śiva had finished, Gaurī awoke from her sleep and at once asked for the teaching he had promised her. Śiva realised that he had been tricked by Mīnanāth and foretold that one day he would completely forget the teaching. This happened through a cunning trick of Gaurī's. It is said she tested the four original mahāsiddha with her sexual charms. Aroused, Mīnanāth could not hide his erection and she cast a spell on him. He would become a slave to his debauchery in a kingdom of women, the prisoner of sixteen hundred Amazonian warriors. It is ironic that one who was known as Adhisiddhācārya, the 'first of the perfected masters' in the list of eighty-four mahāsiddha, was the one to succumb most easily to the charms of Śakti. What is more, he used his siddhi to satisfy his desires by assuming another person's body (parakāyapraveśa siddhi), that of a king. Matsyendranāth's amnesia came about in the lands of Kadalī, the forest of plantains. Kadalī is another name for Rambhā, a celestial nymph. Completely subjugated by the queen Kamalā, Matsyendranāth was so caught up in the game that he forgot his own true identity. He would be saved by his disciple Gorakṣanātha.

"This teaching can be found in the house of each Yoginī of Kāmarūpa. It was brought from the Island of the Moon (Candradvīpa) and its dwelling place is the great belly of the fish (mahāmatsyodarasthiti)..."
MATSYENDRANĀTH, KAULAJÑĀNANIRNAYA PĀTĀLA XXII, 8-12

What does the belly of the fish hold? What is this region of entrails where it seems something obvious is revealed?

"There is a power of emission which is beauty itself, since within it, it contains its power of vibration. May the Yogi rest at the source of this emanation (visarga) that is similar to the fish's belly."
ABHINAVAGUPTA, TANTRĀLOKA V, 57B-58A

In the Śivapurāṇa, Vārāṇasī is extolled as the blest forest, but also as avimukta, that which can neither be abandoned nor forgotten.

"O sage, this sacred place, not even at the time of the great dissolution, is separated from Śiva and Śakti. This is why it is called Avimukta."
ŚIVAPURĀṆA, RUDRASAṂHITĀ V, 30

One day, Pārvatī asks Śiva why he never leaves the Avimukta Kṣetra of Vārāṇasī, where lies the 'sacred place of the liberation of the skull' (Kapālamocana tīrtha). He tells her the following story:

"O Varārohā, there was a superb head of Brahmā which radiated forth as brightly as gold. When this fifth head of the great soul was produced, O Devī, it said unto me:

'I know of the circumstances of your birth.' Filled with anger, my eyes burning, I cut it off with the tip of my left thumbnail. Brahmā said: 'Because you have cut-off my head, of I who am faultless, you will become a Kapālin (skull bearer) and you will be damned. Bearing the burden of having sinned by killing a brāhmaṇa (brahmahatya), you must now go on a pilgrimage to the sacred places in this world'."
MATSYA PURĀṆA CLXXXIII, 84-87

Śiva's wanderings began because he had to find a place to put to rest the skull of Brahmā that he was carrying. After long peregrination, the skull disintegrated in the place known as the 'great repose' (Avimukta).

"By the grace of Viṣṇu, O Sustroni, the skull was smashed into a thousand pieces. I have turned this place that absolves the sin of having killed a brāhmaṇa, into a sacred place. It is a celebrated place within this world, O Devī, like the liberation of the skull of gods (Kapālamocana). He who surrenders his body in this place becomes one with me." MATSYA PURĀṆA CLXXXIII, 84-87

In another myth, it is told how the sage Madhora got rid of the skull of a rākṣasa after bathing in the river Sarasvatī, which here is the symbol of the suṣumṇā nāḍī. Hence the place is celebrated as the 'liberation of the skull' (kapālamocana). Liberation of the skull occurs at the conjunction known as the 'fish's belly' (matsyodarīyoga). In the geographic maṇḍala of Kāśī, the conjunction of the 'fish's belly' was the filling, during the monsoon, of lakes or reservoirs, one of which was known as Matsyodarī, to form a single current between the rivers Varaṇā and Asī. Long ago the Matsyodarī Tīrtha was a big lake but it was drained in the nineteenth century. In the monsoon, the lake became a river that flowed north, joining the lakes of Kapālamocana (where the skull fell), Ṛṇamocana (where debts disappear) and Pāpamocana (where sins vanish), before pouring into the river Varaṇā. In some years of heavy monsoon, the waters of the Gaṅgā flowed abundantly into the Varaṇā and pushed the waters of lake Matsyodarī back in the opposite direction, causing it to flow upstream to its source. The union of these sacred waters was very auspicious, and was given the name Matsyodarī Tīrtha Sangam or Matsyodarīyoga.

"O beloved, when the Gaṅgā comes to Matsyodarī to receive the divine Darśana, bathing at this moment, one obtains liberation. When the Gaṅgā flows in this place and the waters mingle, filled with the current of Varaṇā, it is a truly favourable moment, very rare, even for the gods."
LIṄGA PURĀṆA

"Piṅgalā is the name by which this ardent nāḍī is worshiped. It is also known as the dried-up current (Asī), parallel to the reservoir referred to as the 'quivering sun'. Iḍā is the name by which the moonlike nāḍī is worshiped. It is also known as the river Varaṇā, where the Viṣṇu Keśava temple may be found. The nāḍī that flows between the two is glorified as Suṣumṇā and is known as Matsyodarī. It is worshiped as the current that flows in both directions. There where both currents gather in the lake of the fish's belly, simply bathing here ensures liberation. It is an extraordinary union when the Gaṅgā flows in the Fish's Belly, to the west of Kapileśvara. Bathing in this place endows one with the fruits of the sacrifice of a thousand horses. This place is worshiped as the fluvial syllable of Brahmā."
KṚTYAKALPATARA, TĪRTHAVIVECANAKĀṆḌA,
COMMENTARY ON THE LIṄGA PURĀṆA

In yogic terms, the description of Vārāṇasī, or of the end of dualistic thought, is found in the Śivasaṃhitā.

"The two channels, Iḍā and Piṅgalā, are the true Varaṇā and Asī. The space between the two is called Vārāṇasī. It is said that Viśvanātha, the Lord of the Universe, dwells there."
ŚIVASAṂHITĀ V, 100

Luipā performed the matsyamudrā after settling on the banks of the Gaṅgā to contemplate. In the twilight language of Tantra, the Gaṅgā is the meeting of three rivers: the Gaṅgā itself; the Yamunā, which joins the Gaṅgā at Prayāga; and the mysterious Sarasvatī, which disappears into the plains before reaching the sea. They represent the three nāḍī: Piṅgalā (Yamunā), Iḍā (Gaṅgā) and Suṣumṇā (Sarasvatī). Established on the banks of his own existence, Luipā finds a pile of fish guts giving off a vile smell. He spends twelve years contemplating the entrails of conditioning, concepts and residues of actions that drag their fetid shadows into the present. They become his food, hence his name Matsyantrāda (eater of fish guts). Having begun to consume his own mind, he performs the ritual suicide of the mind. In the fish's belly is heard Śiva's constantly renewed revelation to Umā, the spontaneous display of the evidence of our nature, at the very source of differentiation, between emanation and resorption, interior and exterior, subject and object. This revelation is called Matsyodarīmata, for it is like the stomach of a fish that opens and closes automatically, pulsating without any visible outward agitation. In the same way, Consciousness pulsates without being in movement or becoming.

"In the two realities, internal and external, resides a vibration of Consciousness belonging to the three energies, embellished by that which is generic and by that which is specific; it is endowed with expansion and contraction. Although in reality, this vibration is exempt of contraction and expansion, it manifests itself thus. The yogin whose vision is turned outwards, the visible being perceived within, reaches the supreme kingdom."
ABHINAVAGUPTA, TANTRĀLOKA V, 79

The practice of certain āsana leads to the contemplation of this constellation, specifically the pelvic and thoracic diaphragms. These two hearts are the source of mūlabandha and uḍḍiyānabandha. Although these two bandha are mainly used in advanced prāṇāyāma with retention, they can be unfolded passively in certain āsana. Ordinary breathing only uses the vocal diaphragm. In prāṇāyāma, by establishing jālandharabandha, the vocal diaphragm is made entirely passive. The other two diaphragms, especially the pelvic diaphragm, become the source of the different breathing patterns.

Certain āsana (Vīrāsana, Matsyāsana, Supta Baddha Koṇāsana) are used to cleanse the abdominal cavity, especially the area below the navel (kandasthāna), which stimulates the excretory functions of apānavāyu. Other āsana help to awaken the two diaphragms whilst continuing to rinse out the abdominal and pelvic cavity (Śīrṣāsana, and especially its variations, rope Śīrṣāsana, chair Viparīta Daṇḍāsana, Padmāsana in Viparīta Daṇḍāsana and Setu Bandha Sarvāṅgāsana, which also unfolds Jālandharabandha). But in order to reverse the flow of apānavāyu, two āsana are recommended: Padmāsana in Viparīta Daṇḍāsana and Uttāna Padma Mayūrāsana. The latter is the sovereign pose for this particular action. In this āsana, the energy no longer flows down towards the legs but flows back into the upper part of the pelvis and beyond, like the Gaṅgā that flows upstream during the conjunction of the fish's belly (Matsyodarīyoga).

"The Yogi starts by filling his body with breaths which he stirs up and then retains; drawing the prāṇa, which has a natural tendency to rise, out of the channels where it ordinarily moves; he then lets it penetrate into the middle channel, causing the apāna, which naturally descends, to rise upwards. And finally, prāṇa and apāna rise up through the central channel."
KṢEMARĀJA, PRATYABHIJÑĀHṚIDAYA 18

"When the apāna rises upwards and reaches the sphere of fire, then the flame of the fire, being fanned by this vāyu, becomes lengthened."
HAṬHAYOGAPRADĪPIKĀ III, 66

"When the apāna and the fire join prāṇa, which is by nature hot, then the heat in the body is greatly intensified."
HAṬHAYOGAPRADĪPIKĀ III, 67

"If whilst practising this mudrā, the Yogi is able to unite apāna with the prāṇavāyu, it then becomes Yoni Mudrā."
ŚIVASAṂHITĀ IV, 42

Thus, prāṇāgnihotra, the sacrifice of breath as it is described in the Bhagavad Gītā, may be fulfilled: *"Others offer in sacrifice the exhaled breath into the inhaled breath and the inhaled breath into the exhaled breath."*
BHAGAVAD GĪTĀ IV, 29

This calling back of the energy, or its suction into itself, unfolded by Uttāna Padma Mayūrāsana, is the physiological evocation of the esoteric vajrolī, the practice of which requires *"two necessary things that are difficult for an ordinary man to obtain: one is milk (the moonlike liqueur, amṛtacandra) and the other, a woman (citranāḍī) who submits entirely according to his will."*
HAṬHAYOGAPRADĪPIKĀ III, 84

The movement of the fish (matsyavalana) is evoked in Bhāskara's commentary on the Śivasūtra:
"Comfortably seated the yogi sinks effortlessly into the lake of Consciousness." (III, 17)
"The seat the wise Yogi takes by stimulating the movements of a fish's belly, is the central upwardly rising breath known as: cleansing fire (pavamāna), radiance (śuci) and wrath (caṇḍa). This seat is also the seed, and he who is established in this attitude plunges effortlessly into the lake of Consciousness." (BHĀSKARA'S COMMENTARY)

The heart of these practices is an evocation of the ritual bath, in the incomprehensible.

"We have said before that Iḍā is the Gaṅgā, Piṅgalā is the daughter of the sun (Yamunā), and in the middle there is Suṣumṇā, who is Sarasvatī. The place where all three meet is the most inaccessible."
"He who mentally bathes at the junction of White (Iḍā) and Black (Piṅgalā) frees himself of all blemishes and attains the eternal Brahman."
ŚIVASAṂHITĀ V, 133-134

The Moon of Silence:

The Place of Beheading (Śīrṣacadhasthāna)

"The knife is to cut the six erroneous views into pieces: pride, ignorance, doubt, passion, anger and prejudices. The skull is to end dualistic thoughts which consider existence and non-existence as being different." HEVARAJA TANTRA VIII, 19

"There, there is neither speech nor thoughts. There is neither immanent nor transcendent. There is no access to this sealed silence. There is no place for either Śiva or his energy. If something remains, then that is the teaching."
LALLĀ

The Kula teaching was revealed in the place known as the island of the moon (candradvīpa), mountain of the moon (candraparvata) or hill of the moon (candragiri). In the symbolic yogic map, it is located in different places: the root of the palate (tālumūla), known as the navel of the head, or, as in the Śivasaṃhitā, at the top of Mount Meru (the spine) in the skull. The moon is described as ardhacandra, bindu, the cup of soma or the nectar of immortality, the place of emanation and resorption, but also as the circle of the moon.

"Along the central channel, this path extends up to the cranial vault, there in the moon's circle resides the supreme liṅga of the skull. From above Lampika's seat (the uvula), this liṅga pours out a flow of nectar."
GORAKṢANĀTHA, AMARAUGHAŚĀSANA

For Abhinavagupta, the moon symbolises the heart as being the essence of reality. The phases of the moon, from the new moon (amāvāsyā) to the full moon (pūrṇimā), symbolise the processes of expansion and contraction. It is a reminder of this perpetual breath, the beating and pulsation of the heart, the marrow of life. It is said that each phase of the moon (tithi) resonates with the sound of Sanskrit vowels.

"Vowels which start with A and finish with the bindu are called tithi, or lunar phases because they fill the different quarters of the moon of Consciousness. The power of emission of the moon of Consciousness, which is none other than joy and light, the power of emission of the absolute, is saturated with the resonance of their vibrations."

ABHINAVAGUPTA, PARĀTRĪŚIKĀLAGUVṚTTI 5-9A

In Sanskrit, the vowels are called svara because they shine by themselves with the innate light (prakāśa) of Consciousness that needs no external support, but they are also the wombs (śakti) of the consonants.

"These fifteen are called vowels (svara) because they are of sound by nature and because they shine of their own accord (svayaṃ rājantaḥ), as does Consciousness. They contain the sun and the moon."

ABHINAVAGUPTA, PARĀTRĪŚIKĀLAGUVṚTTI 5-9A

The first three pairs of short and long vowels resonate with the effusion of Bhairava, as the absolute (anuttara), the energy of will (icchā), and opening (unmeṣa).

"At the centre of the junction of expansion
and contraction is the absolute (anuttara: A),
beatitude (ānanda: Ā), energy of will (icchā: I),
maintenance (īśāna: Ī), blossoming (unmeṣa: U),
and resorption (unnata: Ū)."

ABHINAVAGUPTA PARĀTRĪŚIKĀLAGUVṚTTI 5-9A

This nectar of immortality is revealed after the ocean of dualities has been churned and the poison of differentiation has been drunk. It is described as a deep darkness that makes it impossible to distinguish anything.

"In the same way on a dark night, at the beginning of the dark fortnight, while meditating on the darkness, one attains the nature of Bhairava."

VIJÑĀNA BHAIRAVA 87

It is here the dance of concepts, the descriptive and symbolic waxing and waning of the moon, comes to an end. In essence, the moon is always full. This eternal fullness is represented by the 'visarga', which is at the heart and source of vowels, and yet is not included in any of the phases (tithi).

"The germ of emission (visarga Ḥ) is the universal womb, the background to the fifteen lunar phases. Nothing else is necessary."

ABHINAVAGUPTA, PARĀTRĪŚIKĀLAGUVṚTTI, RANIERO GNOLI, PAGE 55

Fundamentally, there is no birth (new moon), death (waning) or fullness (waxing) to be attained. The island of the moon (candradvīpa) is not a place, it does not really exist, and cannot be reached or created, since it is that by which everything is known. Candra is Soma (Sa + Umā), the eternal union of Sa (Śiva) and Umā (Pārvatī).

"There exists a central force (yoni) in the middle of sahasrāra; below is the moon. Let the sage contemplate it. Let him contemplate this ocean of milk. Let him contemplate he who is without mark."

ŚIVASAṂHITĀ V, 145-147-148

In āsana practice, contemplation of the moon is achieved through Viparīta Karaṇī Mudrā.

"Whatever nectar flows from the moon which is of divine form, it is all swallowed up by the sun. Hence the body decays."

"There exists a divine process by which the sun is duped. This should be learned from the guru, and not through theoretical study of the śāstra."
"If one's navel is high and palate low, then the sun is above and the moon below. This position, the inverted pose (Viparīta Karaṇī), is to be learned through the instructions of a Guru."
HAṬHAYOGAPRADĪPIKĀ III, 77-78-79

We have seen how Śīrṣāsana stimulates the constellation of the pelvic and thoracic diaphragms. In Sarvāṅgāsana, Halāsana, Setu Bandha Sarvāṅgāsana and Viparīta Karaṇī it is jālandharabandha that is activated. This bandha is attributed to Jālandhara, a siddha also known by the name of Hāḍipa (the sweeper). Jāla is also the constellation of the throat, and the aforementioned āsana aim to pacify both the vocal diaphragm and the frontal brain.
In the Trikatantrasāra (as quoted in Abhinavagupta's Parātrīśikāvivaraṇa, Jaideva Singh, Page 207) it says: *"Expansion of beatitude is true worship. Everything is pervaded with two mudrā, which are essentially jñānaśakti and kriyāśakti."* This spontaneous worship is expressed through gestures of emptying, of wiping away all gripping of the face. Thus Siṃhāsana cleanses the face of fixed, stereotyped and culturally correct expressions. They are swept away in a complete extroversion, reminiscent of the masks of Bhairava or the face of Kālī. Physiologically, we regain a certain passivity of the facial muscles, as well as space between the jaws, between the temples, behind the forehead, between the ears, along the length of the tongue and in the oral cavity to the back of the throat.
This complete extroversion is coupled with total introversion in Ṣaṇmukhīmudrā. Ṣaṇmukha is the name of the six-headed god of war, also called Kārttikeya, the son of Śiva who was raised by the six Pleiades and thus grew six heads in order to drink their milk. This mudrā is also called Parāṅmukhīmudrā (turned inward), Śāmbhavīmudrā (seal of Śambhu) and Yonimudrā (seal of the womb).
We tackle the world using our frontal brain, projecting an image of ourselves. The projection of this social mask is our window display. In Ṣaṇmukhīmudrā we learn to let the mask melt away. By placing the fingers on the eyes, the eyeballs, which are conditioned to focus, learn to be passive. Here the eyes become defocused, as if watching with the ears. The eyes are brought into contact with the back of the skull, like two little balloons deflating. In this way, the eye sockets become free of all prehension. The first two fingers also teach the top forehead to descend in a circular movement that begins at the back of the skull. This also draws down the eyebrows, the upper part of the nose and the eyelids, which fall like a curtain of darkness over the face. This 'blindness' must be maintained during inhalations as the intake of breath always lifts the gaze and stimulates the forehead region. The thumbs teach the resorption of the eardrums towards the centre back-brain, which goes hand in hand with the withdrawal of the eyes. Sounds are no longer grasped by the ears. The ring fingers touch the outer walls of the nose, thus making the movement of the breath tactile. As we become familiar with the touch of the breath on the nostril walls, the breath becomes more rhythmic and subtle. This contact helps us discover the passage of breath through the sinuses. When inhalation is aggressive, it pushes the opening of the nose upwards and outwards. This area must remain passive. The little fingers are placed towards the sides of the upper lip. Here we become aware of the area between the upper lip and nose, where inhalation is born and exhalation dies. This draws the whole cheek area down, along with the corners of the lips and the lower jaw, as though we are toothless, a bit vacant, like a small baby whose gaze is lost. The tongue moves down to its resting place, neither touching the teeth nor the upper palate.

"Keeping the tongue in the centre of the wide open mouth one should fix the mind there. Uttering the letter Ḥ mentally, one will be dissolved in peace."
VIJÑĀNA BHAIRAVA 81

Our perception of reality is merely the translation performed by our nervous system and our memory. The silence of Ṣaṇmukhīmudrā reveals the tentacles of psychological memory and its resorption into the heart.
Abhinavagupta defines mudrā (mud: joy, rā: to give) as that which reflects our own nature in the body itself. For Kṣemarāja, mudrā means *"mudrayati, where the non-state of states as Consciousness takes upon itself the world's activity as resting within itself."*
This realisation seals the universe as being Consciousness itself, in which *"the mass of all entities is dissolved in the sky of Consciousness, like a small cloud in the autumn."*
KṢEMARĀJA, PRATYABHIJÑĀHṚDAYA 19

For Abhinavagupta, all mudrā are merely the intuitive prolongation of Khecarīmudrā. Khe is the locative of Kha, meaning sky, void or Brahman. It is therefore the absolute. Carī is that which moves.
"Khecarī, although completely immersed in the absolute undifferentiated unity, is that which moves."
"That Śakti is khecarī, who abiding in Kha (brahma) which is identical with herself roams about (i.e. functions in various ways). This khecarī in her universal aspect functions in various ways. She as gocarī brings about a knowledge of objects, as dikcarī effects movements such as grasping, relinquishing, etc., as bhūcarī exists in the form of objective existents. Thus this khecarī exists as gocarī in the form of antaḥkaraṇa (the inner psychic apparatus), as dikcarī in the form of bahiṣkaraṇa (i.e. outer senses), as bhūcarī in the form of objective existents, as blue etc., or subjective existents as pleasure etc."
"Similarly, in the individual aspects, the śakti that are known successively as vyomacarī in the void of consciousness in which the distinction between subject and object has not yet appeared, as gocarī in the form of antaḥkaraṇa in which there is just appearance of knowledge, as dikcarī in the form of the outer senses suggesting the appearance of diversity in which state there is diversity of the knower from the knowable object, as bhūcarī in the form of bhāva or existents in which there is preponderance of clear diversity in the objects, are in reality, according to the principle enunciated, non-distinct from khecarī which abides in the essential nature (anuttara). Thus that Śakti of the supreme Lord is only one."
ABHINAVAGUPTA, PARĀTRĪŚIKĀVIVARAṆA, JAIDEVA SINGH, PAGE 38-39

Svātmārāma sings of Khecarīmudrā in these terms:
"Neither worship the liṅga by day, nor by night. Suppressing the day and the night, the liṅga should always be worshipped."
"When prāṇa, which normally resides in the left and right nāḍī, flows through the middle (suṣumṇā), in that state khecarīmudrā becomes established. There is no doubt about this."
"When the void between the sun and the moon (iḍā and piṅgalā) swallows up the prāṇa, khecarīmudrā is established there."
"Between the sun and the moon there is an unsupported inner space. From this space (vyomancakra) surges the mudrā known as khecarī."
HAṬHAYOGAPRADĪPIKĀ IV, 42-43-44-45

In mudrā, the surrendering of energy is sealed, and is no longer used for internal or external localisation.
"When all agitation ceases, then Lord Śiva reveals himself."
KṢEMARĀJA, SPANDA NIRṆAYA I, 9

The dorsal and cervical region, shoulders and throat are unblocked with certain āsana. The face, and especially the eyes and frontal brain will also be pacified. This helps to establish Jālandharabandha, in which the known is abandoned into the unfolded space of the chest and heart.

"When a Yogi, immersed in the energy, has drunk the supreme wine of Bhairava in profusion and staggers with intoxication, whatever his bodily position, there lies the true mystical attitude, mudrā." ABHINAVAGUPTA, TANTRĀLOKA IV, 200

Jālandharabandha is the renunciation of wanting to understand anything to do with exteriority, be it manifested grossly in an object, or subtly in the body-mind, which too is really only an object. According to Abhinavagupta, Viṣṇu is associated with the cognitive continuum, the flow of becoming, of memory, symbolically located in the throat. Śiva represents the resorption of conceptual speech, of naming, and the site of his contemplation is the palate. Thus, from a physiological viewpoint, Jālandharabandha evokes the gesture of Śiva severing the head of Brahmā, of objectivation.

"Thus, turn away from the various modalities by extracting the sun and moon from their two paths of immersion and dispersion, and devote oneself to the Consciousness of Bhairavian reality."
ABHINAVAGUPTA,
TANTRĀLOKA XXIX, 146-147

"If one does not know the conjunction of the sun and the moon, all things become multiple, like waves on the ocean. When the unique occurs, such separation cannot be found."
SIDDHA SABARI

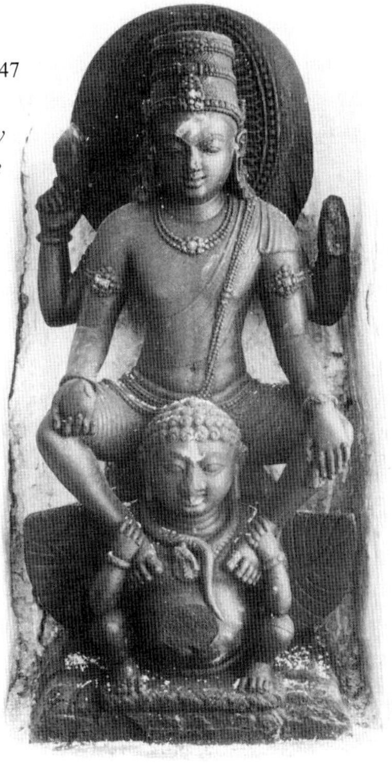

Viṣṇu
7th century
(Gandhareśvara Temple, Sirpur, Raipur, Madhya Pradesh)

Prāṇayāga:
The Sacrifice of Breath

"At the instant of emitting the breath, one should first rest in the emptiness of the heart, and then on the outside as soon as the breath is exhaled (prāṇa). Then, by the grace of the full moon, or inhaled breath (apāna), one grasps the essence of the Self as universal and one loses desire for all things. When the even breath (samāna) arises, one experiences rest, allowing the unifying friction of all aspects of existence to take place. And finally, when the flame of the vertical fire (udāna) rises, one swallows up incitements of subject and object, and also those of exhalation and inhalation, day and night, etc. As soon as this consuming fire is appeased and the diffused breath (vyāna) looms forth, omnipenetrating, one shines forth free of all limitation."
ABHINAVAGUPTA, TANTRASĀRA V

In the Garbhopaniṣad there is a story of a foetus, which of course should not be taken literally. It is said that when the foetus is seven months old, his life story is revealed to him. The more he sees the movie of his existence unfold, the more he becomes a mass of contraction, resulting in a terrible tension due to the fear of separation. The foetus must leave this oceanic feeling of plenitude. Terrified, he becomes very agitated. In whichever direction he goes, he cannot find calm. When he encounters the stomach, he feels burnt by the digestive fire; when he approaches the kidneys, the salt bothers him; and when he is against the intestines, he cannot stand the smell. He thus roves around the womb, only to meet fresh obstacles. In complete despair, the foetus calls to the Lord who reveals the naturally present Haṃsa mantra. The inhaled breath emits the sound 'ham' and the exhaled breath the sound 'sa'. The automatic repetition of this silent mantra, and the space from which the breath is born, calm his fears. Intuitively, he grasps that he is this ultimate reality ('so ham', I am He). When he is forced from the womb, he is once again seized by panic and forgets his true nature. He then begins to weep: *"Kwanh! Kwanh! (ko'ham), who am I?"*

Śaṅkarācārya evokes in a truly poetic manner the essence of the three modes of breathing: *"The dissolution of the phenomenal world is called exhalation, the realisation of 'I am' is called inhalation, and the stability of this state is retention."*

ŚAṄKARĀCĀRYA, APAROKṢĀNUBHŪTI 119-120

Thus the modalities of breathing just point to the savour of tranquillity as they die away into their background. The sole purpose of exploration in āsana is to magnify these modalities so they may culminate and melt into *"the middle breath between the two paths of in-breath and out-breath."*

KṢEMARĀJA, ŚIVASŪTRAVIMARŚINĪ III, 6

This can only happen through the churning action of āsana, which is a prerequisite for understanding the breath and its different colourations. Traditionally, a certain ease in āsana is demanded before prāṇāyāma is taught.

"Jerky movements are a sign of fatigue, loss of attention or want of confidence. If they occur, do not waste time on prāṇāyāma, but practise āsana, which develop the lungs and quieten the nerves."

ŚRĪ B.K.S. IYENGAR, LIGHT ON PRĀṆĀYĀMA, CHAPTER 11, PARAGRAPH 31

Āsana are there to instil rhythmic expansion and extension (āyāma), or clarification, in the body (dehāyāma), breath (śvasāyāma) and perception (indriyāyāma). On the one hand, the groups of āsana help to create mobility and unblock different parts of the trunk, arms and legs, and on the other hand, they awaken different constellations and diaphragms that are the source of bandha or binds. Certain geographies of the body are thus explored and we can begin to understand how they interact with the breath. All āsana cleanse the various cavities of the body in order to find the source of respiratory movements. Certain āsana favour exploration of the different firmaments (vyoman) or spaces.

Śīrṣāsana unfolds two diaphragms or hearts. It is a very important āsana for understanding the suction and spreading of the pelvic floor, which is the heart of mūlabandha, and the suction and spreading of the abdomen for uḍḍiyānabandha. The variations in Śīrṣāsana intensify this action. Sarvāṅgāsana and Halāsana pacify the vocal diaphragm and allow it to spread, whilst unblocking the neck and thus allowing jālandharabandha to be unfolded. Setu Bandha Sarvāṅgāsana awakens all three bandha.

Working with support is essential to this approach, firstly to cleanse certain regions and then to unfold the different colourations of breath into them. Hence, rope Śīrṣāsana, Viparīta Daṇḍāsana on a chair or bench, Sarvāṅgāsana on a chair, half Halāsana with supported thighs, Setu Bandha Sarvāṅgāsana on a bench and Viparīta Karaṇī all become precious instruments for contemplating the different modalities of the breath. The various constellations and their winds become accessible. In practising āsana, we visit the constellation of the pelvis and its respiratory colouration (apānavāyu), the constellation of the abdomen and its respiratory colouration (samānavāyu), the constellation of the chest and its respiratory colouration (prāṇavāyu), the constellation of the throat and lower part of the face and its respiratory colouration (udānavāyu). All these constellations are bathed in the overall breath (vyānavāyu).

Āsana bring us into contact with the backstage of the body, and with its foundations and supports (dhātu), like different sheaths for one and the same energy. The texts speak of seven constituents (saptadhātu): skin (tvak), blood (rakta), flesh (māṃsa), fat (medas), bones (asthi), marrow (majja) and sperm, ova or the vital energy (śukra). Āsana exist to awaken the vital energy, which is the hardest element to awake. It is only when this element emerges that the three famous Sūtra of Patañjali can be understood: *"Āsana becomes stable and comfortable* (II, 46), *when all effort is absorbed in non-effort, the infinite is revealed* (II, 47), *then dualism ceases* (II, 48)*"*. It is therefore this vital energy that opens the door to prāṇāyāma. Patañjali means that it is only once this maturity has been attained that prāṇāyāma can be practised. One may of course practise breathing exercises that perhaps one day will result in the silence of breath and open the gateway to prāṇāyāma.

It should also be added that āsana are very important in creating a certain confidence and stability in not just the spine, but also of the nervous system. This is required for sitting and plunging into the space of the chest. The different groups of āsana explore all aspects of this space. They give elasticity to the diaphragm, which is impregnated with our emotions. Āsana wash this very important junction. It is interesting to note one of the etymologies of schizophrenia: the break (schizo) of the diaphragm (phren, phrenos).

We also talk of piercing (vedha), and especially the piercing of the three junctions or knots (granthi). The brahmāgranthi is located in the mūlādhāracakra, the viṣṇugranthi in the anāhatacakra and the rudragranthi in the ājñācakra. These are places of solidification of the space-time continuum and of identification with existence. The knots are pierced by the unifying interaction of prāṇa and apāna, when their own activity is suspended. Certain agitations and grips in the body-mind must be resorbed in and by the āsana themselves. The body must be imbued with a certain silence.

"The deserted path (Suṣumṇā) becomes the royal road for Prāṇa. Then the mind remains objectless and death is deceived. The deserted path (Suṣumṇā), the great void (Śūnyapadavī), the entry to Brahman (Brahmarandhra), the great road (Mahāpatha), the cremation ground (Śmāśana), appertaining to the auspicious (Śāmbhavī) and the central path (Madhyamārga) are names of one and the same thing."
HAṬHAYOGAPRADĪPIKĀ III, 3-4

In our approach, breathing exercises begin in Śavāsana with support for the back and especially the thoracic area, as well as for the head and neck (see 'Light on Prāṇāyāma', Chapter 19). To begin with, normal breathing is observed, without imposing anything on the breath. Once the breathing has found its rhythm, and has become smooth and unchaotic, the movement of exhalation is lengthened. There is an ever-increasing level of intimacy with the space at the end of the exhalation, known as the outer heart (dvādaśanta), situated in front of the nostrils, and with the inner heart, or the pause at the end of inhalation. This is the gateway to Ujjāyī prāṇāyāma, the basis of all other prāṇāyāma.

Different geometric configurations can also be included to make the breath tactile in particular areas. The breath can thus become triangular, with the apex pointing down or pointing up, cylindrical or from the front to back. In fact, the graphics, writing and rhythms of the breath can take on an infinite number of shapes. The various seed (bīja) mantra of the cakra (Laṃ, Vaṃ, Raṃ, Yaṃ, Haṃ), along with the vowels of the Sanskrit alphabet may also be pronounced silently while exhaling to gain access to certain energy patterns. These same exercises can then be practised in a seated āsana.

The royal pose is of course Padmāsana, which perfectly balances, to the point of silencing the brain, four areas crucial to the art of sitting: the lower limbs, the trunk, the neck and throat, and the head. If it is not possible to remain comfortably in Padmāsana, Svastikāsana can be done using a support under the buttocks in such a way that the knees are slightly lower than the buttocks and the thighs are parallel to the ground. The knees should not be spread too widely as this causes the lumbar spine to collapse. It is better not to use Siddhāsana, even though it may seem more comfortable, because when it is not practised properly the pelvis is not rooted, causing excessive lumbar arching.

If it is not possible to sit on the floor, even with the aid of a support, a chair can be used (refer to 'Light on Prāṇāyāma', Chapter 11, The Art of Sitting in Prāṇāyāma). In all seated prāṇāyāma, with the exception of Bhrāmarī, Śītalī and Sītakārī prāṇāyāma, jālandharabandha must be activated to allow the heart, throat and frontal brain to become completely passive. If prāṇāyāma is done without jālandharabandha, the organs of perception will not be silent and the eyes and eardrums will be tense. During prāṇāyāma, observation of inhalation should be passive, i.e. the breath should neither be pulled in, nor a specific path forcefully imposed upon it. Observation of exhalation should be active to prevent it ending in a state of inertia and collapse. The paths of both inhalation and exhalation end in space. Embracing this space is the art of kumbhaka, or retention. It is not a matter of holding the breath, but of being established in this space, which is also known as omnipenetration (ātmavyāpti) or blazing power of the Self (ātmaśakti). As soon as the kumbhaka is held physically, the space shrinks and the retention must be released.

Kumbhaka are said to be internal (ābhyantaravṛtti, Yogasūtra II, 50-51), external (bāhyavṛtti, Yogasūtra II, 50-51) or independent (kevala or stambhavṛtti, Yogasūtra II, 50). According to Devala, and quoted by Śivānanda in the Yogacintāmani, there are seven types of kumbhaka:

Rechita kumbhaka: retention of prāṇa after exhalation.

Pūrita kumbhaka: retention of prāṇa after inhalation.

Uttara kumbhaka: retention of prāṇa in the chest followed by inhalation.

Ādhāra kumbhaka: retention of prāṇa in the lower cavity followed by inhalation.

Sama kumbhaka: mental retention of prāṇa.

Pratyāhāra kumbhaka: retention of prāṇa in certain regions of the body such as the sole of the feet, genital organs, navel, chest, heart, throat, uvula, middle of the eyebrows, forehead and top of the skull (brahmarandhra).

Śānta kumbhaka: retention of prāṇa followed by exhalation in the above-mentioned regions (from the head to the chest).

The kumbhaka are classified into sagarbha and agarbha. Sargarbha kumbhaka is accompanied by contemplation of the mantra OM according to three modalities:

Sadhūmuka kumbhaka: meditation on the three syllables (A-U-Ṃ) that make up the mantra OM.

Sajvāla kumbhaka: meditation on the syllables of OM and their deities.

Praśānta kumbhaka: meditation on the formless, represented by OM in the central channel (suṣumṇā).

Agarbha kumbhaka is practised without mantra.

In his Kumbhaka Paddhatiḥ, Raghuvīra describes a wide variety of kumbhaka including ekameru kumbhaka, where retention is lengthened whilst surrendering to the Lord (Īśvarapraṇidhāna); dvimeru kumbhaka, where inhalation is lengthened; and trimeru kumbhaka, where exhalation is lengthened. He also describes the forty-seven stages of kumbhaka (ameru) that lead to Meru kumbhaka or Kevala kumbhaka, *"which is filled with the fullness of Brahman and where nothing remains to be experienced."* (Kumbhaka Paddhatiḥ 238)

He adds later, and not without humour: *"Through serious practice of ameru kumbhaka for several lifetimes, it may be possible to reach kevala kumbhaka from time to time."* (Kumbhaka Paddhatiḥ 285)

Nāḍī Śodhana Prāṇāyāma is the hardest prāṇāyāma to practise, as it requires great dexterity in placing the fingers on the nasal walls, as well as total freedom and non-aggressiveness in the right arm and shoulder. It should only be practised after lengthy practice of the other prāṇāyāma (refer to 'Light on Prāṇāyāma', Chapter 22, Digital Prāṇāyāma and the Art of Placing the Fingers on the Nose).

"Nāḍī śodhana prāṇāyāma is the most difficult, complex and refined of all prāṇāyāma. It is the ultimate in sensitive self-observation and control."

Śrī B.K.S. Iyengar, Light on Prāṇāyāma, Chapter 28, Page 210

Kapālabhāti and Bhastrikā should be practised very carefully and judiciously. Unless a master in the subject, prāṇāyāma practice should not begin with Kapālabhāti or Bhastrikā. It is better to prepare the lungs with mild Ujjāyī. Their practise should be stopped as soon as the stimulation specific to these two prāṇāyāma becomes irritation. The sound in Bhastrikā or Kapālabhāti should not change. If it loses its clarity and is forced out heavily, causing the chest to cave, it can become dangerous for the brain and push the abdominal organs and uterus downwards. This is why these prāṇāyāma are not recommended for women, especially those who are pregnant. People with ear or eye problems, who suffer from high or low blood pressure, and those who have a weak constitution or low lung capacity, should also avoid them.
Observation of the breath is called Nādānusandhāna. Nāda means sound and anusandhāna means absorption in listening to the sound (nāda) of the breath. Inhalation, which comes from the rising tide of the Self, evolves the different elements of prakṛti, while exhalation turns them inwards and resorbs them into their silent source.
The breath has to withdraw from worldly activities since it is always involved in the body's voluntary and involuntary functions. In the waking, dreaming and deep sleep states the breath varies. It also changes according to our mental or emotional states. Because it is a constant support for bodily identification, it is an area of great seismic activity, continually subjected to shocks. A certain quietness of the breath is therefore required in order it may serve prāṇa. This is why prāṇāyāma can only take place when resorption of the various body-mind activities comes very close to the frontiers of death.

"The states of waking, dreaming and deep sleep must be abandoned... Here begins the dissolution of the objective world..." Utpaladeva, Īśvarapratyabhijñā, Āgamādhikāra II, 18-19-20

Thus, whilst breathing exercises are open to all, prāṇāyāma, or the sacrifice of breath, concerns only very few practitioners.

"For the man resting thus in this state, both the sun and the moon set in the middle path. The unenlightened yogi remains excluded from this great ether, for he in whom the revelation of his own essence is not completely stabilised is tricked by dream and the other states."
Bhaṭṭa Kallaṭa, Spandakārikāvṛtti 24-25

"The restrain of all modifications of the mind, by regarding all mental states like the citta as Brahman alone, is called prāṇāyāma."
Śaṅkarācārya, Aparokṣānubhūti 118

Mahāśivarātri The Great Night of Śiva, Mystic Blindness

Purification of the breaths (pañcavāyuśuddhi), purification and dissolution of the elements (bhūtaśuddhi, bhūtalaya), ritual of the five M's (pañcamakāra)

"Having engulfed all that is internal and external, the yogin realises that resting thus within him and from him, the wheel of energies is gloriously unfolded."
Abhinavagupta, Tantrasāra V

"For Him, the elements are merely an armour."
Vasugupta, Śivasūtra III, 42

"The body of the adept, soluble like a lump of salt, must be fully burned in the fire of Consciousness coming from my mouth." Lakṣmī Tantra XXV, 47

In the practice of effervescence (kṣobhita), āsana explore and establish the body in its elemental quality.

"All that exists is made of these five states, of the material symbolically referred to as Earth, Water, Fire, Air and Ether. He who understands the nature of these elements merits veneration. The beings of all worlds are made of the same principles. The difference results from their subtle arteries being organised differently."
ŚIVASVARODAYA III, 144-145

The body is freed from mental grip or appropriation, returning to the sensation of its structures. Initially, the elements evolve into their energetic form as organic energies (indriyaśakti), and not as organs projected by thoughts (indriyavṛtti). These organic energies take on their quality of earth (pṛthivītattva), water (aptattva), fire (tejastattva), air (vāyutattva) and space (ākāśatattva) in different parts of the body, and may be contemplated via the specific śakti of different groups of āsana. The dominant tattva of standing āsana is that of earth, which is established in the legs. This dominant quality may change according to the sequence of āsana. The elemental quality of standing āsana done after fast vinyāsa, or after Śīrṣāsana, will not be the same. The mahābhūta are established through an understanding of the five vāyu. The breath takes on different expressions depending on its place and function in the body. Apānavāyu is located between the root of the navel and the pelvis. It is referred to as the descending breath. Its functions are mainly those of excretion and elimination. Its elemental expression is earth (pṛthivītattva), represented by a square, as well as water (aptattva), represented by a circle. It is located in and has the energy colouration of the mūlādhāra cakra, the root cakra, situated between the anus and the genital organs, and of the svādhiṣṭhāna cakra, the 'abode of the self', situated in the region of the genital organs. Their seed (bīja) mantra are LAṂ and VAṂ respectively. Prāṇavāyu resides in the upper part of the chest, from the heart to the throat. It is referred to as the ascending breath. Its functions are linked to breathing and the proper functioning of the respiratory system. Its elemental expression is air (vāyutattva), represented by a hexagram. It is located in and has the energy colouration of the anāhata cakra, 'that which is unstruck', situated in the region of the heart. Its seed (bīja) mantra is YAṂ. Between these two is samānavāyu, referred to as the equalising or median breath, found in the gastric region, from the navel to the region of the heart. Its functions are linked to digestion and assimilation. The liver, pancreas, stomach and digestive fire are revitalised by this vāyu. It links apānavāyu to prāṇavāyu. This equalising relationship is of great importance in prāṇāyāma, when the descending and ascending breaths meet and lose their identity. It is samānavāyu that enables this meeting of breaths. Its elemental expression is fire (tejastattva), represented by a triangle. It is located in and has the energy colouration of the maṇipura cakra, the 'city of jewels', situated at the navel. Its seed mantra is RAṂ. Udānavāyu, or upward vertical breath, is found in the region from the throat to the nose. Its functions are

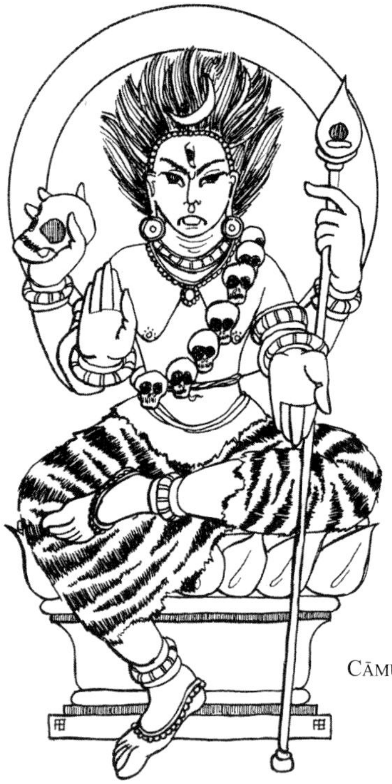

CĀMUṆḌĀ

linked to the act of regurgitation and control of facial expressions and the voice. It also provides support for muscle structure. When the inhaled and exhaled breaths meet in samāna, the vertical ascension that burns differentiation is the action of udāna. Its elemental expression is space (ākāśatattva), represented by a crescent. It is located in and has the energy colouration of the viśuddha cakra, the 'pure', situated in the region of the throat. Its seed (bīja) mantra is HAṂ. Vyānavāyu is the background to the other vāyu and is their main cohesive principle. It is the diffused breath (vyāpti) that penetrates the entire body. It circulates the energy of food and air. Certain other functions of the body are the expression of Upavāyu.

"Nāga is manifested when one belches, Kūrma when one blinks one's eyes, Krikara when one sneezes, Devadatta when one yawns. Dhanañjaya is spread throughout the body. It remains active after death. These ten energies circulate in all the body's arteries. They are the very substance of life." Śivasvarodaya I, 47

From the power of differentiation (māyā) is born space (ākāśa), which in turn generates air, which generates fire, which generates water, which generates earth. The ear, organ of hearing, evolves from the sattvic aspect of ether. The skin, organ of touch, evolves from the sattvic aspect of air. The eye, organ of sight, evolves from the sattvic aspect of fire. The tongue, organ of taste, evolves from the sattvic aspect of water. The nose, organ of smell, evolves from the sattvic aspect of earth. The five vāyu and five organs of action (karmendriya) evolve from the rajasic aspect of the subtle elements (tanmātra). The gross elements in the form of pañcīkaraṇa, which is the mutual combination of these same elements, evolve from the tamasic aspect of the subtle elements. The body is formed from these gross elements and their combinations. Āsana explore the interconnection between the elements and different vāyu.

"Little by little, one becomes aware of the principles of the elements at the limit of their formal manifestation."
Śivasvarodaya III, 152

One aspect of the purification and dissolution (bhūtaśuddhi, bhūtalaya) of the elements is the establishment of the elements in their virile (vīrya) and ascending (bhūtodaya) manifestation. The different groups of āsana teach the intuitive recognition of these elemental qualities and the respiratory colourations they bring to different regions of the body (apānic, samānic, prāṇic, udānic). Then, thanks to the pañcavāyu, an āsana can be approached from a different viewpoint depending whether the breath is apānic, samānic, prāṇic or udānic. The other aspect of bhūtaśuddhi, and which is its main function, is the involution or resorption of all these elements into their source. In fact, these elements are already the source. As is said in the Śivasūtra: *"When the Wheel of Energies fuses together, the universe is withdrawn."* (I, 6)

The hero always contemplates these energies in their totality, and not their fragmented aspect. The successive de-coagulation of the elements burns the different states of Consciousness, which is the background to all these states, including waking, dreaming and deep sleep. This process is of course no more than a description since *"the reality of Consciousness (saṃvittattvam) shines with its own light (svaprakāśa)."*
Abhinavagupta, Tantrāloka I, 10

This complete incineration is described in the Vīrvala Śāstra: *"This Consciousness where all is destroyed and all the thirty-six elements reduced to ashes, should be perceived in the body itself, shining like Kālāgnirudra."* (Kṣemarāja, Śivasūtravimarśinī I, 6), and in the Vijñāna Bhairava: *"One must meditate on one's own fortress as if it were consumed by the Fire of Time, rising from the foot. At the end of this meditation, the peaceful state will appear."* (Vijñāna Bhairava 52)

Bhūtaśuddhi culminates in the ritual of the pañcamakāra, known as the ritual of the five M's, because the names of the ingredients used all begin with the letter M: madya (wine), māṃsa (meat), matsya (fish), mudrā (fermented grain) and maithuna (sexual union). They represent the oblation of our consecrated sheaths in the mouth of death. Thus is accomplished the sacrifice and adoration of the supreme, in the supreme, by the supreme.

"Kula (sacrifice) is the supreme beatitude. Kula is the nature of the Self. Kula is known as the body. Kula is everything, residing in all things. Its splendour is simply tremendous. This sacrifice is only intended for he who is free from all doubt, and who thus sees all things in the same light. Whatever the hero accomplishes in thought, word, or deed, through any activity requiring boldness and heroism, apt to reveal such essence, is called Sacrifice (Kula)."
ABHINAVAGUPTA, TANTRĀLOKA XXIX, 4-5-6

According to the Kailāsa Tantra, the five M's have their origin in the five prāṇa. Symbolically, they therefore represent the mahābhūta. Cereal is the earth, fish is water, wine is fire, meat is air and sexual union is ether. In the coded language of tantra, these terms are explained symbolically.

• **Wine** (madya) is the nectar that flows from non-differentiation. It is also the intoxicating joy of recognising one's true nature, making us stagger as if we no longer see the world. It is also the absorption that arises from such recognition.

• **Meat** (māṃsa) is the fact of considering everything as food for the supreme Śakti and offering it as such. Māṃsa also means speech (ma = tongue, aṃsa = speech). Thus it is the offering of speech, in its gross (vaikarī), intermediate (madhyama) or subtle (paśyantī) expression, to the silence that precedes its utterance (parāvāk). Māṃsa is also the act of consuming the concepts of virtue (puṇya) and sin (pāpa), represented by one's own carcass being consumed in the fire of non-differentiation.

• **Fish** (matsya) is intuition of non-separation, symbolised by the breath. Matsya symbolises exhalation (śvāsa) and inhalation (praśvāsa), as well as iḍā and piṅgalā. Eating fish is to give oneself to the prayer of prāṇāyāma, and to swallow differentiations by means of kumbhaka.

• **Cereal** (mudrā) often refers to a fermented cereal-based drink to which cannabis (gañja) or other aphrodisiac substances, and sometimes menstrual blood, were added. Mudrā also means the woman who participated in the ritual, as well as the mouth of the yoginī (yoni) as the great seal (mahāmudrā).

"The Lord calls the central wheel 'the mouth of the yoginī' since it is upon which the transmission of spiritual lineage is founded, and from which one obtains Knowledge. She escapes duality, cannot be described, and as such is said to move from mouth to mouth. Since it is our own Consciousness, how can we describe it?"
ABHINAVAGUPTA, TANTRĀLOKA XXIX, 124-125

Cereal symbolises nourishment: that of emotions such as fear, hatred, desire, vanity and shame. They have to be feasted upon, fully digested and sealed (mudrā) in that which allows them to be known.

"With the disappearance of these limitations, even anger, etc. appear as of the nature of the perfect divine Bhairava-Consciousness."
ABHINAVAGUPTA, PARĀTRĪŚIKĀVIVARAṆA, JAIDEVA SINGH, PAGE 51

• **Sexual union** (maithuna) is the absorption of subject-object characteristics, in all situations, emotions and mental states, into undifferentiated energy.

"In the deep night of illusion of our daily activities, one must strongly press the two wheels (subject and object) in order to extract the pith. From their copenetration an eminent splendour immediately strikes forth, that of the supreme knowing Subject, transcending the brightness of

the sun and the moon (knowledge and known object)."
ABHINAVAGUPTA, QUOTING A PASSAGE OF THE YOGASAṂCĀRATANTRA, TANTRĀLOKA IV, 131-132-133-134

The brahmacārin is therefore not one who is celibate, but one who abandons himself to Brahman, to the bliss of the resulting union of Śiva-Śakti. According to Abhinavagupta, celibacy for the brahmacārin is the consecration of all actions through the symbolic aspect of wine, meat and sexual union.

"The lineage of the Perfected Beings (siddha) is to be worshiped with ingredients that are both hated by people and forbidden by the scriptures. They must be revolting and despised."
QUOTED BY JAYARATHA, TANTRĀLOKAVIVEKA XXIX, 10D.1

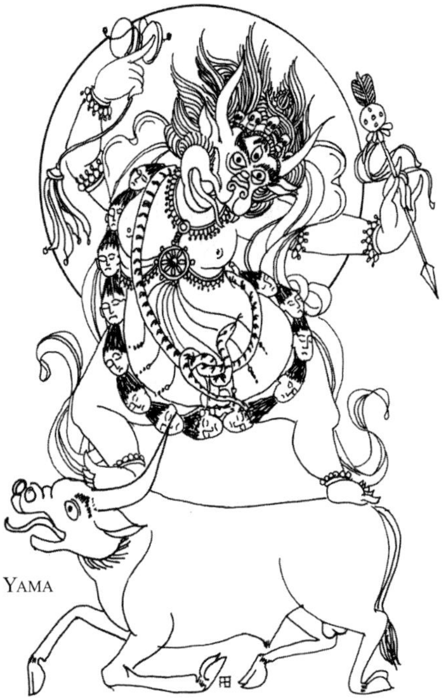

YAMA

Until this sacrifice takes place, we remain merely a social animal (paśu), bound and tied by society's moral codes. These ties are woven by fear and the desire for continuity. They represent the very structure of society, which is no more than the projection of our fear of death. Inner 'de-socialising' begins by recognising and cremating these ties of fear, pity, shame, disgust, family, worldliness, caste or social status, precepts, observances and prohibitions.

This ritual is totally intimate and is therefore completely anonymous and goes unnoticed. No one could suspect the calm madness that inhabits someone who goes about his daily occupations but remains completely estranged from them. Who could comprehend a life lived in perpetual death? It reminds us of the motto of the mystic Sūfī: *"The hordes are their desert, banality their asceticism."* These cremation practices are only meant for those who have heroic (vīrya) inclinations and who have severed the three-fold bind of fear, shame and hate.

As a well-known tantric saying goes:
"Secretly a Kaula, outwardly a Śaiva-Siddhānta, and publicly a practitioner of the Veda; like the coconut that keeps the juice of its nectar hidden inside."
QUOTED BY JAYARATHA COMMENTATING THE TANTRĀLOKA, VOL. 3, PAGE 643

Thus is the plunge into the great night of Śiva (mahāśivarātri), known as mystic blindness, and which is blind to all differentiation.

"Free, without attachment to any ritual whatsoever, without doubts, freed from worldliness, absorbed in the realisation of the 'I am not' and the contemplation of the deities of the body, seeing all that is perceived as the supreme subject, he is made perfect by the khecarī mudrā."
ABHINAVAGUPTA, TANTRĀLOKA XXXII, 20CD-24AB

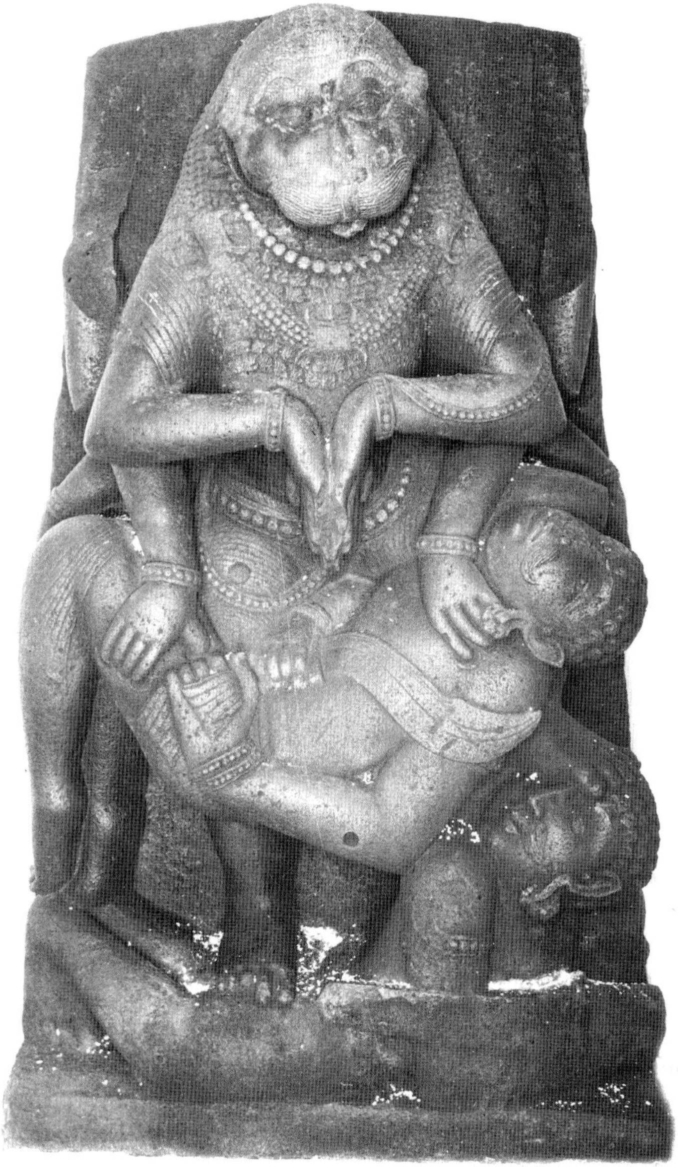

Narasiṃhavatāra
7th century
(Rajivalohana Temple,
Rajime, Raipur District,
Madhya Pradesh)

14

Haunting Nostalgia, Total Helplessness and Facelessness

"Although this world always rests peacefully within Your body,
on the inside it is ceaselessly consumed by the fire of distress."
UTPALADEVA, ŚIVASTOTRĀVALĪ XVIII, 5

"If you are attacked by the squadron of separations and if disappointment cries out to you 'more hope',
with your left hand take the shield of submission, and with your right hand grip the sword of tears..."
HUSAYN MANSŪR AL-HALLĀJ, DĪWĀN, MUQATTA'ĀT 4

"Stop hoping and you will cease to fear"
SÉNÈQUE, LETTERS TO LUCILIUS

"Now is the winter of our discontent."
W. SHAKESPEARE, RICHARD III, ACT I, SCENE 1

"The day will come when a hand of light will strike the wood of the heart,
with such insistence that I will have no choice but to rise and open.
I will be unable to reply to the question I am asked, apart from with a smile:
I have done nothing with my life. I have wasted it as much as possible."
CHRISTIAN BOBIN

"And from the majestic heights of my dreams, I return to being an assistant bookkeeper in the city of Lisbon.
But the contrast doesn't overwhelm me; it frees me. And its irony is my blood.
The nocturnal glory of being great, without being anything!"
FERNANDO PESSOA

In the inner most depths of our gaze there is a deep, ever unsatisfied melancholy that leaves us distraught when faced with the corpses of our experiences. We are left with our mouths half open, as though deprived of food that we can never taste, a feeling of nostalgia for the savour of fullness, satiety and tranquillity. Is this not the unique and true momentum that drives us?

"All beings strive for bliss."
YOGAVASIṢṬHAMAHĀRĀMĀYAṆA VIA, 108.20

This firmament, which we hope to reach by unfolding a universe of destinations, projects, relationships and situations in a hypothetical future, is projected by a past that is already dead. Ironically, this glimpse of the elusive, recalling the past or projecting the future, can only occur in the instant. We try in vain to avert the unexpected and avoid the inevitable with our fortresses of concepts and explanations, with the knowledge we have accumulated and all the strategies we put into place. We can always go back to our yoga practice, our meditation practice, or read the scriptures to try and fill the breech of the real, of the uncertainty, so as not to feel our complete helplessness. Hope entices us with a shimmering of an emergency exit, a sort of life raft, a glorious awakening, an end full of meaning, enabling us to face death head on. But isn't death the moment we become faceless? This unreachable security plunges us into despair! Despairing is another way of hoping, of clinging on. Seeing our expectations brings us back to our conditioning, which continuously translates reality. It is useless to hope to not to hope, to be without expectation. This would only be yet another expectation. All we can do is admit to our complete helplessness.
We recognise ourselves as tranquillity, without need, at the moment a desire is satisfied, when the desire and the object of the desire die. We associate this tranquillity with the object, making us eternal beggars, begging for that which no one can give us. Seekers of material or affective compensation, seekers of an ever fleeing elsewhere, seekers of someone with miraculous answers, seekers of techniques and transformations, seekers of enlightenment, seekers of the ultimate escape, so we may taste the kiss of oblivion once again.
But is there really a seeker or just an impersonal search that wears itself out? Is this not already the presence of grace, the grace of seeing the wall of separation collapse in the course of a glance, a caress, a shock, or through the experience of pleasure, fear or deep sleep? Of all the identities we have taken on, even those in a single day, which can we claim? This sinking is a reminder of what we have always known: identity is a burden and we have no becoming.
All experiences, pleasant or unpleasant, only exist to show us that they are external to us. They are only there to tire the desire for exteriority. This exteriority does not refer to a position in space, but suggests the belief in something different to ourself. This exteriority includes the body as well as all mental states and expansions of Consciousness. From the ultimate point of view, there is no difference in the affirmations 'I am pathetic' or 'I am divine'. These states of Consciousness come before that state by which we are able to recognise them.
We cannot therefore speak of spiritual quest. The entire universe becomes a mirror of this sinking of separation, whether it be in a pub or in an āśrama! We only settle into a certain vulnerability, a certain availability, when this quest dims, comes to an end, when there is complete disinterest in everything which could be added or taken from us, when there is complete absence of manipulation of what we are momentarily as body-mind, as situations, as relationships.
This disinterest creates a fatigue for worldliness. Worldliness makes us believe we would finally be happy if only we could live in the countryside, if we were single or had a different partner, if we studied Sanskrit, if we had another job, if we could remain seated in lotus pose for an hour, in short, if the situation was different to what

it is. There is a point of no return, where watching a football match on TV with your brother-in-law or being invited to a heavenly feast in the company of gods fundamentally boils down to the same thing, and participates to the wonderment of Being.

"In the radiant celebrations that lead to Your splendour, in truth what is there for enlightened beings that is not a miracle?"
ABHINAVAGUPTA, ANUBHAVANIVEDANA 4

This profound disinterest is wonderfully illustrated by the dialogue between Rāma and Vasiṣṭha, taken from the Vairāgya Prakaraṇaṃ chapter of the Yogavasiṣṭhamahārāmāyaṇa. The dialogue is a dialectic and didactic form that is found in many texts, and reflects the dialogue of Consciousness. To paraphrase Abhinavagupta, Consciousness is the question and the answer, being both at the same time. Although the Yogavasiṣṭhamahārāmāyaṇa claims not to belong to a particular school, it is very much influenced by the Trika (Kashmir Śaivism), as well as by Advaita Vedānta and Buddhism. In Advaita Vedānta, the evanescence of the world leads to it being rejected, like an illusion. This is one of the fundamental differences between Kashmir Śaivism and Advaita Vedānta. Advaita Vedānta believes that the universe and everything in it are the effect of māyā, of ignorance, a super imposition that is beginningless and unrelated to Brahman. For Advaita Vedānta, the world is nothing more than a dream, an unreality, like the son of a barren woman. This rejection of the world, the body and the senses has been magnified by Śaṅkarācārya, through his approach for renouncement and through his monastic order. Yet a point of view very similar to that of the Trika can be found in Śaṅkarācārya's tantric and lyrical works. According to Mādhava Vidyāranya, author of Śaṅkarācārya's traditional biography (Śaṅkara Digvijaya XVI, 54-80), Śaṅkarācārya went to Kashmir in the second decade of the 9th century. Concepts about the absolute, as expounded in Śaṅkarācārya's Dakṣiṇāmūrtistotra and in its commentary by his student Sureśvarācārya, are similar to those of the Pratyabhijñā School. There are thus striking similarities between certain passages of Utpaladeva's Īśvarapratyabhijñākārikā and Śaṅkarācārya's Dakṣiṇāmūrtistotra. Śaṅkarācārya's tantric philosophy had a significant influence on the Trika School, and it would appear as though Śaṅkarācārya's trip to Kashmir was perhaps not merely fictional. There is also a local tradition whose thinking is along the same lines. Śaṅkarācārya's inclination for tantrism is obvious, as is highlighted in verse 31 of the Saundaryalaharī, and by the establishment of Śrīcakra in his monasteries (maṭha). Śaṅkarācārya's explanation of vedānta is greatly influenced by tantric concepts. For the Trika, the world appears in Consciousness and is therefore real. Its unreality lies in the belief that it is separate to Consciousness. Māyā, the power of diversity, is also only an emanation of the energy of will (icchāśakti) of Consciousness, and not different to it. The world is merely the Lord on stage.

"The inner self is the stage."
VASUGUPTA, ŚIVASŪTRA III, 10

"Objective existence (the world) is not something that exists separately from Him (Consciousness)."
UTPALADEVA, ĪŚVARAPRATYABHIJÑĀKĀRIKĀ I, 5.15

This may be the reason why aesthetic experience has been explored so deeply in Kashmir Śaivism, especially in Abhinavagupta's works on poetics and dramaturgy. Two well-known commentaries, the Locana commenting Ānandavardhana's Dhvanyāloka and the Abhinavabhāratī commenting Bhārata's Nāṭyaśāstra, have become reference works for generations of aesthetes, affirming that Abhinavagupta made poetry a science. The Yogavasiṣṭhamahārāmāyaṇa presents this point of no return, of extreme wear and dissatisfaction, of objective

Śiva Ardhanārīśvara
11th century
(Karyavarohana Temple, Nagapattinam, Tamil Nadu)

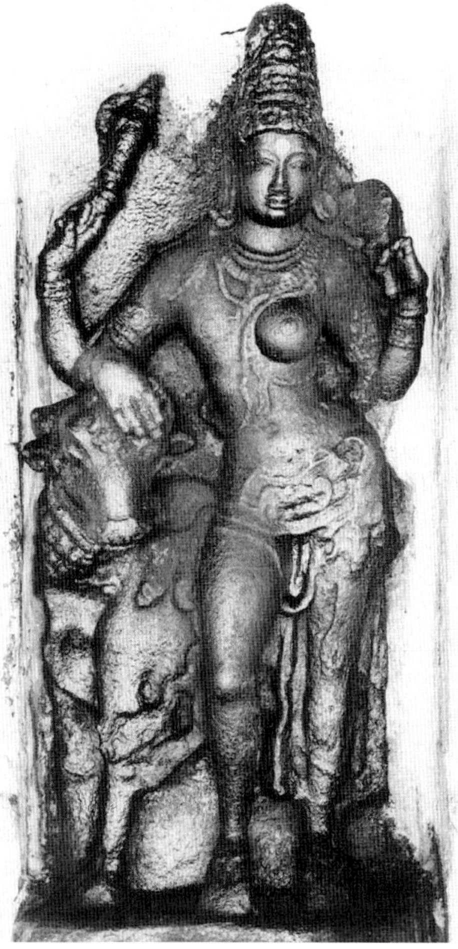

searching or definition of what we may be, in a very poetic and literary way, far from the usual conceptual curtness of some philosophy or other. That which we are can never be described because we are already it, if only through that which we are not. We are not the body, the mind, emotions, thoughts or perceptions, all of which only appear on the screen of our presence. The feeling 'I am not' doesn't stem from separation but on the contrary, from profound intimacy with the various coagulations and crystallisations of our psychophysical clothing. In the feeling 'I am not', there is a fragrance of 'I don't know', since there is no definition by which we can know ourselves.

The Yogavasiṣṭhamahārāmāyaṇa celebrates the union of poetry (kāvya) and sacred text (śāstra) dear to Abhinavagupta and Ānandavardhana. This poetic and literary wealth is found in most Trika texts. In the Vijñāna Bhairava, does Śiva not refer to Devī as *"O Gazelle-eyed goddess"*?

Contemplating the evanescence of the world, which in Advaita Vedānta leads to its rejection, here opens to an inclusiveness of all perceptions since the world too is merely a reflection in Consciousness. Vasiṣṭha is thus able to declare to Rāma: *"Drink, live, make love, for you have obtained the far shore of worldly existence."* (V, 50.75)

"It makes no difference whether the wise man be given, with unbridled passion, to heavy drink, or dance, or whether, on the contrary, he abandons society and retreats into the mountains." (V, 56.53)

These two passages are only meaningful when seeking and desire have been fully exhausted.

"True happiness only really exists when the mind ceases to function. Such happiness cannot even be attained in heaven, just as it is not possible for a house of ice to exist in the desert."

"Higher than a kingdom, than heaven, than the moon, than the state of Maghavan, and even higher than the delight

that arises whilst making love, is the happiness that comes when desire ceases."
YOGAVASIṢṬHAMAHĀRĀMĀYAṆA VIA, 44.26; V, 74.44

Here follows a passage from chapter I of this text on the subject of abandon (Vairāgya Prakaraṇa) that I have freely translated. The young prince Rāma has returned from his travels. Like all young men he wanted to see the world. Being the king's son, he has experienced the best life can offer. He was given the best tutors and the best courtesans. He has wealth, power, youth, beauty and courage, and yet is still not happy.

It is said that the sage Sutīkṣṇa asked the sage Agastya if action or knowledge was the liberator. He replied that they are like the two wings that enable a bird to fly. To illustrate this he told him the following story:
A very long time ago, in a forgotten age, a heavenly nymph by the name of Suruci was seated on a Himalayan peak when she saw Indra's messenger cross the sky like a flash of lightning. When questioned, he revealed the purpose of his mission. A royal sage by the name of Ariṣṭanemi had bequeathed his kingdom to his son and withdrawn to a hillside where he practises terrible austerity. Upon seeing this, Indra requested that I go to him with a group of nymphs and escort him up to heaven. But first, the sage wanted to know the advantages and disadvantages of this place. I replied that in the heavens everyone received rewards for their good actions and lived in pleasure and abundance, but returned to the mortal world once their merits had been exhausted. The sage refused Indra's invitation. Indra then sent me again, telling me to ask Ariṣṭanemi to follow Vālmīki's advice before refusing the offer. The sage was presented to Vālmīki, and asked him the best way to rid oneself of birth and death. Vālmīki replied by recounting the dialogue between Rāma and Vasiṣṭha.

He who feels chained, but asks himself why, is qualified to study this dialogue, since he is neither totally ignorant nor totally enlightened.
Rāma travelled the length and breadth of the country. He then returned to his capital, to the great delight of the entire city. For eight days the entire city of Ayodhyā celebrated Rāma's return.
For a while Rāma attended to his affairs. But very quickly he underwent a profound change. He lost weight, became weaker and his paleness was frightening. Worried, the king wondered what was happening to his son. Each time he asked, Rāma replied that he shouldn't worry, and remained silent. The king didn't insist. Then, not having seen him for several weeks, the king asked Rāma's chamberlain for news of his son. The chamberlain was visibly worried:
"My Lord, since his return, Rāma has not been the same. He does not even see the point of bathing. He no longer enjoys the company of courtesans in his quarters. He does not care for the presents he receives. He drives away the palace's dancers and no longer organises feasts. All of that bores him. He lives like a machine, does things in a mechanical fashion, shut-off from the world like a deaf-mute. He is often heard muttering to himself and moaning: 'What is the use of wealth and property? It is nothing but a dream'.

"For most of the time he remains silent and nothing can distract him. He only takes pleasure in his solitude, lost in his own thoughts. We really have no idea what has happened to our prince, what he is thinking or what he is seeking. He is wasting away day after day. Again and again he moans: 'Alas, we waste our lives in a thousand different ways without asking ourselves why. People complain bitterly that they suffer but nobody sincerely wishes to put an end to the causes of their torments.'

"It is plunging us into deep sadness. We do not know what to do. He no longer has any hopes or desires. He seems to be completely detached from everything. He does not delude himself, he is not mad either, or enlightened. He sometimes appears to be submerged with suicidal thoughts. Lord, only you are able to find a cure for the prince."

The king asked Viśvāmitra for advice. Viśvāmitra replied: "If this is so, then ask Rāma to come to me. His state is not the result of a whim but the reflection of great maturity and wisdom. Let us go and find him and dispel his despondency."
The king ordered the chamberlain to go and fetch Rāma. Rāma prepared himself to meet his father. When he arrived, he greeted his father and the assembled sages. Although still young, they saw the maturity that shone from his face. He bowed before his father, who tenderly took him in his arms and embraced him. "My son, what is making you sad? Depression opens the door to all kinds of misery."
The sages Viśvāmitra and Vasiṣṭha agreed.
Rāma replied: "My father, holy men, I will answer your questions as clearly as possible. I grew up happy in your residence. I had the best tutors. I recently left on a pilgrimage. During that time a thought took hold of me, tearing away all hope. My heart has started to question itself: what is it people call happiness? Can this happiness be obtained with the thousands of impermanent things in this world? All beings are born to die, and die to be reborn, again and again.

"For me, all these transient phenomena no longer have any meaning and are the cause of suffering. People that have nothing in common meet and invent a relationship. Everything in this world is dependent on our state of mind. And if we study this state of mind, even this appears to be unreal. But we are bewitched by it. We chase after a mirage in the desert so we can quench our thirst. Unaware of reality, we wander aimlessly in this thick jungle we call the world. What is existence? What is it that is born, grows and dies? Is it possible to end this suffering? Although I do not weep so as not to upset my friends, my heart bleeds with suffering. Wealth too serves no purpose; it only deceives the ignorant. Fortune is uncertain and changing, and gives rise to many anxieties and causes insatiable appetite. Fortune is blind, both the good and the bad can become rich.

"Be that as it may, one is able to be good, amicable and compassionate as long as one's heart has not been hardened by power. Power even pollutes the heart of scholars, heroes and kind men of soft voice. Power and happiness do not go together. It is rare to be powerful and not have rivals and enemies. Power is the night of fair action, the moonlight of suffering and a squall for the flame of discrimination. A person's good inclinations wither away in its presence. The truth of power is that it chooses those who are already death's prey.

"By the same token, the length of life is merely a drop of dew on a leaf. The length of an existence is only of use to those who have knowledge of the Self. We can imprison the wind, divide space, make garlands out of the waves on the sea, but we cannot wage a penny on how long we will live. Man tries in vain to extend his life, but he only succeeds in extending his own suffering. Only he who knows who he is lives, all others simply exist like donkeys. For one who is ignorant, knowledge of the sacred scriptures is a burden; for one who has many desires, wisdom itself is a burden. And for one who has no knowledge of himself, the body is a burden.

"The rat of time gnaws at our existence without respite. The termites of illness destroy our vital energy. Like a cat eyes a mouse with extreme attention, death fixes its eyes upon us. My friends, I am afraid. I am afraid when I contemplate wisdom's terrible enemy, the ego. It is born out of the darkness of ignorance and blossoms within it. All suffering stems from egoism. It is the 'I' that suffers and egoism is the cause of mental distress. I sense that egoism is my worst illness. With its net of worldliness, egoism traps living beings. All calamities in this world stem from egoism. It eclipses self-control, destroys virtue and equanimity.

"I am abandoning the notion that I am Rāma and I only wish to rest in the abode of the Self. Whatever I have done under the influence of the 'I' was futile. Truth lies in the absence of the 'I'. When I am under its influence, I am unhappy; but when, for a few seconds, I am free of it, I am full of joy. It is the 'I' alone that has built up the social fabric we know, the prison of one's family and its hypocritical

relationships to chain us even further. I thought I was free of it, yet I am miserable. I beg you to help me!

"The mind is as agitated as the raging wind. Whatever it has, it is never satisfied and only becomes more agitated. As a cullender cannot be filled with water, the mind can never be satisfied no matter how many objects it accumulates. The mind wanders in all directions but finds happiness nowhere. The mind is forever restless, like a lion in a cage that has lost its freedom and is frustrated with its current condition.

"Alas, my friends, I am suffocated by illusory needs. Like a river in flood uproots trees, I too have been uprooted. I am being thrown in all directions like a leaf in a storm. I am unable to rest.

"The mind is the cause of this world. The three worlds only exist through it. When the mind disappears, they too disappear. When the mind is submerged by desires, the errors caused by ignorance are innumerable. These desires kill the heart's noble qualities and make us hard and cruel. Desire and its different forms dance a furious saraband in this darkness.

"Although I have adopted different methods of control, they are of no use and I am carried away, like the wind whisks away wisps of straw. All my hopes for detachment have been blown away. Like a bird caught in a net, we are unable to escape, even though we have wings. Even if I drank nectar, my thirst would never be quenched.

"Desire tosses me from one place to another, in no particular direction, tossing me onto conflicting paths, like a wild horse. Desire lays before us a theatre of husbands, wives, children, friends and other illusory relationships. Although I may be a kṣatriya, desire turns me into a cowardly, frightened person. I have eyes by which to see, yet I am blind. Although full of joy, desire makes me miserable. Bewitched by this magician, man is not even able to appreciate the pleasures offered to him, and yet we are all striving for happiness. Desire fills life's stage, upon which happy and unhappy situations are acted out, and this bad actor, despite his flop and failure, continues his performances. Desire ceaselessly fills the sky and plunges into the bowels of the earth because its source is the emptiness of the mind. The light of wisdom may shine in the mind for a few instants, but the psychosis soon regains the upper hand. It is a miracle that sages are able to cut through the mind with the sword of knowledge.

"This pitiful body, made up of veins, arteries and nerves, is also a source of pain. Enchained by the smallest of gratifications and distressed by the smallest of adversities, this body is abject. Who is able to say he possesses a body? It is useless to feel hope or despondency for the body. It is nothing more than a boat given to us so we may cross the ocean of life, from birth to death. But we should not regard it as being the Self. This tree, which is the body, is born in the forest known as Saṃsāra. Here lives the mad monkey of the mind, it is the abode of the grasshopper of worries, constantly eaten by the insects of suffering, it shelters the poisonous snake of desire and the savage crows of anger hide within it. There are a few flowers of laughter; its fruit is good and bad, and the immense vulture of the ego reigns there. This tree is hollow, empty and we can hope for nothing from it, whether it lives for a long time or whether it dies in the next instant. How would it be able to fulfil our hopes? The body is the victim of depressions, emotions and changing states of mind, like a weather vane in a strong wind. I do not care for it! What is fortune, what is a kingdom, what is the body? All of these are mercilessly reduced to nothing by death.

"Let us now speak of childhood. Most people, in their ignorance, find childhood joyful and a happy time. But it too, O sages, is only full of suffering! Helplessness, misfortune, frustrated desires, unable to express oneself, total stupidity, mischievousness, weakness, does all of this not characterise childhood? A child takes offence at the slightest of things

and becomes angry and starts to sob over something petty. I can say without a shadow of a doubt that a child's anguish is much greater than that of a dying man, of somebody old, somebody ill or of any other adult. The state of a child is comparable to that of an animal at the mercy of others.

"A child is the prey of innumerable events that make him perplexed. They are the origin of fears and fantasies. A child is impressionable and easily influenced. He is therefore subjected to his parents and bound by either reward or punishment. For me, childhood is nothing more than a period of submission. Albeit a child may appear innocent, he can also be the prey of fears and neurosis. O sages, I pity those who think that childhood is a happy period.

"What suffering is worse than an agitated mind? And a child is terribly agitated! A child is unhappy if he does not have something new each day. A child's activity can be summed up as crying and complaining. It is heartbreaking for a child not to obtain what he wants. When a child goes to school, conditioning and punishment only serve to worsen his suffering. To calm a crying child, his parents promise him the world, and so he starts to place an importance on the material world and desire its objects. His parents tell him 'be quiet and you'll get what you want', and the child believes it. Thus the seeds of illusion are sown in his tender heart. Although a child feels the hot and the cold, he is unable to protect himself against it. He is in no better situation than a tree. You can see at home how he is scared of everyone older than him.

"When childhood is left behind, the human being enters into adolescence and youth, but the suffering is never left behind. He undergoes great physical and mental changes. His life is full of desire and anxiety. Those who do not lose their innocence during their youth are open to all manner of attack. I am not attached to this period of life where short-lived pleasures open the door to never-ending suffering. But what is worse is that we devote ourselves to actions that cause misfortune to others. As a tree is consumed by a forest fire, so the heart of a youth is consumed by the pain of losing a beloved. Youth is like a hurricane that scatters us. Alas! When our youth has left us, the passions that were awakened and sustained still burn within us. It is easy to cross a great ocean, but it is something quite different to reach the other shore of youth without bringing along our open and purulent wounds.

"In his youth, man is a slave to sexual attraction. He perceives beauty and charm in a body that is nothing more than an aggregate of flesh, blood, moods, bones, hair and skin. But this body never lasts for long. The flesh, which was the source of attraction and desire, is very soon transformed by the withering ugliness of old age, and then consumed by fire or eaten by worms or vultures.

"This is how creation is maintained. Childhood seems like an eternity and our youth leaves us as quickly as it came; so cruel is life! In the same way the wind blows away dewdrops, old age destroys the body. Like a drop of poison that enters into the body and immediately invades it; senility does the same, breaking and bending the body. The spectacle is absurd.

"Although an old man cannot satisfy his desires, they continue to gnaw away at him inside. He only starts to question himself about what he is when it is too late to change the course of his life, his hard and fast habits, or to give a meaning to his existence. How all of this is astounding and stupefying! Those who have come through terrible battles, who have climbed the highest mountains and then settled there, they too have been afflicted with senility and degeneration.

"All the distractions in this world are only an illusion; like a madman who tastes the reflection of a fruit in a mirror! All our hopes are being constantly destroyed by time. Time alone, O sages, ruins everything. Nothing can escape it.

Time creates innumerable universes and just as quickly makes them disappear.

"The different seasons of nature and existence give us an inkling of what Time is, but its essence remains hidden to us. Time is without mercy, inexorable, cruel, greedy and insatiable. It is the greatest of magicians who knows all the illusions. It cannot be analysed and, although divided, it remains indestructible. Its appetite is insatiable. It consumes the smallest of insects and the highest of mountains, and even the king of the heavens. In the same way a small boy plays with a ball, Time plays with two balls: the sun and the moon. It is truly Time that appears as the destroyer of the universe, its creator and its protector; it is also the nothingness of cosmic dissolution. It is Time that creates and destroys the universe again and again. As a huge mountain is rooted in the ground, all-powerful Time is rooted in being.

"Although Time creates an infinite number of universes, it neither tires of them nor rejoices in them. Time neither comes nor goes, neither wakes up nor goes to sleep. Nobody really knows what Time is. All I can tell you is that Time dances in the universe, creates and destroys everything. What hope is there? Everything changes, nothing is permanent.

"All relationships are nothing more than enslavement. Distractions are nothing more than disease, and the pursuit of happiness a mirage. Reality! What reality? The reality of an ant is different to mine. Reality is unreal.

"Intelligence is controlled by the ego, and not the other way round. There is thus neither peace nor happiness for our mind. Being in the company of sages has become a rarity. I see no solution. Nobody appears to be able to achieve the realisation of truth. Nobody is full of the happiness of others and there is no compassion in our hearts. People are becoming more and more half-wit with each day that passes. Weakness is triumphing over strength, cowardliness over bravery, and bad company easier to find than good.

"My friends, the mysterious force that controls this creation destroys armies of demons and even kills immortals and makes transient that we take for eternal. Does there remain any hope for an ordinary person such as I? And so, O sages, it is neither in childhood, nor youth, nor maturity, nor old age that one finds happiness. Although the mind strives in vain for material happiness, it is clear that no object in this world can provide it. Only he who is free from the illusion of separation is happy.

"I do not consider he who is able to conquer a terrible army as a hero, but rather he who is able to cross the ocean of the senses and the mind.

"I do not consider that which can be just as quickly lost as something gained; only that which cannot be lost is gained, and no such thing exists in this world.

"My friends, I am astounded to see men wander in all directions during the day, inventing responsibilities, being wholly involved in destructive activities, spreading confusion throughout the world. I really do not see how are they able to sleep at night!

"Albeit a busy man overcomes his ordeals and adversity, surrounds himself with luxury and security to give him a misleading sense of happiness; albeit that this man surrounds himself with power and revels in his success, death remains by his side, ready to touch him at each instant. In his ignorance, man becomes attached to his spouse, children and friends. He does not know that this world is merely a vast place where innumerable people meet by chance, and those he calls spouse or child are part of these shadows.

"As the speed of a potter's wheel makes it appear motionless,

so this world appears to us as being motionless, whereas it is constantly changing.

"How many aeons have already passed? They are only instants in time because in reality, there is no difference between an era and an instant. Both are measurements of time. For the gods, aeons are instants. What futility, what derision!

"My friends, everything is merely a dream. That which is a crater today was a mountain yesterday, and that which is a mountain today will become a hole in the ground. A dense forest will become a large town and fertile ground will turn into a desert. In the same way, changes are continually having an effect on us.

"The cycle of life and death appears to me as a talented dancer whose dress is made of entities. In her mad choreography she throws them to the heavens, hurls them to hell or spews them onto the earth. All great and good actions, all religious rites are very soon only a memory and an empty promise. Human beings are reborn as animals and vice-versa; as for the gods, they lose their divinity and return as beggars. I can even see the creator, the protector and the destroyer heading towards their own downfall.

"This world and its distractions have a bitter taste. I am fed up with chasing after shadows. I only wish to be at peace with myself. I aspire to neither life nor death. I remain as I am, detached from the fever of worldliness. If I do not become wise now, who knows when I will? Tomorrow never comes, and I already feel the grip of death on my throat.

"O sages, I beg of you! Teach me the secret that will free me from anguish, distress and fear. Through the light of your teaching, dispel the darkness of ignorance from my heart.

"When I contemplate the pitiful fate of living beings, fallen thus into bottomless wells of suffering, I am filled with sorrow, I am confused, I tremble, and the slightest step fills me with terror. I have abandoned everything, but I have no wisdom; half imprisoned, half free, I am like a tree that has been pruned but not uprooted. I ask you, tell me what is this state free from suffering? How can someone engaged in the world and its blazing fire, as I am, reach the supreme and taste peace? What is the state of mind whereby experiences leave no mark?

"Tell me, how do enlightened beings live in this world? How can one free oneself from desire and see the world as the Self with the same detachment one has when watching a blade of grass? How can one live in this world? Teach me this wisdom that will make my mind as stable as a mountain.

"This world is only suffering and death. How can it become a source of joy without the need to act out a role? The mind is nothing but an attic of impurities, how can it be purified? And with what? How can one live without being destroyed by the conflicting currents of love and hate?

"It would appear there is a secret to living in this world without being affected by it, as mercury is not affected when thrown onto a fire. What is the secret? What is the antidote for this mind that spreads out in the form of creation? Who are these heroes who have freed themselves from the illusion? However, if you think I am not ready or able to understand this, then death will be my refuge."

Having said this, Rāma then remained silent. All those gathered in the palace's court were greatly inspired by Rāma's fiery words, capable of uncovering the illusions of the mind.

Who had listened to Rāma? Sages such as Vasiṣṭha and Viśvāmitra, ministers, members of the royal family, as well as the king himself, ordinary citizens, prominent citizens, servants, caged birds, domestic animals and horses from the royal stables, but also celestial beings including blessed sages and musicians of the higher realms. Even the king of the heavens and the head of the infernal worlds had listened to Rāma's diatribe.

The assembled sages said: "The answers to these weighty questions must be drunk like a nectar and merit being heard by all beings in this universe, because when we listened to Rāma, we were gradually overwhelmed by the sensation that happiness does not exist, not even in heaven. O sages, let us gather together and listen to the reply of the supreme Vasiṣṭha. If we do not meditate in our hearts on what Rāma has said, it is we who are the losers, whatever our powers and faculties."

Vasiṣṭha replied: "O Rāma, you are truly the greatest of sages and there is nothing more for you to know. But be that as it may, your knowledge requires confirmation, like Śuka's knowledge needed Janaka's confirmation before he was able to find peace beyond all comprehension. Like you, Śuka also came to this point of no return after deeply contemplating the evanescence of the world. But his contemplation was still tainted by the tugging of the 'I', and the truth was not able to dwell within him. He did of course need to reach this stage of extreme dissatisfaction."

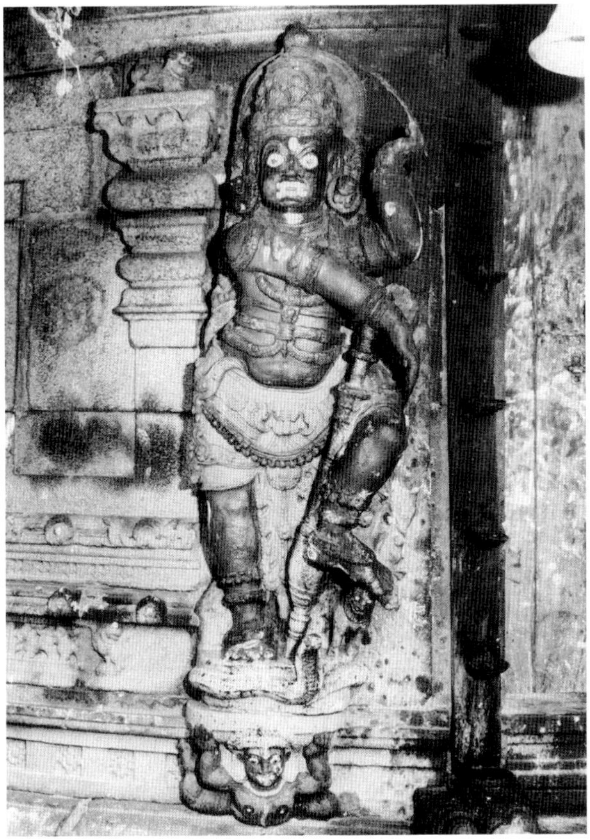

Dravida
17th century
(Chathannoor, Kollam, Kerala)

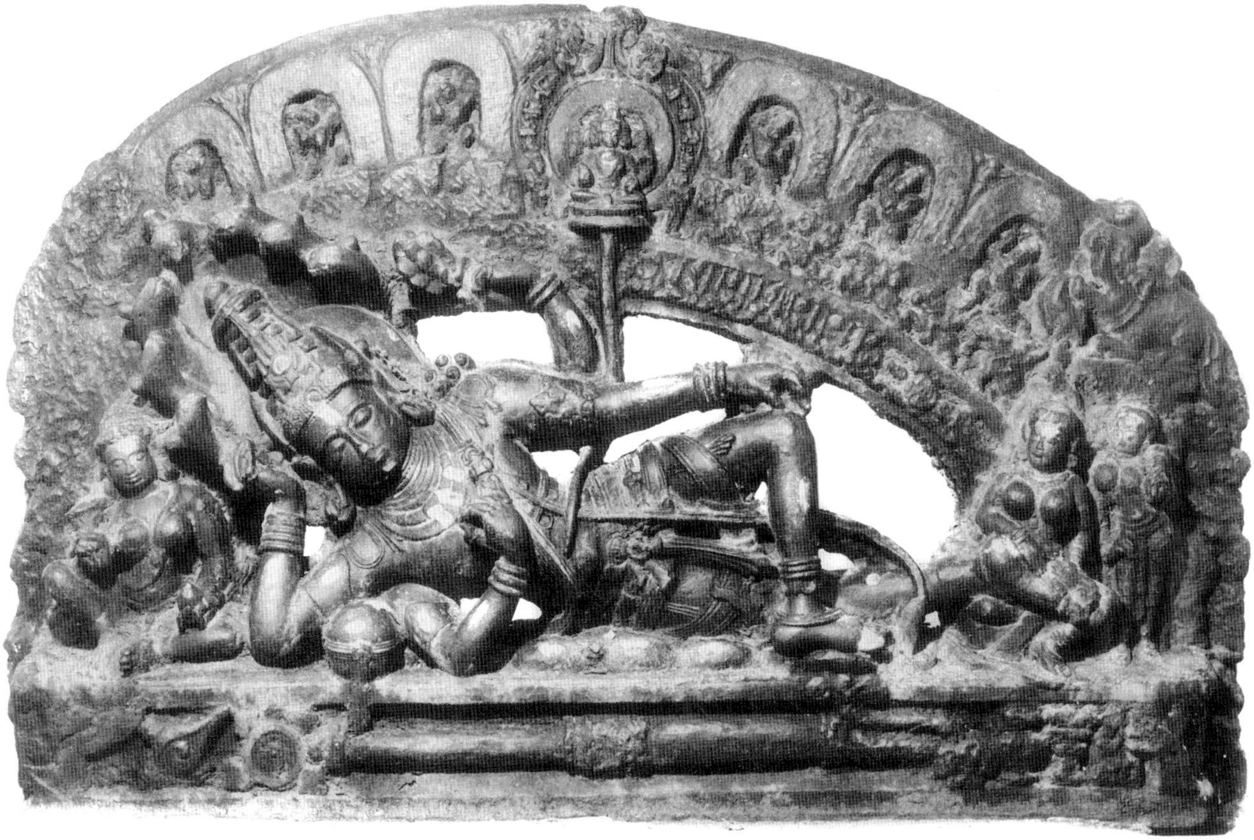

Viṣṇu-Anantaśayana *11th century (Ron, Karnataka)*

15

Waves of Emotion in the Ocean of Tranquillity

"If one makes one's mind stable in the various states of desire,
anger, greed, delusion, intoxication or envy,
then the Reality alone will remain which is underlying them."
VIJÑĀNA BHAIRAVA 101

"Just as when various objects such as pieces of wood, leaves, stones, etc.,
fall into a salt-mine they turn into salt,
so also emotions turn into bliss
when they fall into the pure Consciousness that is our very Self."
JAYARATHA, TANTRĀLOKAVIVEKA I, 2-35

A man staggers, his side pierced by a sword, the pain he bears written across his face. He shines with sorrow, glaring with lucidity, as he watches his world that consisted only of vanity come to an end. But what surprise! Before finally collapsing to the ground, he starts to sing! He sings of his despair to his enemies and friends alike, and his cry fills us with joy. This is the magic of opera and theatre, of lyrical suggestion (dhvani) where suffering is transformed into poetry. This is what Vālmīki relates, when, deeply touched by the suffering of a bird separated from its dead mate, his sorrow roars up as poetic brilliance to curse the hunter that had slain the bird.

"The blessed-one notices a couple of inseparable curlews singing and frolicking without a care in the world. And before his eyes, a hostile Niṣāda with a determination to sin kills the male. Seeing her mate's quivering and bloodstained body on the ground, the female cried out a pitiful song. She had been deprived of this copper-headed bird, her spouse and partner who, love-struck, was uniting with her. The blessed-one cried out: 'Niṣāda, may you never find peace for many a year for having killed this curlew who was abandoning himself to love'. Meditating on these words, he said to himself: 'How have I voiced my grief? These words that surged from me are divided into

four hemistiches of regular syllables and have the rhythm of a musical instrument. Because they were pronounced out of my grief (śoka), this poetic form, and no other, shall bear the name śloka'."
Rāmāyaṇa I, 2

Aesthetic resonance takes us back to the shiver of pure emotion. *"An individual is everywhere; he contains all feelings. The entire universe is his form."* (Abhinavagupta)

The term 'dhvani' was first used by grammarians (vaiyākaraṇa) to describe articulated sound through a non-articulated sound (sphoṭa), which represents its awareness. The concept of sphoṭa is very similar to the all inclusiveness of Consciousness for non-dualist Śaivites. It is attributed to a ṛṣi by the name of Sphoṭāyana, mentioned in the Pāṇini Sūtra. This word is derived from the root SPHUṬ meaning 'to open', 'to unfold', or 'that which develops from itself'. Patañjali speaks of it as the essence of words. Grammarians thus note that a word is made up of successively pronounced syllables. As soon as a syllable has been pronounced it disappears. They hence ask the following question: how can sounds that disappear as quickly as they are pronounced unite to make sense? In the word 'paper', when the syllable 'pa' is pronounced, the syllable 'per' has yet to be pronounced. When the syllable 'per' is pronounced, the syllable 'pa' has already disappeared. How can the whole meaning arise from successive and impermanent parts? Grammarians answer this with the sphoṭa theory and the underlying totality of sense preceding the articulated sound, which can only be articulated because of this wholeness. The following analogy is used to illustrate this: intuitive knowledge of a species is needed in order to recognise an individual belonging to it.
"Consciousness is present even in an instant of perception. Otherwise, how could actions such as running be possible or explicable, when deliberation about one's steps is not possible." Utpaladeva, Īśvarapratyabhijñākārikā I, 5.19

Dhvani also describes the functional, conventional and literal meaning, the sense resulting from relationships between words, as well as the capacity of suggestion in poetic creation. These definitions are unable to pay justice to the essence of the term. Ānandavardhana, as well as Abhinavagupta's commentary, say that rasa is the heart of dhvani. It is therefore not simply intellectual suggestion, or even passing emotions, but a sympathetic resonance of the heart, an inexpressible rapture.

"The word sahṛdaya (having their heart with that) denotes people able to identify with the subject. Since the mirror of their hearts has been polished by the constant practice of poetry, there is a sympathetic resonance of their hearts. It has been said that the realisation (bhāva) of the object, which is sympathetic resonance of the heart, is the origin of rasa. The body is pervaded by it, just as dry wood is pervaded by fire."
Abhinavagupta, Dhvanyālokalocana,
Ingalls, Masson, Patwardhan, Page 70

This resonance can only occur if there is a sympathetic response from the heart (hṛdayasaṃvāda), made possible by this savour that is already within us. This sympathetic response, or vibration of unity, caused by aesthetic experience, is merely the fragrance, the savour (rasa) of the permanent innate emotions (sthāyibhāva, sthāyi: persistent, basic) present in all human beings. According to Abhinavagupta, our ceaseless wandering in objectivity since time immemorial, which includes all experience, is the recipient for the latencies of all possible and imaginable emotional nuances, leading him to say: *"Nothing human is a stranger to us."*
Traditional Indian theatre acknowledges eight of these predominant emotions and their corresponding savours or feelings: love and amorous feeling, cheerfulness and humour, sorrow and pathos, anger and fury, ardour and heroic feeling, fear and dread, aversion and disgust, amazement and wonder. For Abhinavagupta, there is a

ninth savour, which is the source of all the others, the savour of peace (śāntarasa).

"He should unfold the eight rasa in the thrones of the eight deities. And in the centre he should unfold śāntarasa, the supreme God Śiva."
ŚĀNTARASA AND ABHINAVAGUPTA'S PHILOSOPHY OF AESTHETICS, MASSON, PATWARDHAN, PAGE 139

As waves rise up from the ocean, these mental states (bhāva) are only able to rise up from these persistent feelings. As Abhinavagupta notes, there is a huge difference between aesthetic emotion (rasa) and ordinary feeling (bhāva).

"Enjoyment of aesthetic experience consists of transcendental wonder (alaukikacamatkāra), and is decidedly different from ordinary knowledge produced by memory and inference."* ABHINAVAGUPTA, ABHINAVABHĀRATĪ, VOL. 1, PAGE 284

Ordinary emotion is quickly polluted by the feeling of rejection or by the desire to cling onto, depending on whether the emotion is painful or pleasant, thus preventing the possibility of distancing oneself from it. It becomes emotivity. In art, these same states give rise to rasa: the savour being the perception, freed of the affect of these same states. Paradoxically, as the spectator distances himself, the savour of the immediate and joyful evidence of his own substance re-emerges. We can, without fear, be fully open to the gamut of feelings without the agitation caused by emotivity. Abhinavagupta uses two terms to signify their difference: foreign to the world (alaukika) and beyond the world (lokottara). He also stipulates that experience of rasa differs from all ordinary cognition, memory, inference, or consciousness of oneself linked to attraction and aversion.

"Rasa is not an objective thing, which could function as a knowable object."
RANIERO GNOLI, THE AESTHETIC EXPERIENCE ACCORDING TO ABHINAVAGUPTA, PAGE 85

Although Abhinavagupta accepts the different nuances of aesthetic experience, he only acknowledges one fundamental savour, that of the fullness of our own nature. All other savours flow from this fundamental savour. There are three main savours (love: śṛṅgāra; anger: raudra; heroic feeling: vīra) upon which the others depend. They are said to be dependent because they only lead indirectly, through the other fundamental states (sthāyibhāva), to the four goals of life (puruṣārtha): prosperity (artha), pleasure (kāma), function (dharma) and emancipation (mokṣa).

"As the tree comes from the seed, the flower from the tree, and then the fruit from the flower, thus all the rasa are the root from which sentiments (bhāva) are manifested."
NĀṬYAŚĀSTRA VI, 36-38

* *Camatkāra:*
term meaning awareness filled with wonder, rapture, enchantment, but also the clicking of the tongue that accompanies this rapture, or when savouring a delicious dish.

The Amorous Shiver
(Śṛṅgārarasa)

The erotic or amorous (śṛṅgāra) aesthetic savour, whose basic emotion is that of love (rati), is very different to its mundane experience based on the intense attraction between two people. This mundane desire only lasts as long as the other person meets our criteria for security and affective gratification. It is therefore impermanent since the nature of its object is impermanent. Yet the components of the aesthetic savour of śṛṅgāra lie in the dramatisation of the mundane experience. Hence, individuality of the mundane experience becomes union and dissolution of lovers within love itself. The space-time shackle, which is the representation of individuality, dies in the representation of union and separation. This savour can only arise in the heart of the spectator by the symbolic representation of the amorous play of two individuals in union (yoga), in privation (ayoga), and above all in the feeling of separation (viprayoga).
It is said that the representation of love in union alone has no value, like a meal with only desserts, unless tainted with profound nostalgia. Rādhā who sheds tears for Kṛṣṇa, or Rāma who cries out after the abduction of Sītā: *"The effort I make to breathe is a mockery, Jānakī is my life"*, bring about a feeling of absoluteness, beyond time, beyond the person and beyond circumstances.

The same cry can be found in Hallāj's poem:
"Your place in my heart is my whole heart.
There is no room for anything else.
My soul put You between my skin and my bones.
What would I do if I were to loose You?
When I think of You, nostalgia almost kills me.
And my absence from You is grief and sorrow."

Or in Tukārām's poem:
"I am looking for You O Keśava,
With the wishful eyes of a newly married daughter
Who leaves the parental home.
I am looking for You
With the eyes of a baby that misses his mother.
Out of the water a fish twists,
Like a tortured Tukā."

It is the same fervour that leaves us bewildered when confronted with the vulnerability of Juliet's words to Romeo:
Romeo: *"Would'st thou withdraw it? For what purpose, love?"*
Juliet: *"But to be frank and give it thee again!*
And yet I wish but for the thing I have.
My bounty is as boundless as the sea,
My love as deep.
The more I give to thee, the more I have.
For both are infinite.
Parting is such sweet sorrow,
That I shall say goodnight 'til it be morrow."
W. Shakespeare, Romeo and Juliet, Act II, Scene 2

The etymology of the word śṛṅgāra only becomes even more striking. The root ŚṜ means 'to kill' (śṝhimsāyām, according to Uṇādisūtra 'Śṛṅgārabhṛṅgāra' – 423), because this rasa completely eliminates the feeling of personality. According to Ibn'Arabī, who described the forty-four conditions of the lover, the first condition is to be slain and the last is to ignore that one loves.

Fury

(Raudrarasa)

Anger (krodha) is the expression (bhāva) of the rasa of fury (raudra). It is evoked by indignation, intoxication, inconstancy, envy, cruelty, agitation, arrogance and insolence, which act as catalysers for excitement.

Duryodhana's fury towards the Pāṇḍava is legendary. When his mother told him he had everything he needed to be happy, youth and power, and that he should be satisfied, he replied in a bout of madness saying that satisfaction was for slaves! Duryodhana's fury resonates with our own dissatisfaction. This anger reached its peak in the battle between Bhīma and Duryodhana.

"To my mind, nobody is capable of conquering Duryodhana when he wields his club, not even someone immortal. He cannot be conquered when playing by the rules."

VĀSUDEVA, MAHĀBHĀRATA IX, 33.1-27; 58.1-10

Bhīma was only able to win by using a trick that was against all the rules of battle.

"The Pāṇḍava ran towards him roaring like a lion, and using all his strength struck Duryodhana's thighs with his club. The terrible action of Bhīma's weapon struck like lightning and broke Duryodhana's thighs...

"Seeing Duryodhana felled like a tall, uprooted tree filled the hearts of the Pāṇḍava with joy...

"The fiery Bhīma approached the fallen Kaurava king and said to him: 'Idiot! Do you remember how, in the sabhā, you called us cows and made fun of Draupadī who wore only a single garment! Today, you have reaped the fruit of this insult!'

"He then placed his left foot on the head of this lion amongst kings, and with his foot turned Duryodhana's head in all directions. 'In the past, the insane danced around us, calling us cows. And now it is our turn to dance around them and call them cows...'

"The best of the Somaka, doomed by nature to dharma, were discontented to see that a joyous Bhīma, of vile soul, had put his foot on the head of the best of the Kuru.

"Dharmarāja said to Bhīma, who was boasting and dancing like a madman: 'You have fulfilled your debt in this conflict; you have kept your promise by acting loyally, and even disloyally. Now you must stop! Do not crush his head with your foot. Do not violate dharma! This fallen King is your close kin. What you are doing is not proper, O immaculate one.'

"Seeing Bhīma stamping on the head of Duryodhana, the powerful Rāma (Baladeva), the best of warriors went into an extreme rage. He raised his arms, and in a voice made terrible through indignation, shouted: 'What shame, what shame, O Bhīma! Alas, what shame that a blow beneath the belt has been given in a battle fought according to dharma! What you have done has never before been seen in a confrontation using clubs! The treaties are clear. It is forbidden to hit below the belt. But this madman who knows not the treaties, does whatever he wants!'

"His fury intensified when he spoke. Baladeva, his eyes red with anger, looked at the king and continued: 'This man, who is my equal, did not only fall because he was inferior. But we blame the support when that which it supported was lacking in force'."

MAHĀBHĀRATA IX, 33.1-27; 58.1-10; 60.3-46

A paroxysm of anger and hatred can be a gateway to the absolute, as was the case for the ogress Pūtanā who intended to kill Kṛṣṇa. Her perpetual hatred pushed her into using the stratagem of pretending to be his mother and breast-feeding him as a child. It is said she was exempted from all 'sins' when he walked on her body. The demon Agha, brother of the ogress, harboured the same hatred up to the point of loathing. It is said he also obtained union with the object of his hatred when Kṛṣṇa entered into his mouth and suffocated him.

Uddhava considers demons (asura) entirely dedicated to the path of hatred towards Kṛṣṇa as devout.

"I regard the asura as devotees of the Supreme Lord because their minds are fixed on the Lord of the three worlds through their anger, and who on the battlefield, visualise him armed with the sudarśana disc, seated on the shoulder of Garuḍa attacking them."
BHĀGAVATAPURĀṆA III, 2.24

Viṣṇu reassures the worried brāhmaṇa who had cursed his two guardians, Jaya and Vijaya.
"The Lord said: O Brāhmaṇa, know that this curse of yours was ordained by me. My two guardians will be born as non-heavenly beings. Having developed their yoga through concentration intensified by wrath, both will return to me." And then Viṣṇu calms his guardians: *"Go now. Do not be afraid. May you be happy. Although it is within my powers, I shall not go against the brāhmaṇa; this is my will. It was ordained by Lakṣmī, who became enraged when you prevented her from entering whilst I was absorbed in Yogic sleep. You will quickly return to my presence by means of your concentration in me, stirred by your anger."*
BHĀGAVATAPURĀṆA III, 16.25-26-29-30-31

Kṛṣṇa also points out that those who concentrate on him, with bad intentions under the influence of anger, will become his devout followers.

"He who becomes a devotee intending to cause harm, or through hypocrisy, jealousy or under the influence of anger, and who only sees differences, shall be called a tamasic devotee."

But the most striking example is that of Rāvaṇa in the fourteenth century version of the Adhyātma Rāmāyaṇa. When killed by Rāma, Rāvaṇa was instantaneously liberated and reached the eternal Vaikuṇṭha.

"The sky was now filled with the delightful sound of the deva's drums. Showers of flowers fell upon Rāma... The deva witnessed how a light equal to that of the sun emerged from the body of Rāvaṇa and entered into Rāma. The deva said: 'Look at the good fortune of the great soul Rāvaṇa. Even we, virtuous as we are, special objects of Mahāviṣṇu's mercy, are immersed in saṃsāra, characterised by fear and sorrow. But see how this rākṣasa, who is known for his cruelty, who is antagonistic towards Viṣṇu, who is full of tamas, how even he has entered into Rāma before us all.' To the deva who were speaking of this, Nārada said with a smile: 'O deva who know the secret of dharma, listen! Rāvaṇa, on account of his antagonism towards Rāma, was always talking about him, even to his servants. His thoughts were continually of Rāma. Fearing that he would meet his death at the hands of Rāma, he was in the habit of seeing Rāma everywhere, even in his dreams. Rāvaṇa's anger towards Rāma served him far better than a preceptor or a guru. At the end, when killed by Rāma, he was freed of his sins and released from bondage, and become one with Rāma'."
ADHYĀTMA RĀMĀYAṆA II, 77-78

The Viṣṇu Purāṇa considers anger and rage towards Kṛṣṇa as a form of devotion as it provides a continual reminder (kīrtana) of Kṛṣṇa's name and is constant meditation, like an 'amorous hatred'.

"My only love sprung from my only hate!"
W. SHAKESPEARE, ROMEO AND JULIET, ACT I, SCENE 5

Heroic Feeling

(Vīrarasa)

Heroic feeling corresponds to the emotion of ardour. The transient colourations of this feeling are confidence, contentment, joy and arrogance.

According to Bhārata, there are traditionally three types of heroism: generous, religious and that of the warrior. Rāma personifies the perfect hero, having these three qualities in their purest and most uncluttered form.

This ardour (utsāha), whose energy is contagious, abolishes the limits of the possible. It is a source of wonder because it allows us to feel the unimportance of death. How otherwise could the madness of the Japanese swordsman Musashi be explained, who, knowingly, entered into the ambush of a famous sabre school whose reputation was at stake? He had to confront no less than sixty men who, far from being cowards, were accomplished samurai warriors. *"We are here to kill Musashi and we can't be too fussy as to how we go about it. A dead man does not tell stories."*

How can we explain the madness of this man who walked into certain death, a death he was fully prepared to embrace? One of his opponents said of him: *"He fights without a care for his own life. And because he does not fear death, orthodox methods of sword combat have no effect, as reason has no effect when confronted with folly."*

In the Dhvanyālokalocana, Abhinavagupta says that heroic feeling and wonder can combine together, because the glorious acts of heroes create amazement. And what can be more glorious than giving oneself so completely to death that it no longer exists?

Bhārata says: *"The effect of heroism is wonder."*
NĀṬYAŚĀSTRA VI, 41

Abhinavagupta also points out that: *"Heroism and cruelty blend together in a proud and noble hero such as Bhīma, because there is no obstruction between anger and heroic energy."* DHVANYĀLOKALOCANA III, 24

This non-obstruction is the heart of rasa, and especially of heroism. It is this total exaggeration for embracing life that fills us with admiration for heroes. All our pettiness melts away like snow in the sun when listening to Cyrano de Bergerac: *"But we do not fight hoping to win! No! It is far more beautiful when it is useless."*
EDMOND ROSTAND, CYRANO DE BERGERAC, ACT V, SCENE 6

In the tirade that follows, anger and heroism blend together and have a purifying effect:

*"To not please is my pleasure. I love it when I am hated.
My dear, if you knew how one walks better when followed by excited piercing eyes!
...Hatred is a shackle, but also a halo!"*
EDMOND ROSTAND, CYRANO DE BERGERAC, ACT II, SCENE 8

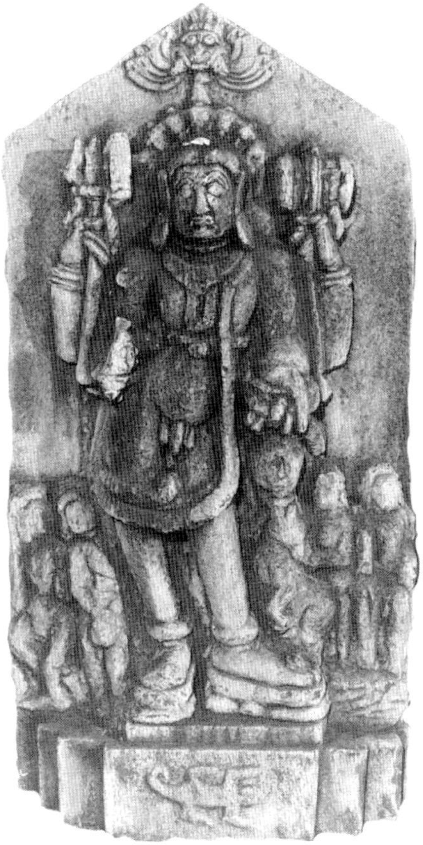

Vīrabhadra

12th century

(Someśvara Temple, Pura, Shimoga, Karnataka)

Disgust
(Bībhatsarasa)

The rasa of disgust corresponds to the emotion of aversion. Its associated transient states are those of agitation, disease, nausea, fainting and apprehension of death.
There are three sorts of disgust. The first plunges us into agitation (kṣobhana), and is linked to the sight of blood, entrails, bones and other horrible visions. The second chills, stiffens or shrinks the mind (udvegin) at the sight of repulsive and putrid scenes. The causes of this disgust are highly relative and subjective. For a surgeon, the sight of blood and bodily injuries does not give rise to the effects mentioned above. It may also be linked to cultural or moral conditioning, like the disgust Muslims hold for pork. A food that delights one palate will cause vomiting for someone allergic to it.
There exists a third type of disgust, linked precisely to the contemplation of the impermanence of objects, making us realise our complete vulnerability and the futility of all human enterprise. This is why some yogis live in crematorium grounds. Others maintain that the whole world is simply one great cremation ground (mahāśmaśāna). This disgust is said to be pure as it disengages us from objectivity. In one famous passage from the Bible, the Ecclesiast expresses this disgust.
"I, the preacher was king over Israel in Jerusalem. I devoted myself to study and to explore by wisdom all that is done under heaven. What a heavy burden God has laid on men! I have seen all the things that are done under the sun; all of them are meaningless, a chasing after the wind. What is twisted cannot be straightened; what is lacking cannot be counted.
I thought to myself: 'Look, I have grown and increased in wisdom more than anyone who has ruled over Jerusalem before me; I have experienced much of wisdom and knowledge.' Then I applied myself to the understanding of wisdom, and also of madness and folly, but I learned that this, too, is a chasing after the wind. For with much wisdom comes much sorrow; the more knowledge, the more grief.
I thought in my heart: 'Come now, I will test you with pleasure to find out what is good.' But that also proved to be meaningless. 'Laughter,' I said, 'is foolish. And what does pleasure accomplish?' I tried cheering myself with wine, and embracing folly - my mind still guiding me with wisdom. I wanted to see what was worthwhile for men to do under heaven during the few days of their lives. I undertook great projects: I built houses for myself and planted vineyards. I made gardens and parks and planted all kinds of fruit trees in them. I made reservoirs to water groves of flourishing trees. I bought male and female slaves and had other slaves that were born in my house. I also owned more herds and flocks than anyone in Jerusalem before me. I amassed silver and gold for myself, and the treasure of kings and provinces. I acquired men and women singers, and a harem as well - the delights of the heart of man. I became greater by far than anyone in Jerusalem before me. In all this my wisdom stayed with me. I denied myself nothing my eyes desired; I refused my heart no pleasure. My heart took delight in all my work, and this was the reward for all my labour. Yet when I surveyed all that my hands had done and what I had toiled to achieve, everything was meaningless, a chasing after the wind; nothing was gained under the sun.
Then I turned my thoughts to consider wisdom, and also madness and folly. What more can the king's successor do than what has already been done? I saw that wisdom is better than folly, just as light is better than darkness. The wise man has eyes in his head, while the fool walks in the darkness; but I came to realise that the same fate overtakes them both. Then I thought in my heart: 'The fate of the fool will overtake me also. What then do I gain by being wise?' I said in my heart: 'This too is meaningless.' For the wise man, like the fool, will not be long remembered; in days to come both will be forgotten. Like the fool, the wise man too must die. So I hated life, because the work that is done under the sun was grievous to me. All of it is meaningless, a chasing after the wind."

Humour
(Hāsyarasa)

The rasa of humour corresponds to the emotion of cheerfulness or gaiety. Absurdity is the catalyst for this contagious emotion, a bit like a good yawn causes others to yawn, or watching someone savouring a delicious food causes salivation.
Abhinavagupta describes two causes of humour: that which is direct or which originates from oneself (ātmastha hāsya), caused by an absurd situation; and that which is indirect, stemming from another (parastha hāsya) and for which the object of absurdity is unknown. Humour stems from upheaval, where the normal framework of a situation is shattered. Humour has always been used to transmit a spontaneous openness that dissolves the decor of our concepts.

Succulent passages can be found in the life of Drungpa Kunley, the divine madman. One day he joins a group of monks in philosophical debate. He butts in and says: *"I too am knowledgeable in metaphysics"*. He then breaks wind and says: *"Which came first, the sound or the smell?"*

Laughter bursts references and unfolds a lightheartedness of non-separation, hence the expression 'to burst out laughing'. Legend tells that when Bodhidharma awakened, he burst out laughing and had a cup of tea. Laughter is sometimes so intense that we laugh until we cry. The object is completely forgotten and we don't know whether to laugh or cry. There is amnesia of the how and why; all answers are forgotten and everything joins together and exudes the same vibration.

Pathos
(Karuṇarasa)

The rasa of pathos corresponds to the emotion of pain, sorrow, grief. Its associated transient states are those of agitation, despair, anxiety, stupor, dementia, depression, disease, indolence and death.
In the Rāmāyaṇa and Mahābhārata, karuṇa is the determining factor for peace and tranquillity. In the Rāmāyaṇa, Vālmīki talks of it from the outset, putting it into verse. It is present throughout, right until the final paroxysm, the irreversible separation of Sītā and Rāma, when Rāma must banish Sītā even though she is with child.

"Fearing shame, I see no way of keeping Janaka's daughter. Just look at the ocean of grief in which I am drowning! There is no greater tragedy than this! Saumitri, at dawn tomorrow, climb onto your cart, driven by Sumantra. Drive Sītā to the country's limits, and abandon her... Upon hearing these words, the virtuous kākutstha, his eyes full of tears and blowing like an elephant, took leave of his brothers."
RĀMĀYAṆA VII, XLV

Rāma must also sentence his brother Lakṣmaṇa to death because of the promise made to the ṛṣi Kāla, who bore a message: *"This conversation must not go beyond our ears if the interest of the gods is to be respected. You must kill anyone who hears or sees us if the words of the greatest of ascetics are to be respected."* Meanwhile, the sage Durvāsa goes to the palace gates and asks to see Rāma. He is received by Lakṣmaṇa, who questions him about the motive of his visit and asks him to wait because he knows his brother cannot be disturbed. Durvāsa then goes into one of his legendary fits of anger.

"Durvāsa, tiger of the ṛṣi, was greatly annoyed by these questions. Staring at Lakṣmaṇa as though he was going to set him on fire, he exclaimed: 'Saumitri, inform Rāma

of my presence immediately, otherwise I will curse all of you, the kingdom, the town, you yourself, and even Rāghava, Bhārata and all your family. Enough is enough! Hurry up! I can no longer contain this indignation within my heart.'
The sage, having just finished a thousand years of ascetic practice, was hungry and wanted nourishment. It was with great pleasure that Rāma offered the greatest of ascetics the food available in his kitchens. But Rāma, remembering the words of Kāla, was filled with despair. Overwhelmed by grief, Rāma kept his head lowered and was unable to pronounce a single word. He just tried to imagine everything around him no longer existed and that his sorrow would die away into a deep silence. When he saw Rāghava with his head down in despair, like the moon during an eclipse, Lakṣmaṇa said, joyfully: 'O powerful king, don't feel sorry for me, Kāla's visit and what ensues is merely the outcome of a plan decided long ago. You must fulfil your promise. Kill me without hesitation.' Vasiṣtha, after having heard the terrible curse, declared: 'Being separated from Lakṣmaṇa is the worst thing that could happen. O Rāma, it is a terrible situation, yet you must banish him. You cannot go back on the promise made to the powerful Kāla. Tiger of men, to preserve creation, you must today separate yourself from Lakṣmaṇa in order the universe may be saved.'
After having listened to these words, approved by all, Rāma turned to Lakṣmaṇa and said: 'I banish you Saumitri in order that dharma may be saved. Whether you choose exile or death, it makes no difference to someone as good as you.' Upon hearing these words, Lakṣmaṇa left hurriedly, his eyes full of tears. He went to the bank of the Sarayu and entered into the water, joining his hands in respect. He then closed all of his body's orifices and held his breath."
RĀMĀYAṆA VII, CHAPTERS CIV, CV, CVI, CVII

After the ritual suicide of his brother, Rāma gave up his kingdom, withdrew into the forest and *"from that day on, followed the path taken by Lakṣmaṇa."*

Similarly in the Mahābhārata, the story of the collapse of what appears to be indestructible, of power in all its forms, of wealth, strength and beauty, fill us with the most intimate of questions, that which is most essential. How can we not question the ways of the world when we learn of the end of these two families, the Kaurava and Pāṇḍava? The civil war was also to completely destroy Kṛṣṇa's lineage, the Vṛṣṇi.

"Having heard the details of the great slaughter of the Vṛṣṇi, the Kaurava king set his heart on leaving the world. He addressed Arjuna, saying: 'O thou of great intelligence, it is Time that cooks every creature in its cauldron.'"
MAHĀBHĀRATA XVII

The Pāṇḍava chose 'the great road' (mahāpatha), the death pilgrimage, where one walks into the Himalaya until annihilation. All these heroes and heroines, these worthy men and women, meet with an unhappy end. Even Kṛṣṇa is not spared from a miserable death, without glory, accidentally killed by a hunter.

Arjuna tells of his grief to Vyāsa: *"Kṛṣṇa is dead. The Yādava have been clubbed to death. It was a horrible slaughter! Not even one of the great heroes escaped. Five hundred thousand warriors wiped out with bludgeons made from blades of erakā grass. There is no joy in living without Kṛṣṇa. Tell me what to do? I am a wanderer with an empty heart. My dearest are dead and I am weak."*

"It was written and was meant to happen. Kṛṣṇa could have stopped it but he let it be. So you have no need to grieve. The hand of Time is behind all things. Kāla is the seed of the universe. Kāla gives and takes back. Kāla gives joy and suffering. One day you are the master, the next you are the servant. One day you are powerless and the next day it could change. Now your time has almost come and you must surrender to the supreme."
MAHĀBHĀRATA XVI

The rasa of pathos gives rise to profound disenchantment with the world as an object, as exteriority. There can be no real questioning as long as our efforts are scattered in the search for satisfaction, running after the phantoms of our projections, too busy fulfilling our lives with psychological destinations that die as soon as they are reached. When this disenchantment comes to maturity, we find ourselves in a state of complete availability where the unique question is able to shine forth. In this questioning there is peace.

"The more worldly affairs go wrong for us and lose their substance, the more our disenchantment will grow; of this there is no doubt." Bhīṣma, Mahābhārata XII, 168.4

For the question 'who am I?' to become a burning question, there must be a blatant hopelessness of all exteriority. From a yogic point of view, we can say that the worse things are, the better they are! The sinking of social, relational and financial structures is a desirable and unavoidable meditation. The failure of worldliness is therefore a gift, a blessing.

"Look at this Oedipus, this expert of famous riddles, who became the first human. There was no one from his town able to contemplate his destiny without feeling envious. But today, into what flood of dreadful misery has he been hastened? Hence, for mere mortals, it is this final day one must always consider. Be careful never to say a man is happy before he has reached the end of his life without having suffered sorrow."
Sophocles' Oedipus, Last Monologue

"The ultimate meaning of the Mahābhārata thus appears very clearly. The two subjects intented by the author as primary are the rasa of peace and the human goal of liberation. The other rasa and human goals are subordinated to these..."
Ānandavardhana, Dhvanyāloka IV, 5a

Abhinavagupta adds that the aesthetic experience of pathos, whose basic emotion is that of grief, is not unpleasant as it is disengaged of all individuality.

Wonder
(Adbhutarasa)

The rasa of wonder corresponds to the emotion of amazement. Its associated transient states are those of joy, agitation and contentment.
Wonder opens and wipes clear the horizon of ordinary perception. The state of rapture, which can lead to the sublime, can occur through the vision of something seemingly impossible that causes stupefaction.
Mundane perception is filtered. All that is not essential to biological, social or psychological survival is smothered. When feeling amazement, this 'reducing value', to use Aldous Huxley's expression, does not operate. An object in its most ordinary state is in essence something extraordinary.

"Draperies, as I had now discovered, are much more than devices for the introduction of non-representational forms into naturalistic paintings and sculptures. What the rest of us see only under the influence of mescalin, the artist is congenitally equipped to see all the time. His perception is not limited to what is biologically or socially useful. A little knowledge belonging to Mind at Large oozes past the reducing value of brain and ego, into his Consciousness. It is a knowledge of the intrinsic significance of every existent. For the artist as for the mescalin taker, draperies are living hieroglyphs that stand in some peculiar expressive way for the unfathomable mystery of pure being. More even than the chair, though less perhaps than those wholly supernatural flowers, the folds of my grey flannel trousers were charged with 'is-ness'. To what they owed

this privileged status, I cannot say. Is it, perhaps, because the forms of folded drapery are so strange and dramatic that they catch the eye and in this way force the miraculous fact of sheer existence upon the attention? Who knows?... For the glory and the wonder of pure existence belong to another order, beyond the power of even the highest art to express. But I could clearly see what, if I had been a painter of genius, I might have made of my old grey flannels. Not much, heaven knows, in comparison with the reality, but enough to delight generation after generation of beholders, enough to make them understand at least a little of the true significance of what, in our pathetic imbecility, we call 'mere things' and disregard in favour of television."
ALDOUS HUXLEY, THE DOORS OF PERCEPTION

The ultimate amazement is the intuitive recognition of one's own nature, where we are left flabbergasted, speechless, without expression, without definition, without explanation.

It is said in the Śivasūtra: *"Wonder is the heart of the stages in yoga."* (I, 12)

In his commentary, Kṣemarāja explains that: *"One is struck with wonder upon seeing something extraordinary. In the same way, there is a pleasant surprise for the great yogi who notices in mute wonder an expansion of his entire complex of senses, as they come fully under the influence of the inner Self which is a mass of Consciousness and full of unique, pre-eminent and ever new delight of I-consciousness, which blossoms forth in the experience of the various objects of perception. He is filled with wonder when, in the intensity of his contemplation, he feels the wheel of energies, as organs, gradually open, come to a standstill or fully spread. This amazement is without end because the yogi never tires of this spontaneous bliss that ceaselessly gushes in his heart. Adhering to this natural state as being Supreme reality is a magical wonder, which is at the heart of the seasons of yoga..."*

A stanza of the Spandakārikā also mentions: *"How can there be the wretched flow of transmigratory existence for he, who, struck by wonder, perceives his own self as the ground of all existence?"*
VASUGUPTA, SPANDAKĀRIKĀ I, 11

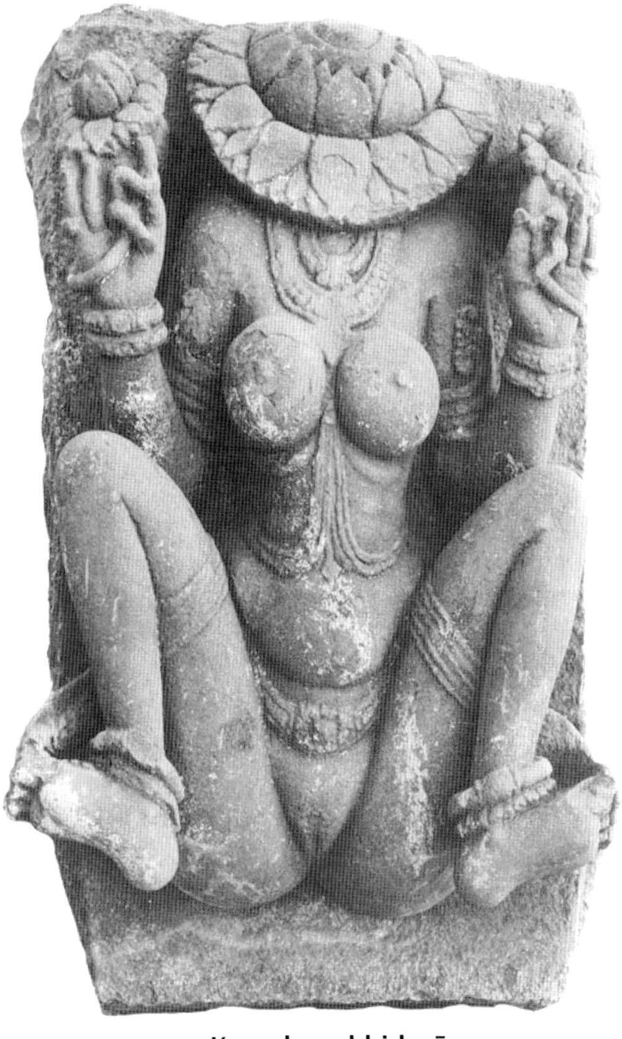

Kamalamukhidevī
7th century (Mahakuta, Bijapur, Karnataka)

Dread
(Bhayānakararasa)

The rasa of dread or terror corresponds to the emotion of fear. Amongst its associated transient states are those of agitation, trembling, quivering, paleness, crying out, stupor and anguish.
Solitary places, the feeling of insecurity, cries of wild animals or enemies, a terrifying noise, the vision of horrible incidents or monstrous creatures all have decisive influences on this emotion. These influences are only pretexts to reveal the fundamental fear that hides behind all other fears: the fear of death, annihilation, of not being. Tantric iconography and some tantric rituals depict evocations whereby the body-mind becomes the offering to wrathful deities.

"Imagine this body, that is the result of your own tendencies, to be a dead, fat, enormous prey that fills the entire universe.
Imagine the radiant intelligence that is within you as being the wrathful goddess yielding a knife and a skull.
Then imagine she cuts-off your head and places your skull like an enormous cauldron on top of three other skulls that act as the feet of a tripod covering the three regions.
And that she cuts-up your body into small bits and throws them into the skull as an offering to the deities..."
Vision of the Corpse and the Wrathful Deity
(Tibetan Yoga of the Ningmapa tradition)

These evocations, which take place in the body itself, are of different intensities. They awaken the taste of death and are expressed in a variety of experiences: sensation of vertigo or of falling, impossibility of moving one's body, images of terrifying forms that eat us raw, terrible noises, being burnt alive, having one's throat cut, being chopped up into small pieces, being suffocated or being unable to breath. The feeling of dread is a contemplation of our finitude. In the yogic ritual, which is in essence an art of death, dread is the meditation on our different grasps and conditionings. All we know about ourselves, our knowledge, our experiences, the world we have built up and projected, all our efforts to continue living by having mental and emotional strategies, will all one day come to an end. These evocations do not need to take on exotic forms, which in many cases are only another way of escaping. They can and must be directly related to our situation in the instant. We do not need to go to India to meditate in a cremation ground (śmaśāna). The image of a supermarket, a Saturday afternoon, the accident and emergency wing of a hospital or a reality television show all provide suitable opportunities. Our wife or husband who wants a divorce and wants to keep the house and all the money in the bank account can become a magnificent wrathful deity. Each insult is like the sacred knife that cuts into our fear and attachments, that guts our arrogance and severs the limbs of our illusions. This sacred fear that leaves us with an absence of knowledge, a vulnerability, is itself tranquillity.

"In a state of fear or sorrow, standing on top of an abyss or while fleeing from the battlefield, the illusion of separation ceases."
Vijñāna Bhairava 118

According to the Vijñāna Bhairava, one of the etymologies of Bhairava is 'he, who, with fear, makes everything resound, and who pervades the entire universe'.

Tranquillity
(Śāntarasa)

The rasa of tranquillity corresponds to the state of quietude. The basic emotion is neutrality (sama) with regards to objectivity. This neutrality (sama) or tranquillity (śānta) comes from realising the insubstantiality of the universe, as well as from being deeply disenchanted (nirveda) with the objects that make up the universe. The desire for tranquillity is in fact at the heart of all our actions, all our experiences and all our desires. When a desire is fulfilled, we savour the restfulness of non-becoming. We attribute this tranquillity to the object, where in fact it simply reflects our own quietude. This is the reason a certain wearing-down of objectivity, of everything external to us, is needed. The body-mind is part of this exteriority. When the thirst (tṛṣṇā) of becoming, of the love of sense objects dies, we can then taste the quietude (tṛṣṇākṣayasukha, happiness from the cessation of desire) of no longer needing to define ourselves, of involving ourselves and of proving ourselves in destinations that are never reached.

"In vain did I milk a bull mistaking it for a cow bending under the burden of her full udder; in vain did I embrace an ugly eunuch thinking him to be a young girl; in vain did I cherish a longing for a piece of glittering glass thinking it to be beryl. All this I did when bemused as I was, I bowed to you, a miser unable to appreciate merit."
STANZA QUOTED BY ABHINAVAGUPTA IN THE ABHINAVABHĀRATĪ, ŚĀNTARASAPRAKARAṆAṂ

Each situation questions us about the essential, about what cannot be abandoned. It is only the clothing of circumstances that can be taken from us. All that we may think ourselves to be, including these thoughts themselves, all that we call 'I', our entire psychophysical structure, is destined for the scrapyard. According to Abhinavagupta, this intuition of the essential (tattvajñāna), through the impermanence of things, is the natural quenching of cognitive thirst.

"It is possible for ordinary people to imagine what it is like from their own experience at the time when the course of desire for all objects of the senses, such as food, etc., has completely ceased because of having eaten to satiation."
ABHINAVAGUPTA, DHVANYĀLOKALOCANA

According to Abhinavagupta, this is the unique and real happiness:
"And the peaceful is indeed apprehended as a rasa. It is characterised by the full unfolding of happiness that comes from the dying of desire. As it is said: 'The joy of pleasure in this world and the greater joy of pleasures found in heaven are not worth a sixteenth of the joy that comes from the end of desire'."
ABHINAVAGUPTA QUOTING THE MAHĀBHĀRATA (XIII, 174.46) IN HIS DHVANYĀLOKALOCANA

In a passage from The Secret of the Goddess Tripurā, Hemalekhā, the daughter of a fairy, initiates her husband Hemacūḍa to the peaceful vision. The prince, worried about his wife's indifference of their amorous games, questions her by saying:
"How can I be happy at your side as long as you continue to despise sensory objects? It is as though I am making love to a wooden doll! And yet nothing arouses my desire other than you! I follow you everywhere like a blossoming lotus follows the moonlight. O you who is dearer to me than life itself, I beg you to calm my mind by making clear your intentions!"

She replies to him by shedding light on the relativity and evanescence of pleasure.
"Please do enlighten me. Once you have, I will abandon all these cogitations, and day after day, I will not cease to devote myself to pleasures in your company...

You said pleasure is good and pain evil. But a one and same thing is able to give both pleasure and pain depending on the place and the instant. How then is it possible to decide something as fixed? Fire can produce different effects depending on circumstances. In winter it is pleasant, in summer unpleasant. It is pleasant for those with a cold constitution, unpleasant for those with a hot constitution. It can also be pleasant in small doses and unpleasant in excessive quantities. The same is true of all things. Man is filled with thousands of desires. How can fulfilling a desire be enough to make him happy? An ounce of sandalwood pulp applied to a man whose limbs have been burnt is not enough to cool him! There is no doubt that a man who kisses a woman he loves senses pleasure; but there is also pleasure in the violence and suffering of embrace. Look how lovers are as exhausted as beasts of burden after making love. That you are able to consider this as happiness leaves me perplexed. You may tell me that a man's pleasure is of higher quality because it stems from the contemplation of feminine beauty. But this is pure imagination, like the union with a woman in dreams. Beauty, my dear husband, is only that which the mind projects and wishes to see. You find me beautiful and this is the reason you enjoy intense pleasure with me. But others succeed in enjoying a similar or even greater pleasure with women you find ugly. So tell me, in these conditions, how in this world can it be decided that one thing is pleasant and another unpleasant?"

Śāntarasa is merely the ocean upon which waves are formed, waves that are never separated from it. These waves may bear different names, take on different forms, but in essence they have the same savour: restfulness in non-differentiation.

"Śāntarasa is that state wherein one feels the same towards all creatures, wherein there is no pain, no happiness, no hatred and no envy. Śānta is the natural state of mind (prakṛti). Other emotions such as love, etc. are colourations of that original state. These colourations arise out of this natural state of mind and in the end merge back into it. The emotions arise out of śānta depending on their particular respective causes. And when the specific causes cease to function they all merge back into śānta."

VERSES ATTRIBUTED TO BHĀRATA AND QUOTED BY ABHINAVAGUPTA (ABHINAVABHĀRATĪ, PAGE 340)

The rasa that spread softness (mādhura guṇa) are the amorous shiver (śṛṅgāra), pathos (karuṇa) and tranquillity (śānta); these cause the heart to melt. The rasa of vitality and force (ojas guṇa) are fury (raudra), heroic feeling (vīra), wonder (adbhuta) and disgust (bībhatsa); these cause the heart to expand and burn. The rasa of humour (hāsya) and dread (bhayānakara) unfold the characteristics of the two guṇa mentioned above, according to the situation. Clarity and lucidity (prasāda) are qualities common to all rasa. In āsana practice, different moods are perceived, through bodily sensation, as the extension of space. No attempt is ever made to appropriate an emotion or an explanation of this emotion. Bodily ramifications of the emotions felt provide a gateway to welcome all that arises from an impersonal viewpoint. The body is thus free to become a stage, a theatre, where we can experiment with these sensations, free from emotivity and reactivity, and then later transpose them into our daily lives.

"When owing to the absence of limitation, the aberration of the modes of the mind caused by the non-recognition of the essential nature ceases, the very states of anger, delusion, etc., appear as only an expression of the Consciousness of the perfect, revered Lord Bhairava Himself. As revered Somānanda has said: 'Śiva is that whose very nature consists in the expansion of His Śakti' (Śivadṛṣṭi III, 94)."

ABHINAVAGUPTA, PARĀTRĪŚIKĀVIVARAṆA, JAIDEVA SINGH, PAGE 40

"Whether it is the state of pleasure (the expression of sattva), or of pain (the expression of rajas), or of delusion

(the expression of tamas), I abide in all of them as the supreme Śiva."
UTPALADEVA'S COMMENTARY ON THE ŚIVADṚṢṬI, VII, 105

"Even the states of anger etc., exist because of their identity with the wondrous play of the divine Consciousness, otherwise their very existence would be impossible. The divine Śakti of the senses themselves carrying out the various play of life are like the rays of Śiva-sun. These states of anger, etc., at the time of their arising are of the form of nirvikalpa, i.e. they are sheer energy of the divine."
ABHINAVAGUPTA, PARĀTRĪŚIKĀVIVARAṆA, JAIDEVA SINGH, PAGE 40-41

Tranquillity lies at the heart of all āsana, and actualising this tranquillity in a pose, even the most dynamic, is the essence of āsana. At the start of the learning process, attention is paid to the different grips in the body, senses and breathing, and to the process of resistance and effort, all of which are chaotic movements that occur when performing an āsana. Little by little we settle into an āsana and make ourselves comfortable with the discomforts it may cause. We become conscious that as soon as there is discomfort, the breathing becomes blocked, the diaphragm hardens, the throat tightens, and the frontal brain, eyes, temples and ears cement. We thus learn, in a tactile way, to connect all apparitions generated by an āsana, pleasant or unpleasant, to space. We then let this attentiveness diffuse, firstly in simple āsana and then in more complicated ones. When a certain tactile maturity has been reached in various postural forms, we are then able to learn how to play with the moods and colorations of an āsana. Can I practise intense āsana, such as certain backbends, whilst developing the savour of introversion experienced in the frontal brain, eyes, ears, tongue and throat that other āsana such as Sarvāṅgāsana, Ardha Halāsana or Ṣaṇmukhīmudrā give? Can I keep the dynamism of the legs in standing āsana whilst in Sarvāṅgāsana, without losing the fragrance of jālandharabandha in the frontal brain? When coming out of an āsana, attention should be paid to the resonance of the āsana as it fades away, and how a sort of spontaneous spreading occurs. Thus, when coming out of a standing āsana, listen to its resonance in Samasthiti. This resonance is the intuitive echo of Śavāsana.

"When waves strongly stir quiet water if one looks attentively one can find the origin of the motion, that is the orientation; or when one makes a fist, one can sense the initial shiver. Some describe it as a kind of swelling."
SOMĀNANDA, ŚIVADṚṢṬI I, 13B-15-16-17

With more mastery, this happens during the pose, and the āsana becomes the echo of Śavāsana. The different moods, attitudes and emotions are thus experienced in the body's theatre as the actualisation of the rasa of tranquillity (śāntarasa). This participates in sinking the illusion of separation. The āsana are unfolded spontaneously, without a doer.

"Having thus perceived one's own body as the recipient of pure Consciousness, all divisions having disappeared, one abides all powerful, identical to the Lord."
ABHINAVAGUPTA, TANTRĀLOKA IV, 119B-120A

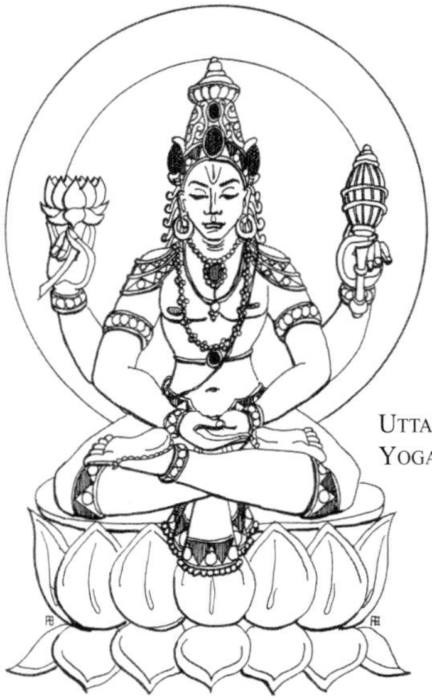

UTTAMA-YOGAŚAYANAMŪRTI

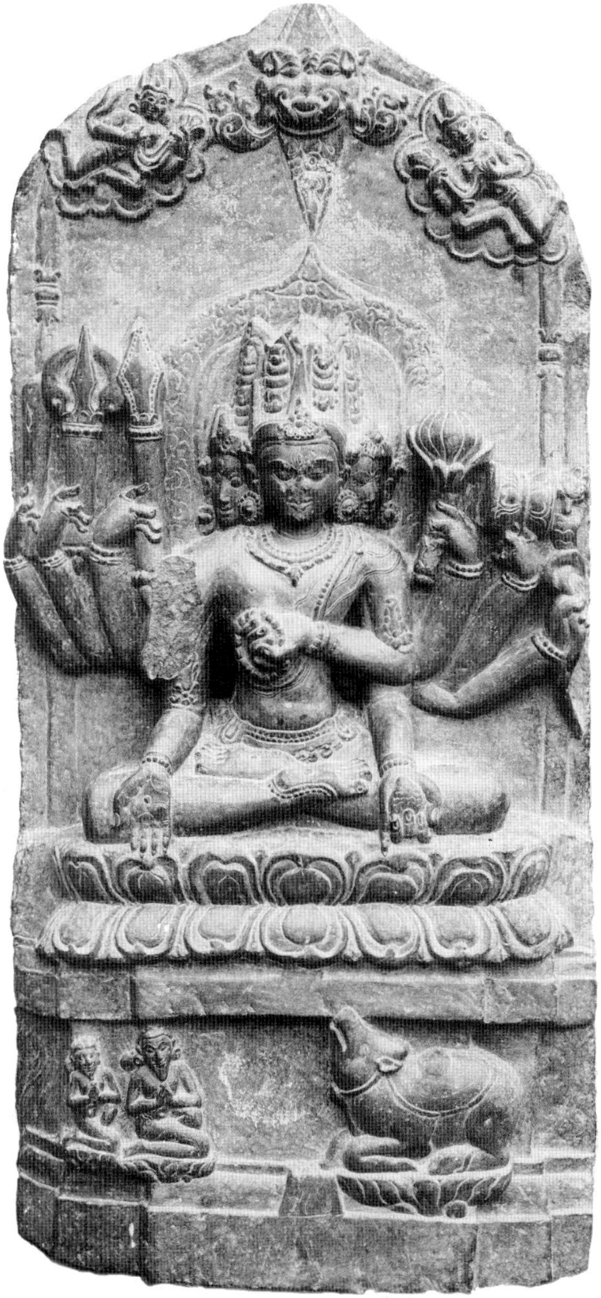

Sadāśivamūrti
10th century
(Hili, Bengal)

16

The Guru-Śiṣya Relationship: The Ultimate Swindle

Tales of Recognition

"The Self who is the natural state of all existents, who is self-luminous, amusing Himself with question-answer which is not different from Himself, and in which both the questioner (as Devī) and the answerer (as Bhairava) are only Himself, enjoys self-reflection."

ABHINAVAGUPTA, PARĀTRĪŚIKĀVIVARAṆA, JAIDEVA SINGH, PAGE 48

"Praise be to He who possesses within Him the three worlds, to this Reality which is His own! Homage to the spiritual master, to Śiva, who is both the way and the goal."

ANONYMOUS

"The manifestations of the self and others, of master and disciple, are merely imaginary constructions. Even the union of the blazing energy of the master and the disciple too is only imagination since they have never been separated."

ABHINAVAGUPTA, TANTRĀLOKA I, 233-234

The dream is gloomy and suffocating. You are being chased by a monster and are terribly frightened. You aren't able to identify it but you recognise it because it has always been there, hidden away in your life, like an inexpressible presence. It scares you to death; all your fears and phobias are condensed into it. It is the Himalaya of terror. You run until you are gasping for breath, hoping to find an emergency exit. Then suddenly you see him. There he is! Calm. Bearing all the signs of a spiritual Father Christmas: the beard of realisation, the thick hair of wellbeing, marks showing his affiliation, a gaze of Valium, barbiturate remarks. He asks you to sit down and then shows you a captivating, hypnotising exercise. The monster is forgotten! In the dream of separation, the guru can take the form of the ultimate distraction, allowing us to forget the total deadlock of our annihilation, the devouring mouth of death that has already swallowed-up a million universes, avatars, prophets and gurus. Yet the monster, guru and disciple are merely part of the dream.

"There is no disappearance, nor origination;
no one in bondage, no one who works for success;
no one desirous of emancipation, no one emancipated.
This is the highest truth."
GAUḌAPĀDA, ĀGAMAŚĀSTRA II, 32

"No individual soul is born,
nor is there any possibility of it.
This is that highest reality where nothing is born."
GAUḌAPĀDA, ĀGAMAŚĀSTRA III, 48

"I do not exist, neither does anyone else.
I only exist as energy (śakti)."
ABHINAVAGUPTA, TANTRĀLOKA XXIX, 64

Far from the caricature of the guru who cements our affiliations and strengthens the ramparts of our identity, there remains a question of existential etymology. One of the etymologies of guru is 'he who is heavy': a weighty reminder of the overwhelming evidence pointing to the lightness of non-separation, of 'what I am not'. The guru is referred to in this way because he his steadfast and unwavering before this evidence. Traditionally, in India, the imprint of this evidence can be found at all levels of existence, right down to the farthest depths of social fabric. Vedic transmission is referred to as nigamana and has a connotation of deduction. Tantric transmission is referred to as āgamana and occurs intuitively.

"The author of all āgama is the omniscient Supreme being. The real sense of the term revelation (āgama) is vimarśa, becoming freely aware of the Supreme Lord, whose light is unbroken and from whom nothing is unknown."
ABHINAVAGUPTA, ĪŚVARAPRATYABHIJÑĀVIMARŚINĪ, ĀGAMĀDHIKĀRA, ĀHNIKA 1

Tantra has thus no need for Vedic confirmation. Its sole validity is that of intuitive experience, and Abhinavagupta describes it as the tradition of experience or intuitive feeling (anubhavasaṃpradāya). Tantra rejects the exclusivity of being qualified by caste, race or sex. It is described as being the fifth Veda because it makes explicit that which was only implicit in the Veda. The revelation of this evidence, whether Vedic or Tantric, is heard (śruti) and is transmitted orally. In the Tantric texts it takes the form of a dialogue between Śiva and Pārvatī. Abhinavagupta explains this dialogue as that of our own Consciousness.

"In conclusion, it is said that this connotes the union of Rudra and Rudrā (Rudrayāmala), i.e. of Śiva and Śakti where there is no division of question and answer, which is the state of awareness of the essential Self (svarūpa-amarśana)."
ABHINAVAGUPTA, PARĀTRĪŚIKĀVIVARAṆA, JAIDEVA SINGH, PAGE 269

This intuition takes on the venerated form of the guru, or ācārya. One of the first functions of the ācārya is to bring to life, in the instant, that which has been transmitted since ancient times. This oral transmission is made doubly sacred by the language of the gods, Sanskrit (gīrvāṇabhāṣā), and by the word of the guru, which is timeless. Both of which participate in the gushing forth and burying of the mystery.
A whole network of manifestations (aṅga) has sprouted from the eternity of this evidence (sanātanadharma) to explore its different facets.

"The Self, made up of the Veda and sacred Revelations, spreads out, ramified into thousands of branches; homage to Him, Śambhu, the miraculous tree that produces an infinite number of fruits." BHAṬṬANĀRĀYAṆA, STAVACINTĀMAṆI 16

• The Ṛgveda sets out the vibratory codes (mantra) of the different energies (deva) of matter.
• The Yajurveda is a guide for officiants and sets out how to use the vibratory codes to prepare rituals of the different energies.
• The Sāmaveda contains chants of the absolute, most of which must be chanted by priests (udgātṛ) during sacrifices for preparing the soma.
• The Atharvaveda is concerned with rituals of magical influence, targeting specific ends.

These four Veda correspond to four deities: sun for the Ṛgveda, fire for the Yajurveda, wind for the Sāmaveda and moon for the Atharvaveda.

• The Smṛti set out moral codes for social functioning.
• The Itihāsa (Mahābhārata, Rāmāyaṇa) transmit Vedic intuitions lyrically, in an easier to understand way.
• The Purāṇa are collections of stories that describe the principles of cosmology (creation and destruction of universes), cosmic ages, and the genealogy of gods, sages and men.
• The Upaveda cover the study of human sciences.
• The Āyurveda, in conjunction with the Ṛgveda, covers medical science, and includes anatomy, physiology, hygiene, treatment of illness, surgery, etc.
• The Dhanurveda, in conjunction with the Yajurveda, is concerned with military and political sciences.
• The Gandharvaveda, in conjunction with the Sāmaveda, explores music and the other arts.
• The Sthāpatyaveda, in conjunction with the Atharvaveda, deals with mathematics, engineering, architecture and urbanism.
• The six Vedāṅga are a semantic, epistemological approach to the Veda:
  - Śikṣā (Ṛgveda) studies the exact articulation, pronunciation and euphony of mantra.
  - Kalpa (Atharvaveda) is the science of rules and of performing the various rituals.
  - Vyākaraṇa (Atharvaveda) studies grammar and is a reflection on language.
  - Nirukta (Sāmaveda) is the study of the etymology of words.
  - Chanda (Yajurveda) is the science of prosody and studies the rules of harmony and intensity, and their relation with mantric syllables.
  - Jyotiṣa (Yajurveda) is the study of astronomy and astrology.
• The Upāṅga are the six philosophical systems commonly referred to as Darśana, or points of view:
  - Gautama's Nyāya, studies reality through logic.
  - Kaṇāda's Vaiśeṣika is the scientific, atomic viewpoint of the universe, and is concerned with the differences (viśeṣa) of the constituents that make up reality.
  - Kapila's Sāṃkhya lists the different categories (tattva) of existence.
  - Yoga Darśana, which here refers to Patañjali's Aṣṭāṅga yoga, describes a practical means to isolate (kaivalya) Puruṣa from Prakṛti.
  - Jaimini's Pūrvamīmāṃsā describes the roles and pertinence of Vedic rituals.

- Uttaramīmāṃsā, also known as Vyāsa's Vedānta, is the study of the Upaniṣads and the ultimate reality. A metaphysical approach of this study of ultimate reality can be found in the Prasthānatrayī: Vyāsa's Vedānta Sūtra, Upaniṣads and the Bhagavad Gītā. The term Vedānta is significant as it means 'the end of knowledge', since it serves no purpose.

According to sanātanadharma tradition, this vast germination can only take place through the seed of Consciousness.

"Verily all this is Brahman. This is born from, dissolves in, and exists in That." CHĀNDOGYOPANIṢAD III, 14-1

The function that transmits this network is called the upaguru. The upaguru teaches a technique, transmits an art, whether it be archery, singing, sculpture, the art of pleasure or of asceticism. The function is therefore more important than the person. In certain cases, the upaguru can also be the sadguru or pratibhāguru (pratibhā: undifferentiated Consciousness, intuition, light). The simple presence of the sadguru reflects our own presence. This reflection is the essence of the sadguru.

"From the point of view of my body, I am his servant; from the point of view of my mind, his disciple; from the point of view of my deepest nature, I am Him."
HANUMĀN SPEAKING OF RĀMA

The pratibhāguru is not imprisoned by a technique, and as such is beyond all functions. Here, reference is not made to a person but rather to an intuition of the essential.

"Pratibhāsa means the light of Consciousness, inclined towards a configuration of reflections (ābhāsa) which rests on a common substratum since all these reflections necessarily rest on one."
ABHINAVAGUPTA, ĪŚVARAPRATYABHIJÑĀVIMARŚINĪ II, 3.6

This intuition can sometimes take on mysterious and very unexpected faces. For example, a couple of untouchables who kill chickens and cook them in a giant pot in front of a dumbfounded Namdev, or a weaver by the name of Kabīr who sings of his madness: *"I've burned down my house, the torch is still in my hand. Now I'll burn down the house of anyone who wants to follow me."* It can also take the form of a butcher who inadvertently touches Śaṅkarācārya, another butcher who teaches a brāhmaṇa in the Mahābhārata, or more recently a beedi seller by the name of Nisargadatta Mahārāj. There is therefore no activity, function or dharma that does not bear the imprint of the essential. This is perhaps why the Master's feet are so venerated.

"Superior to millions of mantra, millions of ritual observances, millions of the greatest sacrifices, is the mere worship of the holy feet (pādukā) of the Guru."
KULĀRṆAVATANTRA

In some āsana, such as the scorpion pose, the feet are in contact with the head. This figure can also be found in other civilisations such as the Olmecs and their Tlatilco acrobat. In his book 'The Art of Yoga', Śrī B.K.S. Iyengar entitles this āsana 'Taming one's own pride'. The pride of believing we live in separation when everything else in the universe is interdependent, of believing ourselves to be body-mind whose apogee is our thinking process, our head. Nisargadatta Mahārāj says that in Marathi, the word for foot signifies the beginning of the instant, where Consciousness gushes forth well before any conceptualisation. Paradoxically, this gushing forth is also a burying. This gushing forth is the Guru himself, who may take on a bodily shape.

"Gururupāyaḥ, the Master is the means."
VASUGUPTA, ŚIVASŪTRA II, 6

The Triśirobhairava explains this gushing forth in the

following terms: *"The energy from the master's mouth is a better master than the master himself."*

Although different types of initiation have been described, varying in their intensity of penetration according to the grace bestowed upon the so-called disciple, they are insignificant because they pertain to experience and hence to name (nāma) and form (rūpa). These initiations are always conditioned by the knowledge-ignorance dichotomy, which is merely a state or change of state. That which allows understanding or non-understanding to be known is without change.

"How can the immutable Self have any knowledge or activity? All external objects depend on our knowledge of them. Therefore this world is void."
Vijñāna Bhairava 134

There is only one initiation: the intuition (pratibhā) that the Guru is our own presence.

"Where there is neither question from the disciple, nor reply from the master, this is anuttara, the transcendent."
Abhinavagupta, Parātrīśikāvivaraṇa, Jaideva Singh, Page 48

His commentary on verse 19 of the Parātrīśikā is very enlightening: *"He who truly knows his real nature (the bījamantra Sauḥ), even if he has not seen the maṇḍala (adṛṣṭamaṇḍala), enjoys eternal perfection. He is a perfect yogi. He is truly initiated."*
According to Abhinavagupta, maṇḍala here signifies knowledge of the system of nāḍī, cakra, prāṇa, etc. Adṛṣṭamaṇḍala is therefore he who is ignorant of this system.
"In the matter of realisation, maṇḍala or the ceremony of initiation is of no use."
Abhinavagupta, Parātrīśikāvivaraṇa, Jaideva Singh, Page 236/238

Ritual initiation is unnecessary for he who is suddenly (evam) touched by the highest of grace. The immediateness and gratuitousness of this grace appears to be at the heart of this initiation.
"This realisation alone is initiation (dīkṣā), what else could dīkṣā be?"
Abhinavagupta, Parātrīśikāvivaraṇa, Jaideva Singh, Page 238

Abhinavagupta explains the nirukta of dīkṣā by two letters: dī (dīyate jñānam), the gift of recognition; and kṣā (kṣīyate pāpam), the destruction of illusion.
For Abhinavagupta, grace is the highest initiation because it is spontaneous. This spontaneity (svayaṃbhu) is the mark of the akalpitaguru, who is not fashioned (akalpita) by knowledge but who is initiated by 'the divinity of his own Consciousness' (svasaṃvittidevībhir dīkṣitaḥ), and whose presence alone radiates intuitive knowledge (pratibhā jñānam). The totally free nature of Consciousness is permanently available, expressing in the instant the five activities (pañcakṛtya): emanation, maintenance, resorption, oblivion and recognition.

"The Self, whose wonderful essence is Light, Śiva, supremely free, through his impetuous play of his freedom, first of all hides his own essence and then reveals it again in its fullness at once or by degrees. And this gift of grace is entirely independent."
Abhinavagupta, Tantrāloka XIII, 103-105, 117b-120a

This availability of grace is masked by the various filters mentioned earlier, which are nothing more than our translation. The guru, or ācārya, fulfils the function of mirroring this availability. This mirroring will vary in intensity according to the translation we make, which depends on the nature of our conditioning, identifications, tendencies and inclinations. It will be qualified as gross (sthūla), subtle (sūkṣma), very refined (sūkṣmatara) or profoundly delicate (sūkṣmatama) depending on the 'transmission' medium used: contact (sparśa), word (vāṇī), vision (darśana) or intuition (pratibhā). According to Abhinavagupta, the guru's function is revealed through four expressions:

• The Akalpitaguru, as we have seen, is the unmade guru who becomes the recipient of the Supreme through the spontaneity of grace.

"Concerning he who follows the intuitive way, the various stages, rules, consecrations, spiritual lineage and initiations are of no use to him. Such a master is inspired directly by God himself. This devotee of Śiva's teachings is, it is said, initiated by the goddesses of his own Consciousness."

Abhinavagupta, Tantrāloka XIII, 140-143a

"He in which intuitive truth manifests itself acquires lordship of all things. He is directly consecrated and initiated by the goddesses of his own Consciousness. Of all masters, it is said he is the supreme. Other masters, those who are fabricated (kalpita), are deprived of all authority in his presence."

Abhinavagupta, Tantrāloka IV, 42b-44a

• The Akalpitakalpakaguru has also been graced, but must refer to the scriptures and certain ritual activities for validation.

• The Kalpitaguru has followed teachings, practised certain purifying disciplines with other masters and then passes them on.

• The Kalpitakalpakaguru is also dependant on other teachers and purifying disciplines, which he does not have to follow rigorously once initiated.

Grace is thus present in all places at all times. As the Lord works in mysterious ways, the guru, whatever his expression, from the most gross to the most subtle, represents the Lord himself. He is thus worshipped as such. The extent of mirroring by the guru varies depending upon how he is perceived. Two types of sādhaka can thus be distinguished: those inclined towards objectivity, the desire to savour the phenomenal world (bhogavāsanā); and those for whom the call of the essential (mumukṣu) is stronger. The āgama describe two types of initiation depending on the sādhaka's maturity and inclinations.

The sāmayī dīkṣā (by convention referred to as sāmayika) is initiation in the various purifying rites (saṃskāra) and ritual activities, including psychophysical cleansing. These initiations may follow an external adoration ritual (bāhyapūjā) or a mental adoration ritual (antaryāga). Their purpose is to dissolve the layers of sediment and the stratums of the psychophysical entity, which merely disguise reality. As long as we continue to identify with our personal history, we only encounter our own projections, and the merest morsel of our daily life, be it the name we bear or the toilet water we use, is nothing more than the theatre of our projections.

"This body is variously coloured (influenced) by material qualities and is the seat of all conditioning..."

Lakṣmī Tantra 41.18-19

When the net of identifications no longer has a personal connotation, when it is no longer the ultimate definition of 'what I am', and when the holes in the net become clearer than the threads, putraka dīkṣā initiation can take place. In order to taste a good wine, one must not be thirsty, nor have the desire to become intoxicated. Within the disciple who becomes the guru's spiritual son (putraka), there is a certain quietude, a certain silence of expectations.

"Spiritual sons have a spontaneous and immediate resonance with the nature of Śiva."

Abhinavagupta, Tantrāloka XIII, 296b-300a

Here, we recognise our own divinity (svarūpa) through non-accomplishment, through the resonance of the guru's presence. The external rite is described in the Lakṣmī Tantra.

"To emphasise enjoyment (bhoga) and release from enjoyment, two final oblations should now be made.

Envisaging the disciple as both differentiated and absolute, the preceptor, who is himself in the state of parātīta, should take butter twice in the sacrificial ladle (sruk) representing the disciple's two states. Then, combining both portions of that butter he should visualise himself as consisting of the sound-Consciousness, the excellent form of Paśyantī, the absolute state of Tārikā, undifferentiated and undisturbed. Identifying the disciple with this state, he should make the final offering of the above-mentioned butter, accompanying it with the recitation of the mantra of Tārā... Next, the preceptor should envisage the merger of both his disciple and himself in Me, the eternal Lakṣmī, in the same way as milk mixes with milk losing separate identity, whilst he throws into the fire the great oblation after the last customary final offering has been made."

Lakṣmī Tantra 41, 51-57

To understand the essence of dīkṣā, we must put aside its external or internal ritualisation since this is still objective. If not placed in its cultural context, the exotic nature of this ritualisation can be simply another form of entertainment. In essence, initiation of what we are is always taking place. Situations within our social framework become the ingredients for a ritual that is beyond us, beyond all control.

"O my heart, before whom to prostrate?
To whom will you say: 'My Guru'?
He is there, so close to you!
He is there, all around you!
He resides in all things.
The Guru is the rice in your bowl,
The Guru is the passion of your soul.
Of your heart which sobs,
The Guru is the tears..."

Baul Chant

The relationship with the guru is what touches our core. *"What is not truly grasped by the heart in a most intimate way is like something that does not exist, such as blades of grass for someone on a passing cart."*

Abhinavagupta, Parātrīśikālaguvṛitti, Page 3, 1.1

This relationship is fundamentally non-relationship, non-separation. The guru as a function is Bhairava, the undifferentiated. He is frightening because his nakedness is so complete that it casts a night (śivarātri) of blindness onto the known. All that we know, starting with the idea that we are a separate entity, is merely a hoax, a fabrication of the mind, which creates thousands of relationships to make us feel secure with our schizophrenia. Our encounter with the guru is that of our own nothingness. When all definition ends, the unique presence of Consciousness, which is nothing more than the screen upon which our existence is projected, is the form itself of the guru, perceived as 'this' or 'that'. It is only the relationship with the vital surge (the guru), at each instant, that can show us our limitations, our agitation. This recognition may be expressed in an infinite number of facets depending on the student's inclinations and psychosocial framework. The framework is used to break identification with the framework.

The upaguru has gone beyond the technique he teaches and can therefore always teach it in a fresh and spontaneous way according to the situation. Śrī B.K.S. Iyengar was once asked how he was able to remain in an āsana for such long periods of time. He replied: *"You do the posture, I am the pose."* When the upaguru teaches, it is always a question of life and death, of urgency. He is always at the sharp edge of the instant.

"What is it to perceive the sharp edge? It is to grasp the moment before the gesture of the opponent. The first impetus of this movement is the energy, or sensation, located at the bottom of the chest. The dynamic of the movement depends on the energy, the sensation and the mood all at the same time..."

Yagyū Munenori, The Life-Giving Sword (Heiho Kadensho)

This exaggeration of urgency shows the student his timidness, half-heartedness and insipidness. There is no place for dilettantism. Miyamoto Musashi, the famous samurai, gives the following advice:

"Devote oneself to the Way without fearing death.
Discern what is true and fair.
Make progress in the Way through practice,
and not through fanciful ideas.
Embrace all arts.
Know how to distinguish the advantages
and disadvantages of all things.
Develop intuitive judgement
and understanding for everything.
Perceive instinctively that which cannot be seen.
Pay attention even to trifles.
Do nothing which is of no use."
MIYAMOTO MUSASHI, THE BOOK OF FIVE RINGS

The pratibhāguru can also transmit knowledge or a technique and have the function of an upaguru. The stories that follow illustrate different facets of initiation, beyond the usual formulas and codifications.

"Even if it is a fault, O God, is it truly a fault if it allows one to reach You? And if it is a quality, is it truly a quality if it does not allow one to reach You?"
BHAṬṬANĀRĀYAṆA, STAVACINTĀMAṆI 47

Whether these stories are true or not is of no importance. They speak of the instant where there is only one vision, with no one looking on. Yet they are merely tales. If taken literally, they become a merry-go-round of exotic destinations and ideal situations, even if they take on a terrible nature. This is how Hollywood's heroes, when in the most dreadful of situations, always seem better than we are at our best. The names too can seem like a string of emotivity for a Westerner. Would it be as meaningful if Marpa were called Smith, a building-site foreman who asked you to shovel earth all day? If you were to clean the toilets in a Zen monastery, you could cling to the story of patriarchs and have the impression you are doing something extraordinarily spiritual and humble. If you were to work for the council as a road sweeper, this romanticism would not exist. We must therefore abandon the carnival and psychodrama of the so-called sādhana in which the seeker and so-called guru indulge. All too often, it is merely a procession of fear, guilt, and of physical and mental dictatorship. These encounters are precisely the end of romanticism, where only the instant itself remains, in its nakedness, without any commentary. When this happens, its silent intensity is such that it occurs almost unnoticed since it is neither knowledge nor experience.
Abhinavagupta says that the droplets of a light shower cannot be distinguished against the continuous background of the sky. They can only be perceived when they fall from a more detailed background such as trees or the roof of a house. In the same way, the supreme Bhairava, because of his extreme subtlety, cannot be perceived directly and never falls within conscious experience.

"Thus the power of grace of the Divine is always and in all experients uninterrupted."
ABHINAVAGUPTA, PARĀTRĪŚIKĀVIVARAṆA, JAIDEVA SINGH, PAGE 14

Ekalavya's Thumb

It looked like it was going to be a glorious day. Was it the light, swollen with the incessant babbling of life, or the exultant joyful silence of each blade of grass that gave the daybreak its indescribable beauty? Bharadvāja, accompanied by other ṛṣi, was on his way to the banks of the Gaṅgā to celebrate the sacrifice of fire (agnihotra). Suddenly he saw her. A divine apparition. A woman who could not be of this world such was her intoxicating sensuality. He now understood the magic of this morning, which already announced the fever of desire. Her robe clung to her wet skin emphasising her shapely figure, full of the arrogance of youth, making him mad with desire. His eyes met those of the nymph Ghṛtācī. Bharadvāja was unable to contain the violence of his emotion. He felt his seed burst out, which he then gathered into a jar known as a droṇa. This is how Droṇa was born. He learnt the art of weaponry from his father and from the hermit Agniveśa, with whom he remained for many years. It was there he met the Pañcāla prince, who became a very dear friend. The prince liked Droṇa so much that one day he said to him: "I am the favourite son of my illustrious father. When I become king of the Pañcāla, my kingdom will be yours. O dear friend, I promise you this. My estate, my wealth and my happiness will be yours also."

At the end of his apprenticeship, Droṇa married Kṛpī, daughter of Śaradvān. From their union a son was born, who they named Aśvatthāmā, because at the moment he was born, he whinnied like a horse.

Learning that Paraśurāma, the sixth incarnation of Viṣṇu, was withdrawing to the forest and giving away all his possessions, he went to find him. Droṇa coveted the Dhanurveda, the ultimate knowledge of archery. He knew that Paraśurāma had obtained his mastery of archery from Śiva himself, and his mastery of the divine weapons after years of austerity and victory over the demons.

Paraśurāma said to him: "I have given my gold and all my other wealth to the brāhmaṇa. My land, which spreads as far as the oceans, and the cities have been given to the Kaśyapa. All that remains is my body and my weapons. Choose one or the other, but choose quickly!"

"I want all your weapons as well as complete mastery of them", he replied.

Paraśurāma gave away not only his weapons but also full knowledge of the rules associated with them and all their mysteries.

One day, Droṇa's son saw a child from a well-off family drinking milk. Having never tasted this beverage, Aśvatthāmā became inconsolable. His son's tears broke Droṇa's heart. He had no option but to admit that although he was an accomplished warrior, and that his mastery of the bow had no equal, he lived in poverty. He was not even able to buy milk for his son.

Aśvatthāmā's friends decided to play a joke on him. They gave him a mixture of flour and water. Full of joy, he cried out: "I have tasted milk! I have tasted milk!" and became the laughing stock of his friends. Seeing this and listening to the scornful comments from his neighbours about his poverty, Droṇa went into a state of despair. So he decided to go and search out his old friend the prince, who was now king.

Droṇa went up to the king full of confidence and addressed him with the following terms: "O Tiger amongst men, I call upon our friendship." "What friendship?" replied the king; "Someone of impure birth cannot be a friend of someone who has noble blood. How could I be the friend of a warrior? My armies are bursting with illustrious military men. Stop making a fool of yourself through your naivety. There is no friendship possible between a poor man and a rich man, between a slave and a king, between a coward and a hero. I have no recollection of such a promise, but I am able to show you hospitality and provide you with food for the night."

Droṇa, humiliated in front of his wife and son, left the palace without a word. The king, Drupada, was not aware that at that instant he had sealed his downfall. This is how Droṇa came to live in his father-in-law's house in Hāstinapura (city of the elephant), the capital of the Pāṇḍava. For a certain time he lived there anonymously.

One day, the young and carefree princes were playing with a ball when it fell into a well. All their attempts to recover it failed. Close by, Droṇa, smiling, was watching them. When they saw him, the young princes were intimidated by his presence. They recognised his status of a high-ranking warrior.

"Shame on you warriors and shame on your ignorance of weaponry. How is it that you of the Bhārata race are not able to retrieve the ball? How is it that you fail at such a simple task? If you give me dinner, I promise not only to recover your ball but also my ring that I am throwing into the well. And what's more, I will recover both of them using these blades of grass."

Yudhiṣṭhira, the son of Kuntī, replied: "Then do so, and by this action obtain from us that which will be of use to you for a lifetime."

"Look at these long blades of grass. By using the power of certain mantra I will make them into weapons with powers you cannot imagine."

The first blade of grass hit the centre of the ball. He then shot the others, which became embedded in each other. It was by using this stratagem that the ball and ring, which Droṇa subsequently offered to the dumbfounded princes, were recovered.

"We bow before you O Brāhmaṇa. Never have we seen such mastery. Who are you and what may we do for you?"

"Go and see Bhīṣma and tell him exactly what happened. He will know who I am."

Bhīṣma had no doubt as to the stranger's identity. Only Droṇa was capable of accomplishing such a miracle. He also knew that he would be the best teacher for the princes. He went to meet Droṇa, and after respectfully greeting him, invited him to the palace. Bhīṣma attentively listened as to how the roundabout paths of providence had brought him to the kingdom of the Kuru.

"O Droṇa, what an honour it is to have you here. Instruct the princes and make them into worthy warriors. From this instant on they are in your care. Your arrival fills us with joy. What an honour it is to have you here. Make this palace your home."

Once settled in, Droṇa solemnly accepted the princes as his pupils. He said to them: "You must promise me that once you have completed your apprenticeship, you will accomplish something that is dear to my heart." Upon hearing these words the princes remained silent. Only Arjuna hastened to accept whatever Droṇa may demand in return. From that day on, the complicity between Droṇa and Arjuna grew and grew.

Droṇa taught them the art of earthly and heavenly weapons. His demands turned them into accomplished warriors. Although they each received the same teaching, Arjuna always proved to be the best. This was not only down to his innate talent for the art of warfare, but also to the profound love he had for his master. Arjuna's devotion let him shine above the others.

Droṇa had given each of his pupils a large narrow-mouthed pitcher to fetch water. This made the task very time consuming. He had given his son a wide-mouthed pitcher, allowing him to accomplish the task in less time and return faster. Droṇa was thus able to teach him secret techniques that he did not share with the others. Arjuna noticed this and in order to fill his pitcher quickly, he used the mantra of Varuṇa, Lord of the waters. He was therefore able to return at the same time as Droṇa's son, Aśvatthāmā, and take advantage of the same teaching. Arjuna's knowledge and excellence was in no way inferior to that of Aśvatthāmā.

One day, Droṇa went to see the cook and secretly said to him: "Never give Arjuna his food in darkness and do not repeat to him what I have just asked of you." Yet one evening, when they were eating their meal, a strong wind blew out the lamps. The princes bustled about asking for light. Arjuna, seeing in this gust of wind the breath of his master, cried out to them: "Silence. Let me eat my food in darkness." Without effort, his hand instinctively found his mouth. And this is how he came to practise in total darkness. Droṇa, seeing him train in this manner, took him in his arms and said to him: "In all truthfulness, no other archer in this world will ever be your equal."

Droṇa continued to teach Arjuna many other fighting techniques: climbing onto a horse or elephant, driving a chariot, and ground combat. He learned how to handle different weapons separately, but also how to use a club, a sword, a spear, different types of knives and arrows at the same time. He also learned how to fight several opponents simultaneously and how to get out of the most desperate of situations. He knew the vital points that would allow him to paralyse or kill an enemy in the blink of an eye. He knew destabilising strategies that would plunge opponents into fear and agitation.

Droṇa's fame grew and many warriors and princes came to him for instruction. One such prince was Ekalavya. He was the son of King Hiranyadhanus, chief of the Niṣāda tribes, a lowly caste that lived in the forests. Ekalavya's father had tried to dissuade his son from undertaking the journey: "Droṇa will never teach you. You are a śūdra." But the young Ekalavya was persuaded that Droṇa was his master and that he would accept him as a disciple. The first time he heard Droṇa's name, he began to shiver. It was a dream that finally convinced him to leave. In this dream, Droṇa presented him with a bow. Faced with his son's stubbornness, Hiranyadhanus gave him his blessing. Ekalavya walked for weeks on end, oblivious to hunger and thirst, carried by his heart and his one desire of meeting his master. When near the palace, he bathed and donned the clean clothes his mother had given him. She had scented them. Their softness reminded him of her presence, her tender gaze. He oiled his hair and marked his forehead. He marvelled at the splendour of the palace and was silenced by the exuberance of the gardens. The guards could not help smiling when they saw him. He was escorted to a room where tens of other princes were waiting. He hesitated upon seeing them. What was a beggar like him doing amongst these princes? He then calmed his fear. The majority of these princes were simply there because they wanted to be trained by this famous master, or because their family had forced them to come. Ekalavya said to himself that very few of them had the sacred fire. Many were accepted simply for diplomatic or political reasons, but Droṇa would see his devotion to follow the path of weaponry. After hours of waiting his turn came. He recognised the Pāṇḍava and Kaurava who proudly surrounded Droṇa. Ekalavya bowed respectfully before Droṇa.

"My life is yours. Accept me as your disciple."

"Moral decorum does not allow me to teach you. You are a śūdra. You should not even present yourself before me. Leave this place immediately and never return."

Droṇa had only used Ekalavya's circumstance of birth as a pretext. The intensity of the look in Ekalavya's eyes could not be mistaken. He would have been able to better the princes under his supervision, and, moreover, to better Arjuna.

Ekalavya didn't say a word. He bowed again before Droṇa and left the palace without any regrets. He had seen his master, and for him, that was enough. That which some were never able to understand after spending a lifetime with Droṇa, Ekalavya's heart had grasped instantaneously. He withdrew to the forest nearby the palace and chose a small clearing in which to settle. Before even building his hut, he moulded a clay statue of Droṇa and placed it on an altar.

At dawn, he took the still hot ashes from the sacrificial fire and rubbed them onto his body from head to foot. After the pūjā to his guru, he started to practise day and

night in front of the statue of Droṇa. With no notion of time, driven by a madness few would be able to understand, he succeeded in mastering the three stages of shooting: fixing the arrow, aiming and releasing; these no longer held any secrets from him.
It was the hunting season and the Kaurava and Pāṇḍava set out on an expedition. One of their dogs picked up a scent and headed into the woods. The princes followed thinking it had picked up the trail of an animal. The dog then stopped and started barking. Everyone saw him, shining like the sun. He was dressed in black rags, covered in ashes, his dreadlocks gathered into a bun. He turned his head towards Arjuna and, without even looking at the dog, shot seven arrows into its mouth before it had time to close it. Arjuna himself trembled in front of such skill.
"Who are you stranger? Where are you from and what is your lineage?"
"O Princes, I am the son of Hiranyadhanus, king of the Niṣāda. I am a disciple of the renowned Droṇa and am devoted to the art of weaponry."
Ekalavya continued to demonstrate his mastery, not only of archery but also of other weapons. The princes hurried back to the palace and told Droṇa about the stranger's skills. For Droṇa this was no stranger. He knew it was the same teenager he had refused to instruct several years earlier.
Arjuna secretly went to Droṇa and said to him: "Remember the day when you took me in your arms and promised me that none of your students would ever be better than me. How is it that this śūdra, who claims to be your disciple, is better than me?"
Unable to go back on his word, Droṇa decided to go with Arjuna to see Ekalavya. All Ekalavya's efforts were transformed into tears of joy the moment he saw Droṇa. He bowed down and said to Droṇa: "Whatever I have accomplished, it is through your grace."
"If you claim to be my pupil, then give me what I am due."
"Whatever you wish."
"If you are my disciple and you wish to offer me something, then give me the thumb from your right hand."
For a moment they became one and Arjuna was envious of this communion. Droṇa could have asked him for both arms. It no longer mattered. Everything that needed to be accomplished had been accomplished. Without hesitation, Ekalavya cut-off his thumb and gave it to Droṇa. He bowed before him again and left without a word.
This is how Ekalavya came to lose his skills and became inferior to Arjuna, who, freed from his frenzy of jealousy, regained his calm. Many of Droṇa's pupils have faded out of memory but we still remember Ekalavya, a bright sun dressed in black rags and covered in ashes that made Arjuna tremble.

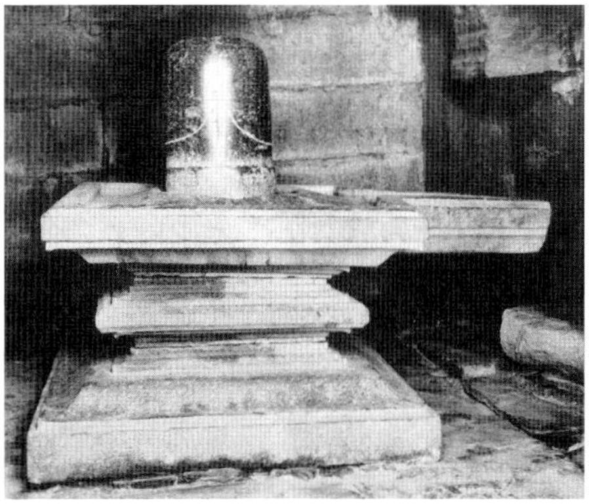

Liṅgapīṭha

8th-14th century (Alampur [Pāpanāśi], Mahabubnagar, Andhra Pradesh)

The Butcher's Song (Vyādha-Gītā)

Mahābhārata, Vana-Parva 3

Kauśika, a brāhmaṇa from a renowned lineage, was an adept of asceticism. He had studied the Veda, Vedāṅga and Upaniṣad, and his knowledge was limitless. One day, whilst practising a complicated ritual where correct pronunciation and intonation of each mantra was of utmost importance, a crow, as black as a moonless night, came and sat on a branch of the tree under which he was seated. The bird gave out a victorious caw that cut the air like a recently sharpened sword, decapitating the brāhmaṇa's concentration as effortlessly as slicing an apple. The crow then excreted on the brāhmaṇa, its faeces splattering on his head like a shower of mockery. Full of rage, Kauśika looked up with such intensity that it hit the crow like a stone. The dead bird fell from its branch into the brāhmaṇa's hands. He could feel the bird's still hot and quivering body. The shiny, silky feathers of the crow filled him with terrible sadness. He suddenly saw its beauty. In an instant, the armour of all his knowledge and austerity was shattered. It was of no use at all when faced with something unexpected in his daily life. What irony! What distress!

He headed off to the village to ask for food, moaning to himself: "Alas! My heart is still filled with anger and hatred. I have killed that poor crow and I can now see my own arrogance." Upon reaching a house, he stopped in front of the porch and, as was the custom, demanded: "Give!" A woman replied: "Wait." Whilst the woman was busy cleaning the beggar's bowl her husband arrived. She gave him all her attention. She brought him water so he could wash himself and then prepared his meal. She dished out his food and stayed close by in case he needed anything else. She suddenly remembered the brāhmaṇa and, embarrassed, brought him his meal.

Kauśika was waiting and angrily said to her: "O woman, you told me to wait and that is what I have done. Why make me wait so long?"

"Forgive me, but my husband came back. To serve my husband is to serve God."

"Do you not think brāhmaṇa merit preferential treatment? Even though he is your husband, this man is of a lower caste. Your pride will be your downfall. Has nobody told you that brāhmaṇa are like fire and are able to consume the entire earth?"

With a piercing look he continued: "I am honouring you by asking for food."

"Why are you looking at me like that? I am not a crow. Why is there so much anger in the eyes of one who is devoted to study and asceticism? I have a lot of respect for brāhmaṇa. I know their worth. I am not arrogant enough to compare myself with them. I know that to be cursed by a brāhmaṇa can destroy several generations. But this power to curse is nothing compared to your inclination for forgiving. That is why I ask you once again for pardon. Not because I fear for my life but because, Kauśika, you will destroy yourself. Despite all your studies, you still have not understood the most important thing. How are you able to know yourself in the difference between you and I? Does the knowledge of separation not come from non-difference? Your virtuous practice is uninitiated. If you wish it to be conditioned by neither time, place nor society, then go and see the butcher who lives in Mithilā."

Dumbfounded, Kauśika respectfully bowed and took his leave. How did this woman, a poor housewife, know about the crow and how did she know his name? But that was nothing compared to the profoundness of her words, which had completely destabilised him. Her look was like an abyss in which his anger and pretentiousness had been drowned.

He spent the day in his hermitage, his head on fire. How could he go and see a butcher? What could a butcher possibly teach him? Simply approaching the butcher's house would tarnish him! But there was one question he couldn't stop asking himself: "How am I able to know myself as being different?" He looked around. His hermitage and existence reeked of separation. Everyday he studied and recited hymns in praise of fear; his own fear of being nothing. He set off without further ado. He crossed many forests, villages and towns before reaching Mithilā, which was governed by the famous king Janaka. He enquired as to the whereabouts of the market and the famous butcher with unhindered wisdom. He was sarcastically told that there was a butcher, and that although possibly famous in his neighbourhood, his unhindered wisdom was hardly likely to extend further than the walls of his house. And anyway, why would a brāhmaṇa want anything to do with a butcher?

Feeling evermore uneasy, he hurried on. The market place was swarming with people, stalls, grocery shops and small dingy cafés. This living palette of colours and odours thrown together higgledy-piggledy made him dizzy. He eventually came across the butcher's stall, which was like a diamond of blood, next to a brothel. Girls called out obscene propositions to passers-by. One of them shouted to him: "Had enough of your prayers have you?"

There was a queue at the butcher's stall. Kauśika watched from a distance. The butcher was impressively calm with an imposing presence. At the same time he served his customers he would slice up large pieces of beef, hang up venison and boast that the bloody flesh was so tender it melted in the mouth. Kauśika was overwhelmed by the man's ease. How was he able to be so at ease amongst this chaos? Kauśika had experience of calmness, but only in the artificial environment he had created for himself. Compared to this butcher he realised that his tranquillity was that found in cemeteries. For Kauśika, everything outside his world disturbed him and he was lost. His eyes met those of the butcher's who, after asking his apprentice to take over the stall, walked over to Kauśika. "I greet you O Brāhmaṇa. You are welcome. I know you have come here upon the advice of that saintly woman. I am also aware that you are not at ease in this place which lacks respect for your function. Allow me the honour of accompanying you to my humble home where you will feel comfortable and then you can tell me your heart's deepest desire."

With the butcher's kind attention, Kauśika's resistance completely disappeared. The arrogance of his life suddenly appeared before him with striking clarity, like an ocean of regrets crashing down on him. He found himself sobbing uncontrollably in the arms of the butcher. He then started to follow this joyfully calm stranger with complete confidence.

As was the custom, the butcher paid his respects to the brāhmaṇa by providing him with water to wash his face and feet, and then sat him down in the best seat.

After a long silence, Kauśika, who now felt he could trust him, asked: "Your profession doesn't appear in keeping with your wisdom. I am saddened that you have such a cruel profession."

"I respect the function I have. It has been passed on from generation to generation in my family. O Brāhmaṇa, do not be saddened because I abide by the duties of circumstance. To serve the mysterious ways of the Lord, which have taken on the faces of my elders, my superiors such as you, and my profession fills me with wonder. Know that I always speak the truth, never envy others and give to the best of my abilities. I speak ill of no creature, large or small. I live life without worries and am happy with what remains after having served the gods, the guests and those who depend on me. A śūdra's function is to serve. This is the way of things. It is only a function. How are we able to know ourselves as this or that? That is the essential question. It is true that I kill animals and sell their meat. I perform a sacrifice, that of the universe itself. Is there a man on this earth who can survive without killing any creature? By the simple act of breathing, do you not sacrifice millions of organisms? In the absolute, is this universe and all it is made of not an oblation to the Lord? My actions are his actions. All action carried out in the ignorance of separation is a sin."

"Then tell me dear friend, what is virtue and what is not a sin?"

"Fully abiding by one's function whilst knowing there is no doer, that is virtue. What is the essential criterion for purity? That which is identical to Consciousness is pure, and everything else impure. But for he who considers the whole universe as being identical to Consciousness, the distinction between pure and impure no longer exists."

At that instant Kauśika knew he had met his sadguru. They spoke for hours, through the night, of the different manifestations of creation. They spoke of karma and its social function, of the three tendencies of nature: tamas, rajas and sattva, of the elements, the different prāṇa, as well as many other things. But for the butcher, there was only the essential: "Know all of this as being an apparition in your own Consciousness. You are clothed in space (digambara)." They spoke until they had exhausted knowledge, until there was nothing left to know or experience.

After having walked in a circle around the butcher, Kauśika bowed before him. They parted company in silence. Glimmers of daylight were starting to appear. Kauśika walked with a joyful stride, savouring the trance of the ordinary for the first time, still carried by the butcher's song.

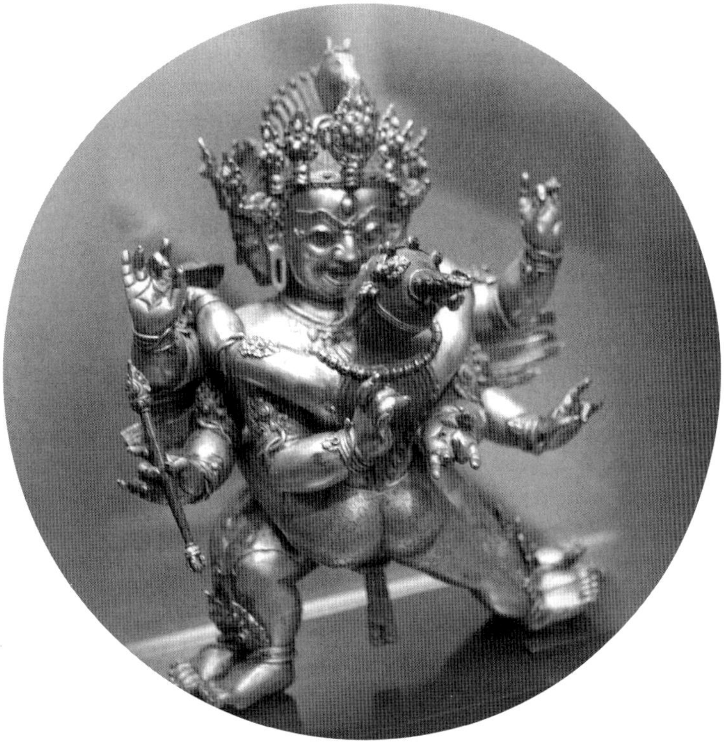

Hevajra with Śakti

The Idiotic Vision

The sage Ṛbhu had taught his dear disciple Nidāgha in these terms: "There is neither one, nor two. There is no mantra, no tantra, nor anything like that. There is no hearing (śravaṇa), no reflection (manana). Deep meditation (nididhyāsana) is only a misunderstanding. Both types of samādhi do not exist. The measurement and that which is measured do not exist either. Ignorance does not exist and neither does lack of discrimination. There is no dharma, purity, truth or fear. There is neither guru, nor disciple. There is neither birth, nor death. Only the Self exists. Be assured that you are this Self and that there has never been a non-Self."

Although Nidāgha showed great maturity and immense devotion to his master, his conviction was not yet sufficiently strong. He returned to his hometown and chose to dedicate his life to ritual practices.

But Ṛbhu loved his disciple as much as his disciple venerated him. From time to time, despite his great age, Ṛbhu went to town to observe Nidāgha, without him knowing, to see if he had gone beyond his ritualism and practices. One day, he came across Nidāgha watching a royal procession. With Māyā's help, Ṛbhu had taken on the form of a simpleton and he asked Nidāgha what was going on. Nidāgha replied that the king was going through the town in a procession.

"Ah! It's the king. Magnificent. But where is he?"

"Look, he is on the elephant."

"You say that the king is on the elephant. I can see both. But who is the king and who is the elephant?" asked the idiot.

"What!" exclaimed Nidāgha, "You can see both but you do not know that the man above is the king and the animal below is the elephant? You are wasting my time."

"Please don't be so impatient with an ignorant man. What do you mean by above and below?"

Nidāgha turned red with anger. "You can see the king and the elephant. One is above and one is below. But despite this, you want to know what above and below mean. If you cannot understand the obvious with the use of simple words, I will teach you by example."

Nidāgha climbed onto the villager's back and triumphantly shouted to him: "I am the king above and you are the elephant below. Is it clear now?"

"Not yet", replied the simpleton. "You say that 'I am the king above and you are the elephant below'. When you say the king, the elephant, above and below, I understand. But tell me what is meant by 'I' and 'you'."

It is said that at that instant Nidāgha recognised the presence of his master Ṛbhu as awareness free of all differentiation.

The Wall of Jñāneśvar
or The Nakedness of "What Is"

In the first quarter of the day of Brahmā, fourteen Indra were born. They all finished up in prison. This is how the mysterious play of fate unfolded. One day, Nārada appeared to them. Moved with joy, they sang love songs to him. One of the Indra was called Cāṅgdev. Although his cell was gilded, he was tired of his long imprisonment and asked Nārada: "I'm awfully tired, please tell me what I should do to free myself from this place forever."

The son of Brahmadev answered: "You must go into the world of mortals. You must become mortal. There is a great and holy city known as Paṇḍhari. There, the supreme Viṣṇu will appear before you standing on a brick. Those who live in the city of gods and other paradises know no freedom. Go and dress yourself in the different clothes of existence and become that which you already are. This is impossible to do here."

And so it was. Cāṅgdev became the son of a brāhmaṇa couple, Viṭhobā and Rukmiṇī, who lived at Puṇyastambha on the banks of the Gaṅgā. The child showed all the signs of being a prodigious incarnation. He received sacred initiation at the age of eight, and when the time came was married. His achievements (siddhi) filled all those who came near to him with wonder. He knew the fourteen forms of knowledge and the sixty-four arts. The ins and outs of the mind and its control held no secrets for him. When he reached one hundred years of age, death beckoned. Placing his Consciousness outside of his body for a few moments, thus disappointing the god of death, he brought his body back to life. Fourteen hundred years passed by. He didn't age and death had no hold on him. He was now very famous and regarded as a saint. People came from far away to hear his sermons and listen to him sing the praises of the Lord. He accepted many thousands of disciples. He was sought after for his teaching and was followed and worshipped. However, he had not yet found his sadguru. He was in the same position as a dietician who eats whatever he likes but prescribes a draconian diet to others, or that of a brāhmaṇa who has not washed himself but teaches ablution mantra to others. He said: "I have looked everywhere in the world of mortals and cannot find a guru worthy of me. I have not met anybody with equal powers, let alone someone with greater powers."

One day he heard about the great Jñāneśvar who was supposedly the incarnation of the absolute and who lived humanly at Āḷandī. Cāṅgdev said to himself: "I will go to him as a student. But first of all, let's see what he's made of. I will write to him and await his reply." Thinking about what he was going to write, he said to himself: "By respect, and if I wish to receive his teaching, I cannot address him as though he is younger than me. I must write to him as though he is my elder, yet Jñāneśvar is younger than I."

This is how he came to send a blank letter, without a message. Jñāneśvar received the message, which was brought to him with much ceremony by a stream of disciples. When he saw the blank page, Jñāneśvar exclaimed: "Fourteen hundred years have past but still he is blind. He is sterile like a fruit tree that doesn't bear fruit, like a lake without water, like an impotent man in a harem, like a woman who dresses up for a non existent lover, like one who renounces but is not indifferent to worldly things, like the immense fortune of a man who is not generous; all of this is only good for the fire. Of what use is speaking about compassion when one's own heart is dry? If a cloud does not pour out its water, it roams the sky in vain, just like Cāṅgdev."

Having said this, Jñāneśvar writes back with his own hand: "All things are nothing more than the reflection of our essential nature. All creatures shine with the same brilliance and hence it matters not whether we are young or old, have a family or are alone. The Self is neither short nor long. It is never far or near. When the sky is saturated with clouds, the space of the sky remains the same. Although phenomenally all things change, the Self is changeless. For the earth, the sun rises and the sun sets. But in reality, the sun never rises because it never sets. All that is perceived in the universe can be found within the body. We have played a trick on ourselves. Since nothing has been forgotten, there is nothing to be remembered. Whatever the seed of this universe may be, you are it."

Cāṅgdev was overcome the instant he read the letter. The words of Jñāneśvar had set his heart on fire and he felt impelled to go and meet him straight away. Straddling a tiger, the symbol of supreme power, he set out surrounded by hundreds of disciples. At that time of day, Jñāneśvar liked to sit down on an old crumbling wall. He liked its coolness and the wrinkled face of its old stones. In the distance he saw Cāṅgdev surrounded by a sea of disciples, riding a tiger and using a furious cobra as a whip. Jñāneśvar said to himself: "A guest is about to arrive. I must pay him my respects." The wall then started to move and went to meet Cāṅgdev! The wall did not literally move, but it was as though it did when Cāṅgdev saw Jñāneśvar in all his simplicity, ordinary looking, conspicuous by his absence of embellishments, make-up and personality.

Cāṅgdev saw the wall of 'what is', in all its nakedness, come to him. He felt ridiculous on his tiger, accompanied by all the artifices with which he surrounded himself. He still had something to prove. He still wanted to be recognised. All the arrogance within him melted like ice in the sun's rays. He bowed before Jñāneśvar and they then both sat down under a Banyan tree. Cāṅgdev listened to what Jñāneśvar had to say and was filled with joy. Even now, the Banyan is called the tree of rest. For the first time after all these years of wandering, Cāṅgdev was able to rest, freed from the jaws of becoming.

Jñāneśvar invited Cāṅgdev to his home. Muktabai, Jñāneśvar's sister, was taking her bath. Realising this, Cāṅgdev went out of the house. Laughing, Muktabai exclaimed: "I've caught you in your ignorance, you who still knows not your sadguru." Cāṅgdev came running back in, and bowing before her asked: "Tell me, mother, how do you know this?" She replied: "When you turned your back it became clear to me. If you were receptive to the omnipresence of the sadguru's grace, you would not have had to fight against such thoughts. If you had seen me through a hole in the wall, would you not have considered my body in the same way, but without having felt the need to leave? Cows go wherever they please without being dressed; does this disturb you? I am like one of these animals."

Cāṅgdev then humbly asked Jñāneśvar to accept him as his disciple. This is how the great Cāṅgdev, who possessed immortality and infinite powers, found himself completely naked before an old crumbling wall. There was a stream of light on the wall, and Cāṅgdev had never seen anything so beautiful, so simple.

Not Fully Baked!

In accordance with Nārāyaṇa's wish, Śuka and Uddhava became avatars in the world of mortals. Śuka would become known by the name of Kabīr and Uddhava by the name of Namdev. These two singing madmen were intoxicated by devotion, one shouting Rām and the other Pāṇḍurāṅga. But for now, let's talk about Namdev. His birth was a mystery; how were an old tailor and his old wife able to conceive a child? From an early age, Namdev's devotion to Viṭṭhala was limitless. One day when his mother asked him to take an offering of food to Viṭṭhala, he was driven to despair when the statue did not accept the food. In his innocence he took everything at face value. Upon hearing his despair and pleas, Viṣṇu started to eat. This is how, each day, Namdev spoke with Viṣṇu. In time, Namdev married and had children. He found it difficult to adjust to family life. His mother made fun of his devotion: "You pray to god all day long while your family live in misery." In the small temple he moaned: "Why have you abandoned me in the sad ocean of existence?"

"What is wrong my friend?" asked Viṣṇu.

"It's my mother, and the burden of my miserable existence that I can no longer bear."

"Do not hold back. Tell me how you live. What is bothering you?"

"If someone has your blessing, what more could he wish for? Yet I am still confronted with a paradox. Your home is the paradise of Vaikuṇṭha; I live in a tumbledown hut. The eight great achievements (siddhi) are your slaves; in my shack we are surrounded by rats. You have divine finery that shines like the sun; my children have only rags. The snake Śeṣa is your bed, on the ocean of milk; we don't even have a straw mattress. You eat off gold plates; we must settle for leaves. Our only comfort is your name."

Viṣṇu started laughing and said to him: "We are one, my friend. Nothing you do, or don't do, can separate us. Like salt in the ocean and salt on the table are not different, like the sun and its rays, we are one. O Namdev, although the lamp and its light are one, they may appear different; likewise, your love and mine are the same. Like the sweet taste of sugar cannot be separated from the sugar itself, your thoughts and mine are the same. The water of the Gaṅgā and ordinary water are of the same substance; the same is true of our nature. Like the sound of a bell is one with the bell itself, the same is true of us. So don't be worried, do what you have to do, free from any notion of duality."

Upon hearing these words, Namdev started crying and said: "I am your Bhakta. I want to sing your praises. Give your blessing that this may be."

Viṣṇu replied: "Let it be so."

Namdev's reputation as a devout person grew and his songs delighted people's hearts. One day, along with other well-known Bhakta of Mahārāṣṭra, he was invited to visit Gora, the famous potter and great mystic. Gora had asked them to come and bless his humble home. Gora received them with the honours they were due. He gave each of them a seat and washed their feet. Jñāneśvar was present, as was his brother Nivṛtti and his sister Muktabai. There was also Sopan, Savata and other Vaiṣṇava. Jñāneśvar then said to Gora in a mischievous tone of voice: "You have put the pots on their stand. Tell us which have been baked and which have not." Gora touched the heads of all those present with his potter's stick. They all remained silent while he did this. But when Gora touched Namdev's head, Namdev became annoyed: "Why did you touch me so?"

Gora cried out: "This pot is not fully baked, it is still soft."

Muktabai said to Gora: "I know of your skill. Jewellers are experts in their field. A good doctor recognises someone who is going to be ill. And you, being a good potter, you know whether a pot is baked or not."
Everyone burst into laughter apart from Namdev, who left the gathering brokenhearted. Did he not consider himself to be the most devoted of devotees? He returned to the temple and gave in to his sorrow. He sobbed: "O God, I have been humiliated and insulted. My heart is full of rage." Pāṇḍurāṅga started to laugh and, taking him into his arms, asked: "Who has insulted you. Tell me without hesitation!"
"O Hṛṣīkeśa (Lord of the heart), we may share with others the compliments we receive, but it is preferable to keep criticism to oneself."
"I know how you feel my friend. Don't keep this poison in your heart. Don't be ashamed and speak out in complete confidence."
Namdev told him what had happened. "Everyone accepted the test in silence. But I was frightened and became annoyed with Gora. Everyone started laughing at my reaction and Gora said that I wasn't yet fully baked. This made them laugh even louder. I have never been so humiliated."
Viṣṇu, looking tenderly at Namdev, said to him: "What Gora said about you is true. He who does not recognise himself in the presence of the sadguru, who has not taken refuge in the guru, is considered as unbaked. That is what Gora meant."
Upon hearing these words Namdev felt as though he was going to faint, like salt that dissolves when water is poured onto it. Full of sadness, he said to the Lord: "I came here with an aching heart hoping to find consolation in your presence. But on the contrary, you speak to me as they do. Why do you make me suffer in this way? I now have no place where I may rest. If the ground falters, how can a tree remain standing? If a mother abandons her child, who will look after him? If a king does not act fairly, how can his subjects be happy? Why do you sadden me in this way? In the three worlds, only You can help me."
The Lord of Paṇḍhari said to Namdev: "Your heart and mine are the same. Like honey hidden in the sap of a flower, nothing separates them. You are my life. Please do not say that you are sad. Go this very instant and take refuge in a guru and put an end to all your ideas of difference."
Namdev replied: "O, support of all worlds, why do I need a guru when I am so close to You? It seems so futile to carry out religious ceremonies, austerities and sacrifices, and to offer gifts in the hope of receiving initiation from a guru so I may obtain the love you already have for me. If there is already sugar, why go to the shop to buy more? If one's belly is already full, why bother going to a restaurant? He who already has a treasure does not need to go off in search of it. You breathe life into the three worlds, you are the guru of gurus, you are my only refuge. You and I are so close, why do I need a sadguru?"
"Listen", said Viṣṇu, "when I was the avatar Rām, I went to Vasiṣṭha as a disciple and questioned him about the ultimate knowledge. When I was Kṛṣṇa, I searched out Sāndīpani with devotion and reverence so he may instruct me in the essential nature of reality. So, my precious friend, accept all forms that present themselves as being me. Go and find your sadguru and free yourself of this subtle notion of difference that is still within you."
Namdev said: "Who should I go and see?"
"I will appear before you today. When you recognise me, you will have found your sadguru."
Namdev was walking under the burning kiss of the sun, still feeling pain and humiliation. He was headed for a place where he liked to go and rest. But when he got there, a strange couple of untouchables had taken over the place. Intrigued, he watched them from a distance. A cauldron, its base glowing red, was sitting over an enormous fire. The man was wearing only an apron, blackened by the blood of the chickens his wife was handing him. He cut off their heads without hesitation and with great pleasure. The ground was covered with

feathers and excrement. Namdev also saw four dogs, as black as night, tied to a tree. They were so ferocious that they were tearing each other apart.
Although the cauldron was only of average size, it seemed as though it would never be full. The man turned to his wife and cried out: "The thirty-six chickens are not enough. This wretched cauldron is still not full. Bring me the dogs." Without hesitating, the woman went over to the dogs and dragged them to the cauldron as though they were mere puppies. The man cut their throats without even looking at them. Laughing, he cried out to his wife: "This blasted cauldron is still not full. It wants even more. Bring me that idiot over there who's watching us, he'll do. Quickly! Let me cut his throat as well."
Namdev watched as this hirsute woman with bulging eyes, dripping with blood and guts, rushed towards him. He had never been so frightened in his life. He started to run as fast as he could and didn't stop until he was about to collapse with exhaustion. When he pulled himself back together, he realised that he hadn't understood what he'd seen. This couple were Viṣṇu and Rukmiṇī. The thirty-six chickens symbolised the tattva, killed and sacrificed in the devouring fire of Consciousness; the dogs, the four Veda, representing all knowledge; and he, Namdev, was the support for all this objective knowledge. What is left when everything, including our identity, has been killed?
He noticed a small śaiva temple that he had never seen before and decided to go and meditate. Was it to gather his thoughts or to look for consolation? He pushed the door open and in the late afternoon light that rushed in like a myriad of cheerful children, he saw an old man resting his feet on the liṅga. His blood boiled. He felt a devastating rage within him but controlled it so as not to depart from the image he wanted to give of being an even-tempered and wise man. Addressing the man with a trembling voice, he said: "Old man, are you not aware that you are committing a terrible offence towards the sanctuary of Śiva, and towards Śiva himself?"
Without looking, the old man muttered: "Listen lad, I am very old, almost crippled and half blind. Help me shift my legs so I do not offend Śiva and, more importantly, so I do not anger you."
Namdev was taken aback in disgust. He would defile himself by touching the filthy feet of this low caste. He could hear the echo of Gora's voice saying to him 'not fully baked'. Gora was right. He was not fully baked! He did as the old man asked and the old man said to him: "Nam, I can still feel something under my feet. Look and see what it is."
Namdev was surprised that the old man knew his name. But the fact he had shortened it to Nam, and in doing so insinuating he was not yet ready to bear the name of god, annoyed him even more. Namdev lifted the old man's feet up again and was stupefied to find another liṅga. He repeated this over and over again, and each time there was another liṅga under the feet of the old man, who said: "Lad, tell me where Śiva is not so I may finally rest my feet in peace."
At that moment, Namdev knew that in Visoba Kechar he had met his sadguru. As if by magic he remembered what Viṭṭhala had said about him. He knew of nobody in the three worlds as indifferent to the world as Visoba Kechar. This is how Namdev, sobbing at the feet of Visoba Kechar, received his teaching. When he next met Gora, who again examined him with his stick, the saintly potter cried out in satisfaction: "Ah, he too is now fully baked!"

The Advice of the Weaver Kabīr

"O Yogi, reflect upon this wisdom:

Those who climbed aboard the boat were drowned,
and those with nothing crossed to the other side!

Those who didn't keep to the path reached the town,
and those who followed the road lost their way!

We have all been bound by the same shackles,
who therefore is bound, and who is free?

Those who took shelter were drenched,
and those outside remained dry!

Those who were injured remained joyful,
and those who were spared are in agony!

Those who have lost their eyes contemplate the entirety of the universe,
and those with eyes to see are blind!

Says Kabīr, the world appears topsy-turvy!"

The Twenty-Four Guru of Dattātreya

"Salutations to Śrī Gaṇeśa.
Through the will of Īśvara who frees us from fear, the mind is inclined towards Advaita.
In the supreme Self and through Him all is contained.
How can I worship it, this Ātman, which is without form, indivisible and eternal peace?
The universe is the work of the five elements: merely a mirage.
In truth, all things are Ātman. There is neither distinction nor absence of distinction, neither existence nor non-existence. All of this appears to me as a marvel."

Thus starts the Avadhūta Gītā composed by Dattātreya, the lion of the Vedānta as he is named in the Jīvanmukta Gītā, the son of Atri, the incarnation of the three gods, the one who is followed by four dogs representing the Veda. He takes on frightening or disturbing forms so he may be left in peace. Datta sang to Rāma of the secret of the goddess Tripurā. To the superficial eye, he who is described in the Dattātreya Stotra as absolute and beyond all definition, only appears, by the magic of the Lord, as a drunkard fond of the company of prostitutes.
King Yadu, expert in dharma, seeing the ascetic brilliance of a joyful drunkard in the company of an ageing, toothless prostitute, asked him: "I can see great intelligence within you. Your appearance is deceptive. Tell me about the fire of your presence that nothing is able to hide. Explain this, as only this is of interest to me."
"O King, I have accepted many teachers by intuition. Listen to the names of those whose wisdom I have accepted into my heart, and which has let me roam carefree throughout the world. The earth, air, space, water, fire, the moon, the sun, the pigeon, the boa, the ocean, the moth, the bee, the elephant, the honey collector, the stag, the fish, the courtesan Piṅgalā, the osprey, the child, the young girl, the blacksmith, the snake, the spider and the larva are my twenty-four guru. From them I have learnt the invaluable and that which cannot be passed on by words.

"O King, hear my song. The earth has taught me patience, stability and firmness, even in unhappy circumstances such as when ill-treated. When one understands that those who act in this way have no choice and are themselves instruments of fate, one does what one has to do without deviating. Being a disciple of the mountain, which is a part of the earth and whose forests, pastures and rivers serve living beings, without distinction, I have learnt to accomplish all my activities for the good of all. Also being a disciple of the trees, which let themselves be cut down and uprooted according to man's whim, I have learnt to be a servant and that my function only has value in the service of others.

"From the wind, in the form of vāyu, which gives life to the body but is not dependent on it, I have learnt to breathe without fixing myself or becoming attached to the objects that, momentarily, the breath inflates and brings to life. Like the wind that carries both good and bad smells but is not identified to them, the avadhūta who learns from the wind is not fooled by the odour of the body and its different sheaths.

"Like the space of the sky is not affected by the clouds that are part of it, I have learnt to watch the clouds of the body-mind take shape in the space of my Consciousness.

"The freshness, babbling and incessant movement of spring water purify one's vision of all that clutters it. By escaping the dams of definitions and the stagnant waters of concepts, the avadhūta becomes a friend to all. The simple presence of his endlessly flowing nature purifies those who, instant by instant, watch themselves flow in his stream. This is what I have learnt from water.

"From fire, I have learnt the brilliance and fervour of consuming everything. As fire feeds on its fuel, I feed on everything offered to me. And, whilst accepting all that is offered, nothing resists the consuming fire of Consciousness. Like a fire that lies dormant under the ashes, the avadhūta remains anonymous amongst men. But if the situation requires, he is able to break out in an instant and embrace everything he touches.

"The different stages of existence, that start with birth and end with death, belong to space-time, which is nothing more than a mental creation and does not concern Ātman. The quarters of the moon, its rising and falling, are only a point of view seen from our planet and do not affect the moon itself, which is always full. This is what I have learnt from the moon.

"Although the sun's rays evaporate water, the sun is not affected by water, even when it rains. In the same way, the avadhūta, although appreciating or disliking the objects of the senses, according to circumstance, is not dependent upon them. For those who identify with the body-mind, Consciousness, although it knows no separation, may appear multiple. In the same way the sun is one, it may appear multiple when reflected. This is what I have learnt from the sun.

"There is no security in this world. Psychological dependence is an abyss of torments. Believing that somebody can give us love and comfort is a sad joke. This is what I have learnt from the tale of a pair of pigeons: A pigeon that was passionately in love built a nest for himself and his companion. They lived happily there for many years. Carried by their love, they were joyfully lost in their conjugal life, uniting their vision, their bodies, their emotions and their hearts. They experienced flights of passion and the fever of tight embraces. He satisfied all his desires and spent his time attending to all her wishes, whatever the effort required. In due course she laid her eggs, watched on in wonderment by her companion. By the incredible magic of the Lord were born wonderfully formed baby pigeons, covered with a down of endless softness. Their parents were filled with joy and tenderly looked after their fledgling, delighted with every step forward they made. Hypnotised by the charms of the Lord, they wove bonds of love and anxiety for their offspring. One day, having left their nest to go and look for food, a hunter, seeing the young birds alone, threw his net and caught them. When they came back and saw their offspring had been captured, the female, heartbroken and full of pain, went after them and was also captured. The pigeon, realising he had lost that which was most dear to him, lamented: 'I have been deprived of my love, of she who was more than just a presence, who filled every moment of my life. Is there a pain greater than losing one's own flesh and blood? I have lost everything. I am nothing now. What is my miserable life without them?' In desperation, the pigeon rushed into the net as well. Everything is evanescence, impermanence. Who are those we refer to as wife, husband or child? This is how the essential question was put to me by a pair of pigeons.

"From the boa, I have learnt to be contented with the food that is offered to me. I have also learnt from the boa the art of digesting everything, even the largest prey, without effort. The avadhūta thus digests all situations without being concerned by them.

"Although a storm may agitate an ocean's surface, from its depths I have learnt tranquillity and absorption in the unfathomable mystery of my Being. An ocean does not overflow when rivers flow into it, nor does it dry-up when rivers run dry. In the same way, the avadhūta does not get carried away by excitement when his desires are satisfied, nor does he become depressed when the same desires are not satisfied.

"From the moth that burns in a lamp's flame, I have learnt the mesmerising power of desire.

"Like the bee that produces its honey after having gathered nectar from different flowers, small or large, the avadhūta extracts the essence from all situations of existence to produce the unique sweetness of non-differentiation. He does likewise with religious treatises. But unlike the bee, the avadhūta does not need to create a hive around him through fear of the future, or to try and gather the honey of his own nature in a system or codification.

"In the rutting season, an elephant will pounce on any female used as bait to capture him. I have learnt from the elephant that desire, by its strength, creates its own prison. The woman or man I may fervently desire today can turn into a shrew or tyrant as time takes its toll.

"From the honey collector, who is mesmerised by the myth of security and lives in fear of tomorrow, I have learnt the futility of his fight. Money that is accumulated is only handed back as tax, stolen by corrupt bankers or lost in judicial hearings and on medical care. When we reach retirement, we have a thousand worries gnawing away at us and are too tired to really appreciate it. The honey collector is my guru. He has taught me that true wealth lies in the instant.

"The stag, which lets itself be captured when hunters imitate its call, is also my guru. The avadhūta does not expect anything of objects, of that which is external to him, of the world and what it contains, or even of his own body. There is no experience or destination that attracts him.

"I bow before the fish that lets itself be caught by the bait on a hook. It too has taught me that when man listens to the tongue of becoming, he runs from one lure to another, only to find the hook of suffering. He who still craves a certain type of nourishment, whether it be a type of food or an experience, only encounters the hook of frustration.

"I also bow before Piṅgalā, the saintly prostitute. Piṅgalā was a very beautiful courtesan. Every evening she would get ready and dress up with irresistible lures before offering herself to passers-by. But in the cold solitude of the night she knew that those who came to her did not really know her and were only interested in the mask of her charms. That which in the beginning made her unhappy became an instant of joyful discovery. It was the Lord himself that wore the mask of the prostitute and of her client. I have learnt from her the highest form of detachment: that there is no one to be attached to. Did she continue or did she stop? This is of no importance because Piṅgalā's home will forever be amongst the mahāsiddha. Listen to what she sang to me the last time we met: 'Satisfied and subsisting on that which Providence provides, I surrender to the Lord who is my own Self. Who other but my own Self could accept me as I am, I who have fallen so low in saṃsāra.'

"I bow before the osprey which, hounded by other birds that covet its sustenance, escapes their attacks by abandoning its bit of meat. He who understands this savours the tranquillity of having no possessions.

"The innocent child is also my guru. Like for the child, the world is a playground for me. Completely ignorant and carefree, I come and go as I please, knowing that my mother is looking out for me.

"A young lady was entertaining guests, one of whom may

choose her to be their son's wife. Being the only one in the household and not wanting her guests to know she was preparing the food like a servant, she discreetly made her way to the kitchen. But any movement she made was betrayed by the clattering of bracelets that she wore around her wrists. So she broke the bracelets until there was only one pair around each wrist. But even this pair of bracelets made a noise. She broke two more bracelets. The two remaining bracelets then made no more noise. I bow before her because she taught me that when several people, or even just two people, suffering from the illusion of separation live together, there are only quarrels and conflicts. Thus I wander alone in the world, encountering only myself.

"I bow before the blacksmith who was so absorbed by his work that he didn't even notice the royal procession passing by in front of his smithy. For the avadhūta, the procession of the world may pass by but he his always absorbed in the Ultimate Reality.

"The snake is also my guru. The snake travels alone, withdrawing into holes in rocks or in the ground that it encounters by chance along its path. In the same way, the avadhūta withdraws into the cave of his heart and does not spend his time trying to build a residence of projects. The avadhūta goes through life in complete anonymity and silence, like the snake that cannot be recognised by the trace it leaves on the ground.

"I also bow before the spider. Like the spider, which creates or retracts its web from its own substance, the Lord does the same with this universe.

"I bow before the larva, my guru who initiated me in non-duality. When caught by a wasp, its survival instinct creates such symbiosis that it ends up resembling the wasp. This could not be accomplished if separation between beings really existed.

"This is how, O King, by silently listening to these preceptors, that intuitive wisdom has risen up within me like a life source. And now, let me tell you how my body has been the greatest teacher of all. It is the body that enables the fruit of holy indifference to ripen. It is subjected to birth, decay and death. It is merely an object like any other, sinking in the ocean of existence. But he who listens to the body is able to explore the very substance of this universe, which is in no way different to it. The body is a sensation, like the fragrance of a flower. For the avadhūta, the body is merely a reflection in the ineffable. This is why he is not attached to it. When the time comes, he will let it fade away, like when after a long day, one joyfully surrenders to sleep. This is how, O King, I am able to wander, free from destination, without a care."

Luipā, Eater of Scraps

Whilst hiding in the belly of a fish, Luipā, also known as the great Matsyendranātha or Mīnanātha, received the secret teaching that Śiva had revealed to Gaurī. Since then he had been wandering like a madman in the mass grave of the world. Although he had received the very essence of the teaching, he had not yet digested it. One day, whilst crossing a town like one might cross a field of ruins, his intuition led him to an inn that was also a brothel. As soon as he entered he was immediately enticed by one of the prostitutes whom he recognised as Śakti. He paid his respects to her. The supreme Ḍākinī silently scrutinised him for a while. She then said to him: "Although your cakra are limpid, a knot of arrogance, the size of a pea, still remains in your heart."

She then gave him an earthen bowl filled with putrid and foul leftovers. Laughing, she said: "O great siddha, here is your sustenance for today."

When Luipā left the inn, he threw the food into the gutter. The prostitute was watching and shouted out mockingly: "If you are still imprisoned by the illusion of having a choice between good and bad food, how can you claim to know the ultimate reality?"

These words hit Luipā head on, and he replied: "O divine slut, you have shown me my profound stupidity. How could I have been so arrogant?"

He settled down in a mass grave on the banks of the Gaṅgā to digest the ultimate teaching. His companions in this madness were the jackals and vultures that were fighting over the remains of smoking corpses. He stayed there for twelve years, begging for his food from fishermen, and only accepting the entrails that were usually thrown to the dogs. This is how he came by the name of Luipā: 'Eater of Scraps'.

Luipā ate the entrails of existence such as they were offered to him. This food was merely the nectar of non-differentiation.

From time to time he could be heard singing:

"Rub honey into the muzzle of a wild dog,
And it will madly devour all it sniffs.
Give the guru's secret to an uninitiated idiot,
And his mind and lineage will be destroyed by confusion.
For he who after having silently listened, understands the unborn reality,
A simple insight of the guru's intuition will destroy the concept of illusion,
Like a mad elephant charging into hostile ranks, yielding a sword in its trunk."

The Infinite Staging of the Guru

or How Gorakṣanātha Thought He Could Free Matsyendranātha

Gorakṣanātha learnt from another siddha, Kānupā, that his guru was going to die in three days' time at Kadali, where he had become a petty king in a kingdom of women. This is what Gaurī had predicted when she cast a spell upon him. He would become the slave of his debauchery in a kingdom of women, prisoner of sixteen hundred Amazonian warriors, having forgotten he had been Ādinātha, the great Matsyendra. Saraha illustrated this episode in one of his songs:

"By taking a women from lower Bengal, you lost your way.
To the left and right are the canals of differentiation.
Saraha says: unity resides in the centre.
She (differentiation) devours her husband and amuses herself in the Sahaja; she loves and she hates.
Sitting by her lover, her heart corrupt, this is how the Yoginī appeared to me."

Before Gorakṣanātha left, Kānhapā wished him a good journey with a monotonous chant:

"The true self is forever fulfilled.
Do not be saddened when the body's clothing and mind's make-up leave us.
How could we not exist?
Only an idiot is sad at the end of a show.
Do breaking waves cause the sea to dry up?
One who is ignorant does not see the butter in the milk.
In the ultimate reality, nobody comes and nobody goes.
In this knowledge, act out this divine play without hesitation."

Before rushing off, Gorakṣanātha thanked him: "Your song has warmed my heart."

The presence of men was forbidden in the kingdom. He therefore had to think quickly of a subterfuge. He disguised himself as a woman and passed himself off as a musician and dancer. He was not immediately granted permission to see the king and was asked to wait at the entrance to the reception hall. Gorakṣanātha started to play his drum, which caught the attention of Matsyendranātha. He ordered the musician to be brought in. After years of separation, Gorakṣanātha was filled with joy to see Matsyendranātha, but his sadness was just as great. Matsyendranātha was sat on his throne, surrounded by women, one of whom was perched on his left leg, another on his right leg. They were giggling and teasing him. The one who appeared to be his queen gave him wine to drink from a golden goblet. He had grown old. His hair whitened his temples with fatigue and the burning presence foremost in his look all those years ago had completely left him. His two young children, a boy and a girl, were constantly squabbling near the throne. He seemed to be overcome with a terrible lassitude, and although he was king, he appeared tyrannised by a thousand worries. Matsyendranātha's days were coming to an end. He was about to die forgetful of who he really was. Gorakṣanātha cried to himself in silence: "How strange fate can be and how the power of the absolute has no mercy. There is no end to māyā. I can see its hold, even on the great Matsyendranātha, the foremost siddha, he who awakened me from my torpor when I was sleeping under the manure of my illusions."

He was unable to speak, because if he had he would have been immediately discovered and killed. So he started to play his ḍamaru, like Śiva had done when he played the Maheśvara Sūtra, resonating his drum fourteen times, revealing the vowels known as svarajana, because they shine of their own accord. This is what Gorakṣanātha said to him without words: "Wake-up Matsyendranātha, Gorakṣanātha is here." Matsyendranātha came out of his torpor but this was not enough for him to leave the kingdom to which he was so deeply attached. Gorakṣanātha, seeing his Guru was still hesitant, dragged him and his two children away. He killed his children in front of him, dismembered them, cleaned their skin of all blemishes and laid them out to dry. Matsyendranātha took him into his arms and said: "Iḍā and Piṅgalā are at peace once more, only the central pulsation remains."

Before leaving the kingdom, Gorakṣanātha transformed the sixteen hundred women and their queen back into what they had always been: imaginary bats. Later on in the day, they stopped at an inn and decided to spend the night there. In the middle of the night, Gorakṣanātha took the hand of his master and said to him: "O venerated guru, my heart is about to explode with joy. I have found you again, but above all, you have found yourself again."

Matsyendranātha turned to him with a mischievous look in his eyes, and Gorakṣanātha started to realise the farce he had played upon himself. Matsyendranātha said to him: "The body may suffer from loss of memory, paralysis, coughing and other pains, but this is our sort as long as there is a body. But even amidst distractions, he who remains at his source is never abandoned by the effusion of the Self. As this reality cannot forget itself, it needs no reminder."

Gorakṣanātha bowed before his master and said: "I thought I'd saved you, but it is you who has freed me. In my infinite ignorance, I still identified you with the body. Wonder of wonders, the play of the guru knows no limits."

The Butcher Ding's Principles of Hygiene

The butcher Ding was cutting up a buffalo in front of Prince Wenhui. His body was moving in time to the sound of his knife and the noise of the meat falling onto the stall, conjuring up a sweet melody. In a choking voice, Prince Wenhui said: "Magnificent! How did you gain such mastery?"

The butcher laid down his knife and replied: "What pleases your servant the most, is the Way. This is how I am able to progress in my art. When I started, I saw nothing more than a buffalo. After three years, I no longer looked at it as a whole. It is now the mind of your servant and not his senses that are at work. As my senses are inactive it is my mind that acts. I comply with the laws of nature by cutting along existing interstices, separating at the main joints, following the natural constitution. The rule of the art is to not cut the tendons, and even less so the large bones! A good butcher only needs to change his knife once a year. Others break and change their knife every month. Your servant has been using the same knife for nineteen years. I have cut up thousands of buffaloes and my knife still cuts as though it has just been sharpened. In each joint there is a space, and the blade of the knife has no thickness. That which has no thickness slices easily through that which has only space. There is therefore more space than is needed. This is why, after nineteen years, my knife cuts as though it has just been sharpened. I observe where the problem lies each time I come across a joint, temper my fear, fix my gaze, slow my movement, move my knife only a fraction and no sooner divide the joint as though it is a clod of earth. I put down my knife and stand up straight. Motionless and satisfied, I look at the four sides. I then clean my knife and put it away."

"Magnificent!" said the prince, "Thanks to this butcher's words, my life is preserved!"

Tales from Zuangzi, or The True Classic of Nanhua

Huairang's Brick

Mazu practised meditation at the monastery dedicated to teaching law. There he met the abbot Rang, who saw straight away that he was a good teacher. One day, the abbot asked him: "Reverend, for what purpose are you sitting in meditation?"
Mazu replied: "To become Buddha."
The abbot Rang took a piece of brick and started polishing it.
Mazu asked: "Why are you polishing that piece of brick?"
"I am polishing it to make it a mirror."
Mazu exclaimed: "How can one obtain a mirror by polishing a brick?"
The abbot Rang answered: "If one cannot obtain a mirror by polishing a brick, how can one become Buddha by remaining seated in meditation?"
"Then what should I do?" asked Mazu.
The abbot Rang replied: "If the cart isn't moving, should one whip the buffalo or the cart? Do you wish to learn to be seated in dhyāna or to be seated as Buddha? If you wish to practise meditation, you should be aware that dhyāna is not a matter of seated position, nor of any position. If you wish to attain the nature of Buddha, you should be aware that the Buddha has no specific characteristics. Within dharma, which has no abode, there is neither gain nor loss. If you are seated as Buddha, you kill the Buddha. If you are attached to the seated position, you will not obtain the absolute truth."
Mazu was delighted with these words, as though he had drunk the most exquisite of nectars. He asked: "Tell me about creation and destruction?"
Rang replied: "He who considers the Way in terms of creation and destruction, accumulation and dispersion, does not really see the Way. Your own nature is devoid of characteristics. How can there be accomplishment or non-accomplishment?"
Mazu served his master for ten years, each day penetrating further into the wonderful and mysterious meaning of reality.

Biographical Accounts of Master Chan Mazu Daoyi from Jiangxi Province

There Is No Tree of Enlightenment

A day when Huineng was selling wood at the market, he came out of one of his customer's shops and heard a man reciting a sūtra. As soon as he heard it, his mind became enlightened. He asked the stranger what he was reciting. He told him it was the Diamond Sūtra (Vajracchedikā Sūtra). The man then told him he had come from the Tung Chan monastery, where Hung-Jen, the fifth patriarch, was the superior. He often went to the monastery to listen to the talks of the fifth patriarch, who encouraged both the laity and the monks to recite this sūtra. Huineng decided to visit the monastery and arrived after travelling for thirty days. He offered his respects to the patriarch, who asked him where he was from and the purpose of his visit.

"I am from the district of Hsin Chou in Kwangtung province. I have made this long trip so I may pay my respects to you. I wish only to become a Buddha."

"How can a native of Kwangtung hope to become a Buddha?"

Huineng replied: "Although I come from the South and others may come from the North, directions are of no importance when it comes to Buddha Nature. I am physically different to Your Holiness but there is no difference in our profound nature."

Although he would have liked to continue speaking to Huineng, the fifth patriarch dismissed him because other monks were looking on: "You have too much spirit. Go to the stables and don't say another word."

Eight months went by before the patriarch crossed his path again. At this occasion he said to Huineng: "Your intuition is profound, but I cannot speak to you. It would cause jealousy and you may be harmed."

There were over a thousand monks in the monastery. One day, the patriarch addressed his assembly: "You are still only concerned about accumulating merit and virtue. This is of no help if you live in the illusion of separation. Question your own heart and write me a poem about this. He who unveils the essence of the Ultimate Nature will receive the patriarchal robe and will be initiated. He will become the sixth patriarch. He who recognises himself in this function will never again forget it, even when in battle." The congregation of disciples withdrew. They agreed to let Shen-Hsiu, their instructor, write the gāthā.

Shen-Hsiu was undecided: "Because I am their instructor, they expect me to write my stanza. And none of them will want to compete against their instructor. If I don't do it, how will I know the depth of my understanding? I do not seek the patriarchate, but I cannot let the opportunity of being initiated pass me by. It is truly a delicate situation."

He composed his poem, but was incapable of showing it to his master. Instead he decided to display it on a wall. "If he is pleased with it, I shall tell him that I am the author. If though the master does not approve of it, I will have wasted many years in this monastery receiving tributes I don't deserve."

The patriarch summoned Shen-Hsiu and asked him if he was the author of the poem. Shen-Hsiu replied that he was. "Your stanza shows that you have still not seen your own nature. With an understanding such as yours, there is little chance of succeeding in the search for the supreme understanding. One must be capable of knowing spontaneously one's own heart and one's own nature, which, because it is not produced, cannot be annihilated. Go and think about it again. Submit another poem. If it shows you have crossed the threshold of enlightenment, I will hand you the robe and dharma."

Dahala *10th century*
(Madhya Pradesh)

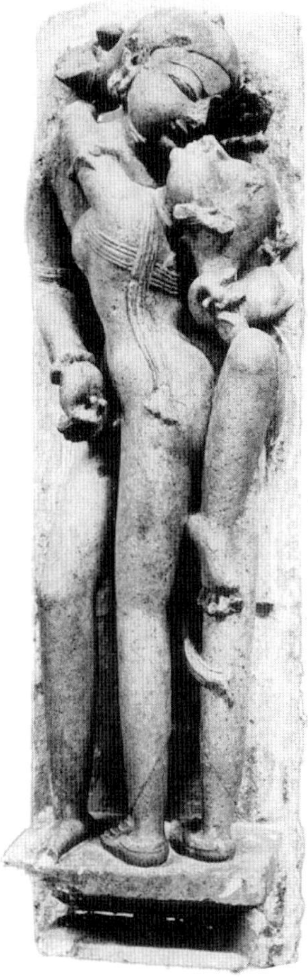

For several days Shen-Hsiu felt as though he was being tortured, and he was unable to write a new poem.

One day, whilst it was still early and the air cold, Huineng was on his way to the stables. He went up to the poem that was on display. He lit up the characters with his candle, but as he could not read, he was not able to decipher them. He called out to a monk and asked him to read out the poem.

"Ah! So you want me to read our instructor's wonderful poem. Everyone knows he will succeed the fifth patriarch. Shen-Hsiu is a great man. What about you? Would you not like to succeed Hung-Jen? You would no longer have to work in the stables or kitchens. Come closer and open your ears."

"The body is the enlightenment tree,
The mind is a bright mirror in a stand.
Take care to wipe it all the time,
And allow no dust to cling."

Huineng smiled and asked the monk if he would write something for him:

"Fundamentally no enlightenment tree exists,
Nor the stand of a mirror bright.
Since all is empty from the beginning,
Where can the dust alight?"

Huineng succeeded the fifth patriarch who secretly handed over the robe and interpreted the Diamond Sūtra for him.

He said to the patriarch: "Who would have thought that Self-Nature is intrinsically pure? Who would have thought that Self-Nature is intrinsically free from creation and annihilation? Who would have thought that Self-Nature is intrinsically self-sufficient? Who would have thought that Self-Nature is free of all changes? Who would have thought that all phenomena are merely manifestations of Self-Nature?"

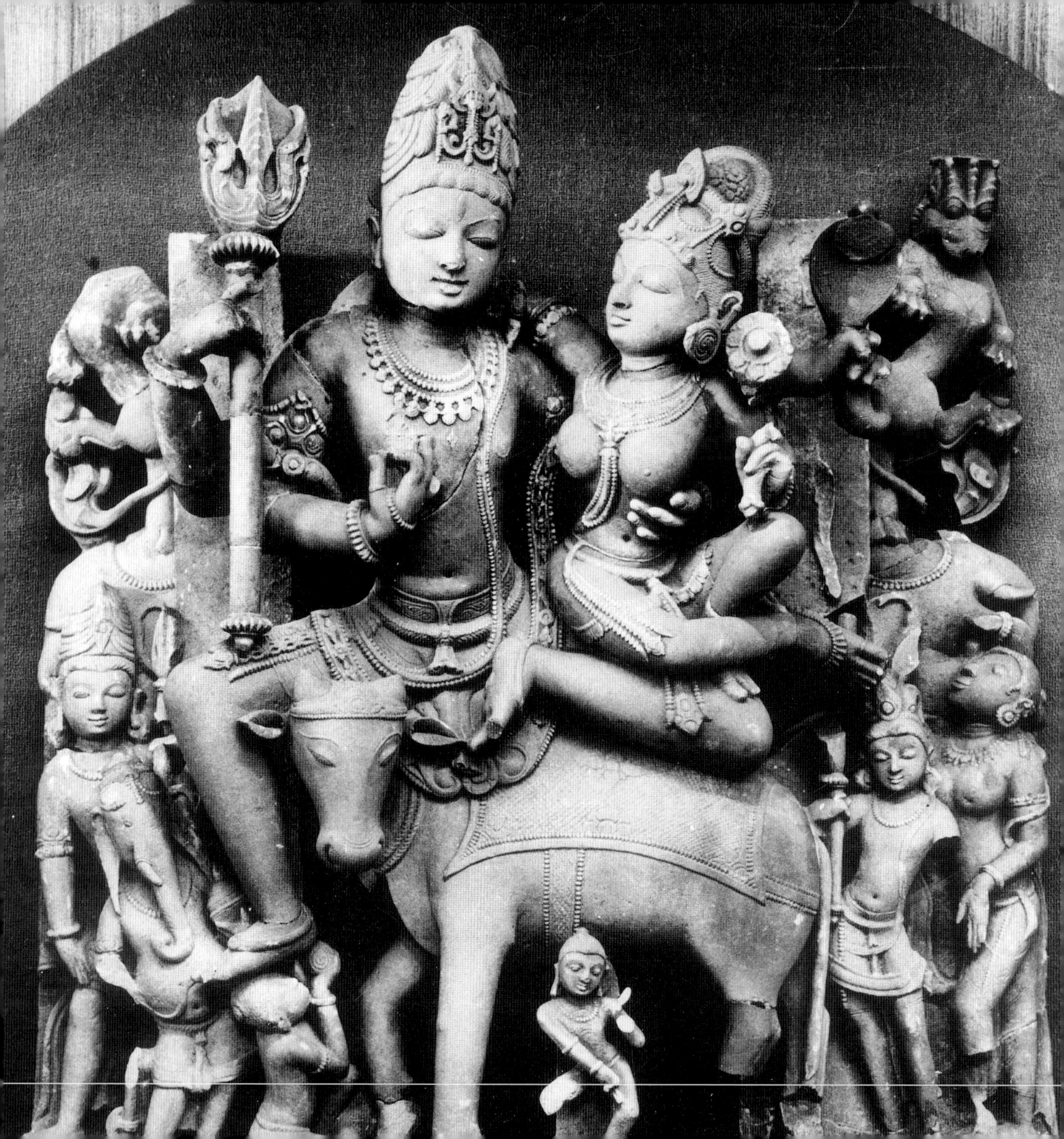

Umāmaheśvaramūrti *10th century*
(Hinglajgarh, Madhya Pradesh)

17

The Practice of Non-Practice

"One only obtains the joy of Your embrace by abandoning the effort of meditation and one's practices. Such is the true worship of lovers. May it be mine forever!"
UTPALADEVA, ŚIVASTOTRĀVALĪ XVII, 4

"All forms of practice can be summed up as learning to kill dragons."
WEI WU WEI, OPEN SECRET, PAGE 46

"The yogic practice is recommended in order to remove the false identification of the experient with the embodiment and not for attaining the status of the experiencing consciousness that by its very nature is always luminous."
KṢEMARĀJA, PRATYABHIJÑĀHṚDAYA, COMMENTARY ON SŪTRA 15

In its essence, practice is the recognition of our own Presence, from which all activities ensue and are expressed. There is therefore no activity or practice able to favour or prevent this Presence. States of Consciousness may be modified, but they remain merely states. That by which we are able to know ourselves in these states remains forever inexpressible, and cannot be objectivised as experience.

"Deliverance is in reality nothing other than the unfolding of our own essence, which is non other than the Consciousness of oneself. The energies of activity, knowledge and will do not add themselves to Consciousness since nothing exists without prior Consciousness, and one cannot hold or support existence outside the Consciousness of a subject with qualities."
ABHINAVAGUPTA, TANTRĀLOKA I, 156-157

Intuition of Presence and Establishing Practice in This Background

"Whatever is prescribed or whatever is forbidden, yoga based on members (aṅga), like control of the breath and so on, all this is a sham. These systems are not worth an iota of ours, which is innate. O Sovereign of the Gods, let the heart adhere resolutely in reality. This alone is prescribed, no matter how it is attained." MĀLINĪVIJAYA TANTRA XVIII, 74, 78, 79

Without this intuition, practising is like performing gymnastics of betterment in the jaws of becoming, which spew out promising destinations and wonderful goals like those in a tourist guide. In order to observe this dynamism of intention and projection passively, without nourishing it, it must be illuminated by its source.
"The upsurge is Bhairava." VASUGUPTA, ŚIVASŪTRA I, 5

The desire to investigate, which may take the gross form of psychological effort aimed at harnessing or improving, is already in essence the intensity of our own Presence. Replacing this effort in its source enables a certain grasping to be washed away, allowing it to rest in its primordial upsurge.

"The stage is the inner Self."
VASUGUPTA, ŚIVASŪTRA III, 10

Like actors who play out their roles on the same stage, the intuition that the background is our own Presence allows the different states of Consciousness to be explored, without putting the emphasis on these states.

"Even though differing states like waking, sleeping, etc. occur, the Spanda principle remains identically the same. The Spanda principle never departs from its own nature as the perceiving subject." SPANDAKĀRIKĀ 3

This intuition is actualised through passive observation, where the sensory organs participate in this non-grasping. It is transposed into āsana practice by ensuring the eyes, tongue and eardrums always remain neutral. Whatever the intensity of an āsana, it must be spread out and not localised in the aforementioned regions. The skin itself must mirror this organic spreading.

"The senses are the spectators" (ŚIVASŪTRA III, 11), and thus become witnesses to the offering of the body and its different sheaths.

"The body is the ritual oblation."
VASUGUPTA, ŚIVASŪTRA II, 8

The observation of agitation, of muscular, organic and mental grasping, is done in the space of one's Presence, where they are like currents freed from the notion of a practitioner identified with a body-mind. The different techniques used will be done so in the spontaneity of the instant, and will no longer be the source of fragmented activity.

Starting the Day with the Fragrance of Deep Sleep

"At the hour of Brahman I remember the Ātman tattva that fills my heart, that is the core of existence, whose nature is intelligence and bliss, and which eternally knows the three states of Consciousness but is beyond them as the fourth. I am that indivisible Brahman and not the cumulation of elements. At the hour of Brahman my mind sings of He that language cannot describe, but who by His grace gives language the ability to describe Him. He that the Veda describe as 'neither this, nor that', this God of gods we know as 'Unborn', 'Unchanging', 'Primordial'."
ŚAṄKARĀCĀRYA, THE HYMN OF DAWN (PRĀTAḤ SMARAṆA)

At the moment of wakening, whilst still between the sleeping and waking states, a certain tranquillity lingers. We have not yet donned the clothes of our qualifications and intentions. Savour this tranquillity for a few moments, like moistening the mouth with a good wine so it may reveal all its flavour, or like the fragrance of wet soil that fills the air once the rain has stopped. The bedroom is perhaps still in darkness, devoid of shape. Far away, there is the sound of a solitary car in a deserted street. There is the lament of dustbins being manhandled in the freshness of the night's end, heralding the start of a new day. The body is left to reappear, emerge, as though space is donning its clothes and taking shape. We can only marvel at this mystery.

Ending the Day by Burning It

"When beings are tired of action, of living, knowing, playing and suffering, and seek true rest through dreamless sleep, they return to the Lord of sleep, to immobility, to the abode of joy, where the universe rests and sleeps."
ŚRĪ ŚIVATATTVA II, 1941-42

The day has been long, with its procession of rituals and repetitive actions. It is late and the house is bathed in a cathedral silence. We take off our clothes without regrets, as if ridding ourselves of an unwelcome witness. Ablutions are performed and a last glance thrown at the mask reflected by the mirror. We return to our bed with the pleasure of someone about to taste the kiss of oblivion, our body shrouded by the softness of the sheets. The day is contemplated like an old abandoned village whose history was forgotten long ago. There is the sensation that things happened by themselves and that they no longer concern us. Our identity, role, functions and projects are left to joyfully die away. Abandoning ourself to the waves of exhalation, the body is deposited like a cloud without substance, disappearing into the depth of the sky.

Consecrating Your Practice with the Heart by Paying Homage to Your Lineage

"Immortal, matchless family, made of dazzling emission, that of the union of the couple formed by the father with the body of plenitude and splendour and by the mother whose brilliance, with ever renewing emissions, sprouts from the pure creative power of energy, completely dazzling my heart."
Abhinavagupta, Tantrāloka I, 1

A good way to start practice is with quiet sitting. Such sitting is simply an outer symbol of the essence of āsana. One of the etymologies of āsana is 'to be seated'. It is therefore the establishment of all we think we are into the background of Consciousness. The arms and legs are considered as subsidiary extensions (upāṅga). The organs of action must be surrendered. We then take refuge in our lineage, or family (kula). Symbolically, the family is the expression of spanda in the siddha lineage and the expression of the universe in the body itself. When we take refuge in a teacher or lineage, we bow before the Heart of our own Presence. As Abhinavagupta says: *"The Heart is the Self of Consciousness."* A stone has more heart than practice without heart. It is the Heart of Presence that illuminates practice and not the opposite.

"Only the light of the heart truly exists. It is the agent for creative activity, and as it blazes, the universe unfolds."
Maheśvarānanda, Mahārthamañjarī 11

Making the Practice Mat a Cremation Ground (Śmaśāna)

The practice mat should be laid out as though it is our funeral pyre. The fire of āsana is used to burn the residue of muscular and organic tensions, as well as mental conceptualisation and bodily identification. The differentiations projected by the inner organ (antaḥkaraṇa): intellect (buddhi), mind (manas), ego (ahaṃkāra), are reduced to ashes.

"There, located on the inner (antara) path, is the cremation ground called Aṭavīmukha. The leader there, as formidable as the Lord of Death (Kṛtāta), is called Śaṇkhapāla, Protector of the Conch. Demons and the leaders of the deities and siddha in the Sky serve him and at night a troupe of Yoginī plays there in the light of a lighted lamp. The congregation (cakra) of Yama (the Lord of the dead) is present there where Yoginī and heroes meet. Then union (melāpa) takes place between them on Rudra's day at an auspicious time (suṛkṣe). The field (viṣaya) is Kulakaula that engenders the union of heroes and Yoginī. Concealed, the great Lord Siddhanāta resides there."
Mark S. G. Dyczkowski, Manthānabhairavatantram Vol. 4, VI, 154cd-155ab, 155cd-156ab, 156d-157ab, 157cd-158ab (Page 133)

Witnessing the Body-Mind as the Shadow of Consciousness

Contemplation of the embodiment puts us in contact with its primary nature, that of sensations. In the intimacy of these sensations, movements of emanation and resorption are discovered that shatter the concept of body localisation and shape. All sensations stem from the foremost sensation, that of existing, without colouration. Tanū is one of the Sanskrit words meaning body. It comes from the root TAN (tanoti), 'to spread', 'to extend', 'to pervade', and from which the word tantra is derived.

"If one evokes, just for an instant, the absence of duality in any part of the body, vacuity shines forth. Freed from all dualistic thoughts, one attains the non-dualistic essence."
VIJÑĀNA BHAIRAVA 46

Practising in Abandonment Resting in the Essence

According to Patañjali's well-known sūtra (abhyāsa vairāgyābhyāṃ tannirodhaḥ, I.12), psychological memory dissolves in practice (abhyāsa) and detachment (vairāgya). Abhyāsa comes from the prefix ABHY, meaning 'movement towards', 'aspiration to', followed by the root ĀS, meaning 'to sit'. It is therefore the aspiration to become estab- lished in one's own essence. This burning call to become immersed in one's own tranquillity is referred to as abhyāsa, as defined in sūtra I.13: *"Practice is the unfolding of energy aimed at establishing the mind in its source."*

This aspiration to one's own essence must blossom in abandonment. It will otherwise become intention, projection into the future and a progressive approach.

Vairāgya is made up of 'vai-vi', which has a privative meaning, and rāg, whose root is RAÑJ, meaning 'to colour', 'to tint'. Vision without commentary, without colouration, when perception stays with 'what is', is referred to as vairāgya. Vairāgya is the absence of passion (rāga) and thirst (tṛṣṇā) for exteriority as an experience, whatever the experience.

Postural and breathing techniques are unfolded to explore our own nature, but also to abandon this desire in its source. Everything encountered in the process of practising is welcomed into our awareness, where psychophysical phenomena are able to spread in complete freedom and be burnt in the instant. Obstacles are thus no longer difficulties for which there is success or failure since they are free from comparison and competition.

Giving Yourself Daily to the Consecration of Embodiment

or how to *"resorb activities of separation into the body"*
VASUGUPTA, ŚIVASŪTRA III, 4

We only think our existence, which is nothing more than a maze of opinions, prejudices and conflicting theories. Our existence is therefore the activity of separation, the bite of differentiation that creates a world of objects external to us, which, in our profound isolation, we try to control. Returning to bodily sensations is the first step in going from a 'thought' life to a 'felt' life. The challenge of āsana and the awakening they provide chip off the sticky varnish of the 'thought' body and take us back to bodily sensations through muscular, articular and organic extension. Whatever the perception encountered, it becomes a resonance in the body. When the perception is unpleasant the throat tenses, the teeth clench, the diaphragm knots and the breathing becomes blocked. In the beginning, spontaneous spreading of the body is only observed when coming out of an āsana. This spreading will later happen in the āsana itself. Perception is therefore not archived or labelled; its echo can be felt in the body as space and spreading. This spreading, or engulfing by successive waves, devours the notions of body, mind and separate entity, leaving us with a sensation (sparśa) of space, which itself vanishes into non-sensation (asparśa), of not being localised as 'this' or 'that'. Daily consecration of the body, through the simplicity of actual sensation in the instant, allows the body to be sensed as a sensation that appears and disappears in the space of one's Presence. This sensation can take the form of gross and subtle bodies, as well as the different states of Consciousness: waking, dreaming and deep sleep.

Traditionally, we speak of contemplating the dissolution (layabhāvanā) or practising the engulfing of different spheres of objectivation, from the grossest to the subtlest. This engulfing is achieved by dissolving a sphere (kalā) into its essence. The earth element (nivṛttikalā) is thus resorbed into the sphere containing the twenty-four elements from earth to prakṛti. This sphere (pratiṣṭhākalā) then dissolves into the third sphere, referred to as vidyākalā, and which unfolds the six armours (kañcuka). This in turn is resorbed into the fourth sphere, śāntakalā, where subjectivity is found, represented by the elements from śuddhavidyātattva to śaktitattva. This sphere then dissolves into the bindu: Śiva.

"When entire objectivity rests in pure Consciousness, there for us is worship."
ṚJUVIMARŚINĪ

The Heart of Āsana

The exploration of āsana and breathing techniques is a prolongation of the intuition of peace experienced during deep sleep. The different postural attitudes allow this savour to be actualised organically. One of the first fragrances of this actualisation is stability (sthira). As we have seen, āsana help add vitality to this organic awakening and reflect the stability (sama-samasthāna) of the limbs, muscles, organs, senses, breath and mind. This stability is the spontaneous and ever-gushing (nityodita) vibration of the inclusiveness of Consciousness, which enables the different levels of embodiment to be actualised. The āsana are accompanied by ease, hence the sūtra:
"The Seat (āsana) should be firm and comfortable."
YOGASŪTRA II, 46

It is a subtle marriage of vigilance and surrender.
"When in the company of others, act as if you are alone; when alone, act as if you are in the company of others."
CHINESE PROVERB

It is therefore clear that āsana does not refer to a posture, but to the plunging into the great lake of Consciousness (mahārada) as undifferentiated awareness.

"Resting all objective experience within oneself is what is meant by 'I-feeling'. This 'resting' or sitting is called Sovereignty of Will, primary doership and lordship because of the annihilation of all relational consciousness, and of dependence on anything outside oneself."
UTPALADEVA, AJAḌAPRAMĀTṚSIDDHI 22-23

Comfort in Discomfort

"Perfection in an āsana is achieved when the effort to perform it becomes effortless and the infinite being within is reached."
YOGASŪTRA II, 47

Āsana reveal discomfort because of bodily stiffness and resistances. In the beginning, the practitioner is submerged by tension, as though in a stifling heat wave, and is oblivious to the fact this tension is localised in certain regions (shoulders, eyes, throat, tongue, diaphragm) that should remain neutral, as should the breath. It is a bit like going home after a bad day and taking it out on your wife, husband, children or dog. Neutrality in these regions lets the various resistances spread out in passive observation. Hence, all effort has its source in and disappears into non-effort. If tension is observed passively, we are not the tension but the space from which it appears, spreads out and disappears, like wrinkles in a cloth that disappear when they are ironed out. Ultimately, effort as psychological intention must die away, devoured by intuition of the infinite.

When Acting Disturbed No Longer Bothers Us

All that arises in the process of practice, and which reflects the tyranny of opposites, is washed away by the background of Consciousness. What happens is not frozen as an event, as this always awakens the thousand-headed monster of concepts: body, mind, pleasure, pain, life, death, etc. On the contrary, the sensation, whether it be pain or pleasure, and its bodily actualisation, is given all the space it needs. We remain with its intrinsic quality of silent energy, like a wave that rises and falls in the ocean from which it is never separated.

"The vow (vrata) is the contemplation of all things as being the Lord and being certain of this at all times and in all places, of the evidence of this similarity without calling upon some other means of liberation; as it is said in the Nandaśikhā: the supreme vow is universal equality."
ABHINAVAGUPTA, TANTRASĀRA IV

That which can be disturbed will be disturbed, and is not worth worrying about. Presence, from which all turbulence stems, is forever present.

The Way of Technique

When a Beginner, Practise Your Scales!

The way of technique is complete immersion in the art one practises, so as to get to know not only the whole, but also the parts. Simple introductory series are done to start with. Their aim is to teach postural emanation through various groups of āsana (see Chapter 12: *Consecration of Embodiment and Rituals of Fullness*). The name of each āsana should be known, as should its place in the group of āsana and its interaction with the body. One should get to know different sequences and combinations of āsana (vinyāsakrama) and the technicalities of each āsana. Their intrinsic qualities must become clear (stimulating, pacifying, heating, cooling, cleansing, nourishing, etc.), as must their use according to needs, seasons, or for specific cases. In Iyengar Yoga, the use of props in different groups of āsana must be integrated. In the way of technique, one becomes a craftsman who knows not only which instruments to use according to the situation, but also the qualities of the material with which one is working. Certain series of exercises should be practised. These must become spontaneous and second nature.

- The breath follows the movement of the body.
- The awareness observes the movements of the body and the breath.
- Each movement is circular and harmonious.
- The end of one movement is the start of another.
- Root oneself (sthānaṃ).
- Align the different parts of the body in the unity.
- After effort, always return to the natural state (sama).

Immersion in the way of technique requires unwavering loyalty to the approach for which one is inclined, and may take twenty years or so of serious and devoted practice and study. The mixing of styles should be avoided as this will only add to the confusion and delay intuitive symbiosis where one becomes the technique, and thus surpasses it. The whole is not the result of an accumulation of constituent parts.

Beginning with What Is Accessible

"Where there is inclination, precept is found; where there is no inclination, prohibition is found. For us who consider the sacred texts as an outpouring of the heart, that is discrimination." MAHEŚVARĀNANDA, MAHĀRTHAMAÑJARĪ 7

The practitioner, apart from often encountering physical stiffness, will also encounter mental contraction. The āsana will reveal limitations. The practitioner should neither consider his body as a country to be conquered nor the āsana, which in essence are merely an offering, as an army. Our conditioning for competition and comparison makes it all too easy for us to get stuck in this attitude. This only serves to maintain psychological tension, or more precisely a tension of separation. This tension, which we continue to nourish in our activities and perpetuate during āsana practice, resonates essentially with non-doership. The various techniques for performing āsana cannot be imposed on a body that is not ready to receive and integrate them. It is necessary to start with preliminaries for each āsana that take into account circumstances and the body's reaction. The practice must be unfolded gradually, like an opera singer who starts by singing scales. Accessible exercises are therefore done to start with to create a welcoming state of ease, the fragrance of which is then present throughout one's practice, even in the most advanced āsana.

The Practice of Cleansing and Churning

"Away with all other knowledge! This God, the Terrifying Churner (Manthānabhairava), churns this Truth abounding in nectar, as He churned the oceans of the four torrents."
MAHEŚVARĀNANDA, MAHĀRTHAMAÑJARĪ 68

The so-called cleansing practices are generated by different groups of āsana. They are aimed at giving back mobility to joints, muscles, organs and the breath. They also allow disengagement from bodily image and sharpening of perception. This process takes time as the ramifications of our habits are deeply anchored in the body's memory. Cleansing practices unfold a churning process in which the āsana's organic and energetic responses start to be felt. One must learn to evolve the āsana from a specific action and unfold it in waves throughout the body, without forgetting the first action. There is therefore no chaotic mental jumping from one part of the body to another. The chosen action in an āsana upon which the emphasis is placed is its bindu, and from which the āsana is unfolded like the emanation of the Śrī Yantra. Emperor penguins have to cope with extremely low temperatures. They congregate in a circle to keep warm; and it is of course much warmer in the centre than at the periphery. They create a rotation whereby they move from the centre to the periphery and from the periphery to the centre. Churning techniques follow the intuition of this energetic, organic and instinctive movement that occurs in concentric circles, by waves. Since breath cycles support this rhythm, it is important they are clear in these techniques. One makes do with only a few breath cycles in the beginning, later leaving the breath to shroud the āsana completely. The clarity of breathing rhythms in specific actions must be accompanied by clarity in the regions to be penetrated. Āsana can thus be churned in an apānic, samānic, prāṇic or udānic fashion, but also by the various sonic forms of cakra and tattva.

Vital Points: The Guardians of Śakti

"Meditate on the rising Śakti in the form of lightning, as it moves upward from one centre to the next..."
VIJÑĀNA BHAIRAVA 29

Certain vital points (marman) have to be positioned in order the body may be immersed in its intrinsic energy. It is like opening the window to let the sun shine in. One must learn to direct energy into the root of the big toes (pādāṅguṣṭha) and awaken the space between the big toe and the second toe. The remaining toes, including the little toe, as well as the space between them, must open. The heels must be firm and rooted. The middle of the inner edge of the arch of the foot must lift up like the vaulted roof of a cathedral. Another important junction is that of the knees. The front of the knees from the top of the shinbones should be sucked up and be in contact with the back of the knees, which are fully open. Speaking of the knees, Śrī B.K.S. Iyengar says: *"The 'divider' must be full of life."* The channels for transmitting this awakening between the feet and knees are the shinbones, which must remain in contact with the calves, themselves fully open, especially on the inner side. The front of the thighs remain in contact with the thighbones, which move back to be in contact with the back of the thighs. There must be no aggressiveness in the lower back. When the vital points have been established in the legs it becomes easier to understand the work of the tailbone (mūlabandha), which leaves the lumbar area in a neutral state. The abdomen and the diaphragm must be softened and widened. Āsana have a toning effect on the muscles, but this is only a secondary effect and of little importance. The organic lifting action of the pelvic (mūlabandha) and abdominal (uḍḍiyānabandha) floors has nothing to do with how toned one's abdominal muscles are or the size of one's belly. The chest should be widened and opened, and the armpit area spread broadly from the back to the front like two wings. The awakening of the knees participates in awakening the chest. When the chest opens, there is a certain passiveness in the eyes and the front of the brain. Organically, the opening of the chest corresponds to the sensation of 'I am'. To open the chest, the shoulders must be freed and the trapezius muscles and the skin of the back must be allowed to flow downwards, like water. The inner side of the shoulder blades, back ribs and latissimi dorsi should accompany the dorsal area as it moves towards the sternum. Certain areas must remain completely neutral. A fear reflex often causes gripping of the shoulders and trapezius muscles. Do not frown, but rather let the skin of the forehead flow from the hairline down towards the eyes, like water flows when taking a shower. Let the skin of the temples connect with the back of the skull. The eyes must learn not to focus, as though looking with the ears. The eyes should be kept in contact with the space at the back of the skull. As with the eyes, the eardrums too are often gripped and should also be directed to the cavity at the back of the skull, as in Ṣaṇmukhīmudrā. From its joint, the lower jaw should drop away from the upper jaw. The teeth should not be clenched and the tongue and root of the tongue should rest downwards. In this way, the back of the throat and neck become like a column of space. This region is known as the 'well' or the 'cave of the throat' (kaṇṭhakūpa). One thus becomes familiar with the so-called effervescent and pacifying energies.

Abandoning Technical Righteousness and Remaining in the Functionality of Āsana

As the semanticist Korzybski said: *"the map is not the territory."* The technique is only a pointer. It is not the terrain. At the start of apprenticeship, technique is important because it allows us to codify attitudes for entering into, holding and coming out of āsana. At this stage there is no room for improvisation or creativity. The technique makes the organs of action and perception vigilant and awake, and allows us to rid ourselves of chaotic movements and certain agitations. Techniques of different āsana must be known and become second nature in order they may then be surpassed. Techniques can very quickly become a straightjacket, whereby the movement is no longer felt but imposed. We are then no longer in contact with the situation. We ceaselessly try to reach an evermore perfect technique, and are therefore always frightened of making mistakes. This obsession for postural righteousness must be abandoned. When maturity comes, an āsana is not tackled technically. Instead one observes the resistances encountered and how they can be organised. It is therefore essential to read one's own terrain. Am I at the beginning, middle or end of practice? What is my condition in the instant? Āsana will reveal constraints. From this observation certain priorities become clear, which take into account the reactions of the body, the breath and the different mental attitudes at a given instant. We must remain functional in order to observe them and give them all the space needed for this observation. If the legs have to be bent in an āsana in order to stay functional, whereas the technique requires them to be kept straight, we naturally tend towards functionality.

"In all things, unless one is in harmony with rhythm, one hesitates between quickness and slowness... Concerning tactics, what can be qualified as profound? What can be qualified as superficial? According to the art or the case,

one talks about 'ultimate principle' or 'secret transmission' and there is a depth unknown to the beginner. But when it comes to principles whilst exchanging blows with an opponent, it is futile to say that one should fight superficially or sever profoundly... In all ways, there are cases where profundity is valid and others where a beginner's level is more than adequate." MIYAMOTO MUSASHI, THE BOOK OF FIVE RINGS

Not Becoming Cluttered with the Psychophysical Effects of Āsana

The tensions and grips revealed by āsana are always linked to the sensation of space, the background in which all elements and states appear and disappear. Emphasis is never placed on what happens, thus allowing the sensation to be freed from all mental appropriation and not be sclerosed as an event. Whatever the subtlety of the mental modifications encountered by the practitioner, these are only states. The exploration of the different colourations of these modifications cannot be selective. It must be open to profound inertia (tamas), all forms of agitation (rajas) and luminous expansions (sattva). Hence we no longer seek a specific frame of mind that only favours well-being. Whatever the subtlety of this state of well-being, it remains merely a modification (vṛtti). The peace created (śāntavṛtti) by a neurophysiological modification is artificial and does not last. It is not true tranquillity (śāntasvabhāva).

Returning to the Essential

Over time, many of us appear to lose the heart for practice, the initial thrill. Practice becomes routine, something we have to do out of duty towards a system. Practice is then simply an accumulation of information and instructions. We forget the poetry and are only interested in the words. It is interesting to observe that when we are no longer stimulated by a goal-orientated practice, we are confronted with a meaningless routine. But this could well be a necessary passage allowing us to ask ourselves the essential question: what was the initial thrill, what triggered my commitment to a practice? The question 'who am I?' urges us to explore the texture of our embodiment. It is said that this texture and that of the universe are woven by Consciousness. This exploration of our own nature is highly intimate, and out of respect for this intimacy, all desire to achieve whatever goal we may have must be put aside. All of us seek this intimacy because our deep down desire is for tranquillity.

Resonance With and Libations To the Different Śakti of the Body-Mind

To intuitively understand āsana as a stable and tranquil seat, certain libations must take place. Resonance is established with the body (śarīradhvani), breath (śvāśadhvani) and the different modalities of breathing, senses (indriyadhvani), speech (vācdhvani) and mind (mānasadhvani). All that arises is therefore used in this ritual of offering. The different inclinations of the body, i.e. its constitution in the instant, are used to unfold a tactile understanding of the effects on the breathing, the mind and the body itself. The different inclinations of the breathing are used to understand the effects on the body, the mind and the breathing itself. The different inclinations of the mind are used to understand the effects on the body, the breathing and the mind itself. Their confluence and interaction are visited with ever increasing intimacy. These interactions occur through the senses and are manifested as internal semantics, a unifying vibration.

"At the end of sexual union, a sound gushes from the throat of the beloved. This sound is a spontaneous resonance (dhvani), uncontrollable, that requires neither meditation nor concentration. If one becomes absorbed in it, one becomes the master of the universe." KULAGAḤVARATANTRA, QUOTED BY ABHINAVAGUPTA, TANTRĀLOKA III, 146-148A

The Vision Precedes the Gaze (Antardṛṣṭi, Antarmukhī)

"Through the intuitive vision (dṛṣṭi) of his own freedom, the yogi realises with certitude that his Consciousness is pure and that the body, the breath, etc. are merely reflections, like that of a face in a mirror." ABHINAVAGUPTA, TANTRĀLOKA V, 11B-12A

The eyes are conditioned to focus and they fix a perceived object as a form with certain characteristics, separated from the perceiving subject. In yoga, the eyes are used to draw us back to the vision that precedes the gaze, and which is not dependent on the eyes. We merely gaze at the expansion of our subjectivity. There are traditionally nine external points of focus (bāhyadṛṣṭi): the tip of the nose (nāsāgradṛṣṭi), between the eyebrows (bhrūmadhyadṛṣṭi), the navel (nābhidṛṣṭi), the thumb (aṅguṣṭhadṛṣṭi), the hand (hastagradṛṣṭi), the big toe (pādagradṛṣṭi), the sides: extreme right and extreme left (pārśvadṛṣṭi), upwards or the sky (ūrdhvadṛṣṭi). These points of localisation are there to cleanse the eyes of their desire to flit around. For beginners, the execution of an āsana is all too often localised in the eyes, especially the inner corner of the eyes. This localisation is due to tension when 'executing' the āsana, which then becomes merely a posture. It is a frontal perception, manifested by projecting the face forwards and contracting the organs of perception. The practitioner's perception should be of a more tactile nature, located in certain areas of the eyes: the floor of the eyes, the roof of the eyes, and especially the outer corner of the eyes. The gaze then becomes panoramic and the eyes remain in contact with the space at the back of the skull. In essence, the dṛṣṭi is like being at a vantage point where traffic can be observed, but without being in amongst it. There is nothing to watch, but everything to see. In the Dhvanyāloka, the dṛṣṭi is the imagination (pratibhā) of the poet. For Abhinavagupta, who comments this text, the vision (dṛṣṭi) is the illuminating intuition (pratibhā).

"And so this vision is said to be new and wonderful."
LOCANA III, 43B

Bhairavamudrā is characterised by the inner vision (antarmukhī), which is not turned inwards but which precedes any inner or outer (nirmukhī) gaze.

"Attention should be turned inwards (antarlakṣya), the gaze should be turned outwards (bahirdṛṣṭhi), without the twinkling of the eyes. This is the mudrā pertaining to Bhairava, kept secret in all the Tantra."

Once the Rules Have Been Learnt, Break Them Without a Care

Once the basic principles have been established, we must try and understand our constitution in the instant. To do this, there must be a total absence of dogmatism and an inclusive approach of one's self in one's environment. In essence, there are no rules. We simply have to stay connected with the intelligence of the sensation in the instant. No two bodies are the same and hence there can't be one single approach. What is valid for one person will be an obstacle for someone else.

Abandoning Postural Variety to Contemplate Inner Vibration (Spandasamāveśa)

In the preparatory phase, the postural garland is used to establish the body in a state of alertness and vivacity. The different groups of āsana and their sequencing provide the vocabulary of inner semantics. A variety of āsana are also used to provide our perception with different supports that satisfy and stimulate the mind. Without this, the practitioner succumbs to inertia and boredom. The more mature practitioner, on the contrary, will seek boredom and the absence of stimulation. Long series with a wide variety of āsana (which can also have their use) do nothing more than intensify outer dynamism. In order to contemplate inner energy flows, the series should be minimalist. An āsana will be used and practised in different ways and from different points of view. One or two other āsana will be added to provide some free time, before coming back to the chosen āsana (iṣṭāsana) and immersing fully into its specific inner vibration.

Playing Truant From the Posture To Reveal the Spontaneous and Natural Āsana (Sahajāsana) To Your Constitution

Once the posture has been established, it is left free of all conditioning. External dynamism is reduced to a minimum. Even the slightest effort to improve the pose must be abandoned. Nothing else is corrected; nothing else is imposed. We simply become a witness to the spontaneous movement of the body, of the breathing, of the perception.

"Whatever your position, stay there, without moving either outwards or inwards. Thus, with the radiating Consciousness alone, swallow the multiple diversity of becoming." JAYARATHA, TANTRĀLOKAVIVEKA II, I.3, PAGE 29

The Way of Intuition: Forgetting all Techniques

"When gripped by illusion and deceived by the discourse of the ignorant, he who puts his trust in a bad master must then give himself to intuitive reason, and even he is lead to the true master. This illuminating intuition is nothing other than pure Knowledge, which is one with the will of Parameśvara." ABHINAVAGUPTA, TANTRĀLOKA III, 33-34

It is said that in ancient times, at the end of their apprenticeship, practitioners of martial arts, calligraphy or any other traditional art would retreat to a hermitage to forget everything. If this is not possible, especially nowadays where traditional arts have become a profession, then the practice itself becomes the hermitage. Many years of apprenticeship are of course needed in which the way of technique has been completely worn out. We will have already learnt to practise according to our natural rhythm and sensitivity, and according to our own structure. No matter who our teacher is, he is not able to do this for us. Having trodden the paths of the way of technique, we suddenly see the uselessness of it. We have accumulated piles of technical notes and have enough recordings of the master's teachings to fill another lifetime. We have been dissecting a poem for many years without having really understood its meaning, and all that remains is a corpse. It is now time to fast and empty ourselves of āsana techniques. We no longer fear the absence of accumulated knowledge; on the contrary, we slide into this absence of borrowed knowledge. Āsana are no longer explained anatomically, physiologically, or even with yogic concepts. There is no more talk of quadriceps, kneecaps or cakra. The different regions are now only in expansion or contraction, heavy or light, hot or cold, dry or humid, light or dark. We leave place for sensation, without expressing it, without explaining it. If, in one of these moments of intimacy, we are asked to explain an āsana, we would be incapable of doing so. We become completely ignorant of what we are doing.

Whilst rimming a wheel in the courtyard, a wheelwright questioned a scholar who was reading:
"What are you reading?"
"The teachings of the sages."
"Living sages?"
"No, ancient sages."
"Then it's rubbish!"
The scholar became angry and the wheelwright explained:
"In my trade, it is not possible to work in a way that is too refined or to work with too much force. But when I am making a wheel, without my knowing how, it turns out

perfect! You need a certain 'knack' that cannot be explained. I was not even able to pass it on to my son. Are those who have gone before me better able to explain their 'knack'? If it is not the case, your books contain only rubbish."

The Single Stroke of Āsana

"The single brushstroke is the origin of all things, the root of all phenomena; its function is manifest for the mind and hidden within man, but the commoner is unaware of it."
SHITAO (THE MONK 'BITTER PUMPKIN') ON PAINTING

We all have intuitive knowledge of the subtle body. When we see a tree swaying in the wind, we sway with it. When we marvel at a dancer's lightness, we dance with him. When we are in our car, we take on its size. The quiver of āsana starts in the subtle body. The subtle body 'brushes' the āsana in a single and unique movement, which, paradoxically, is beyond space-time. The body then simply follows and responds to this unique stroke of space. If we are in the fullness of sensation, external limitations (stiffness, frustration, etc.) or aptitudes (suppleness, enthusiasm, etc.) of the body-mind are of little importance. In certain instants of grace, we can feel the āsana's single stroke of space, which has neither beginning nor end. For the rest of the time, one gives oneself to one's art without expectation.

Open Heart Surgery Without an Anaesthetic

The exploration of āsana and situations encountered whilst practising should be done with an open-hand attitude. Competition, comparison, intention and goals to be reached are all barbiturates that send us off into the dream of separation. This 'open heart surgery' is not something that can be accomplished because it is not in the field of doing. It arrives like an unexpected slap in the face. As for its technical transposition, we learn to encounter āsana, with their entire palette of effects, naked. Stiffness, tension and their emotional and mental prolongation are given all the space they need. During apprenticeship a lot of energy is wasted building ramparts of resistance, like a thief who locks himself in his room, frightened he may steal from his own house. Observe how the refusal of 'what is' predominates, and how we continually prevaricate with reality. During this phase, the dynamism of intention and psychological effort is minimised. Bodily or mental goals are no longer sought and the virtual body, which is merely the projection of psychological memory, is left to collapse into itself, in a sigh of silence.

Nourishing the Rākṣasa

"Troupes of flesh-eating, mischievous spirits,
My stretched skin covers the three worlds.
I placed my flesh, my blood, my bones there as an offering.
What weakness to think of all this as being mine!
Rejoice with all your heart at this offering.
Swallow me raw.
But if you prefer, cook me and savour each bit of flesh.
Eat until every bit is finished."
THE OFFERING OF SACRIFICE TO SPIRITUAL BEINGS
(TIBETAN YOGA OF THE NINGMAPA TRADITION)

As we cross the different levels, referred to as gross and subtle bodies, energies are expressed that may take on the form of either wrathful or peaceful deities. All too often it will seem as though we are a playground for ogres and ogresses. The cleansing and churning practices invite these energies to feast upon our body. We begin very simply by letting any resistances felt within the body be spread out and resorbed with cycles of exhalation. Later, we penetrate more deeply into the sensation of offering the muscles, joints, bones, organs, nervous system and brain. These different localised energies are left to eat themselves up. This phase of practice reverberates in more subtle states, such as that of dreaming, where it becomes much more significant than in the waking state. There may be the sensation of complete immobility, of no longer being able to move our body, or of not being able to see. We hear noises of the end of the world and experience terrifying visions. Death rears up its head in terrible forms: falling from a breathtakingly high height, being crushed, burned alive, having our throat cut or being unable to breath. The experience is often too intense and we will wake up with a start. Then, for a few moments, we can contemplate the sensation of the dream as it is carried over into the waking state. We may sometimes accompany a fall or suffocating sensation until its end. All differentiations then return to their source, the Presence.

"I began as a bloom of cotton, outdoors.
Then they brought me to a room where they washed me.
Then the hard strokes of the carder's wife.
Then another woman spun thin threads, twisting me around a wheel.
Then the kicks of the weaver's loom made cloth.
On the washing stone, washermen wet and slung me about to their satisfaction, whitened me with earth and bone, and cleaned me to my own amazement.
Then the scissors of the tailor, piece by piece, and his careful finishing work.
Now, at last, as clothes, I find You and freedom."
LALLĀ

Attitude of Non-Profit in Āsana

"Although apparent phenomena manifest as diversity, yet this diversity is non-dual. And of all the multiplicity of individual things that exist, none can be confined in a limited concept. Staying free from the trap of any attempt to say 'it is like this', or 'like that', it becomes clear that all manifested forms are aspects of the infinite, formless, and indivisible from it, are self-perfected. Seeing that everything is self-perfected from the very beginning, the disease of striving for any achievement is surrendered. And just remaining in the natural state as it is, the presence of non-dual contemplation continuously spontaneously arises."
VAIROCANA, THE SIX VAJRA VERSES (OF DZOGCHEN)

Practice can become another materialism, another mundane event, in which we are completely captivated by our make-up. This identification with our make-up means we practise from the point of view of either accumulation or renunciation. There is a deep-felt sensation that something is lacking, which creates a 'stingy saver' attitude. Āsana are thus performed according to their effects, to give us more of this or less of that. Yet the idea of a body-mind, and of being a separate entity acting upon them, becomes very porous when immersed in sensation. First there is an inclination that stems from the desire for tranquillity. This inclination is what pushes someone to enrol in the army, to become a banker or to practise a traditional art. When an art is practised with the heart, we realise there is no choice. It is of no fundamental importance whether we drive a bus or make pizzas. It is said that yoga is skill in action; whether it be the skill of an acrobat, a musician, a rickshaw driver or a sword master. This skill, this ease, does not put the emphasis on the person who possesses it, but on the contrary, it reveals the total absence of the doer. This intuition is accompanied by a certain passion for that which is useless. This is what lets us give ourselves full-heartedly to the art, without a reason. The more reasons we have for practising an art, the more reasons we have for abandoning it. Without this passion there is a risk of becoming a collector of techniques, of going from one method to another, from one teacher to another. What reason could there be to explain the madness of doing the same exercises for years on end, other than the intuition that there is nothing to be gained and nothing to be lost?

"When your mind is empty, all things appear to happen by themselves. At the beginning you know nothing and there are no questions to clutter your brain. Then, as your practice

progresses, thoughts appear providing as many barriers, and all things become difficult to accomplish. When the content of your study has fully left your mind, and when the practice too has disappeared, then you are able to acquire with ease the mastery of all techniques, without being hindered in the slightest by your apprenticeship, and at the same time without deviating from it. It is when you are conforming to the real, without even being aware of it, that you are able to act this way."
YAGYŪ MUNENORI, THE LIFE-GIVING SWORD (HEIHO KADENSHO)

Functional Liberty of the Organs of Action and Perception
(Yama, Niyama)

"The organic functions of the body are the vow"
VASUGUPTA, ŚIVASŪTRA III, 26

"The five restrictive rules of non-violence, truthfulness, non stealing, continence, non-hoarding, and the five disciplines of purity, etc. are of no use for revealing Consciousness."
ABHINAVAGUPTA, TANTRĀLOKA IV, 87

The world is merely the projection of how our mind translates it. We only encounter our own universe. In the exploration of āsana, intimacy with different grasps in the body makes us realise how we construct the world as an external object. The various mental states we encounter give rise to as many filters that colour our vision. When the body settles into a certain space, where the articular, muscular, organic and cerebral silence can be felt, the world is no longer an external object but becomes the extension of bodily sensation. From this understanding ensues a completely functional way of being, of wandering joyfully in a world that is no longer a psychological world. This functionality is the essence of Yama and Niyama, which become an organic response. It is without regret that I shall digress from an orthodox explanation, even if it means deviating from the usual meaning. I shall therefore not present Yama and Niyama as they are often defined, as commandments and disciplines to be adhered to. I shall instead present them as a constant reminder in each situation of how we grasp the world, of our fears and of our constant agitation.

Yama

Non-Demand (Ahiṃsā)

We broach situations by demanding, by having certain expectations. We can see the violence that exists if we demand situations to be different from what they are, or if we demand people or the world to correspond to our expectations, to change, to improve. We are also able to observe the perpetual tension created if we apply the same demands to ourselves in order to have a different body, a different mind, different abilities, or in order to conform to some ideal or other or to project ourselves into different destinations.

What Is (Satya)

By silencing our demands we are able to remain with the 'what is' of each situation. Everything that arises is the 'what is'. It cannot be escaped. We remain with the source of the event, and even if we run away from the situation, this distraction itself then becomes the 'what is'. A psychological costume no longer needs to be worn and we realise we are always trying to don such a costume to escape the nakedness of 'what is'. It is like trying to shake-off our shadow! The 'what is' of any and every situation is satya.

Non-Need (Asteya)

All our actions seem to be motivated by the bitter taste of lacking. We are always bound for somewhere. We accumulate and seek experiences in the hope they will give us satisfaction. We try to steal from situations that which can never be given: our own fullness. Whatever the experience, it is only lit up by our Presence. The instant a desire is fulfilled, there is a calm return to our Presence and the realisation that there was never anything missing and nothing is needed. Experience is merely a corpse.

Totality and Inevitability of 'I Am-ness' (Brahmacarya)

All the definitions we may have of ourselves, all the dual notions and differentiations we cultivate, stem from the sensation of existing, of being. All commentaries, discursive thoughts, perceptions, sensations and emotions bring us back to the evidence of being. Circles on the water's surface that move away from a stone's impact bring us back to its point of impact. The ineluctability of 'I am-ness' is also found in its negation, like saying 'there's nobody here' when in a dark room.

Non-Appropriation (Aparigraha)

We grasp the world as an object in order to make sense of it. We appropriate the object of our perception because we want it to meet our expectations. But the object no longer has meaning and content when seen as united in the act of perception on the background of Consciousness. We may come across a book full of knowledge that we are eagerly seeking, then, all of a sudden, we realise that it is our own Presence that enables this knowledge to shine forth. This is true for all knowledge contained in all books. We therefore let the object of our desire die in this intuition. This does not of course stop us from reading the book!

"When there is neither grasping nor abandon, the 'I' shines forth. There is no separation between object and subject. This may be observed through ordinary experience."
TRIŚIROBHAIRAVATANTRA, QUOTED BY JAYARATHA IN HIS COMMENTARY ON TANTRĀLOKA V, VERSES 130-131

Niyama

Clarity (Śauca)

Postural flow cleanses the skin, the cells and the respiratory, circulatory, digestive, excretory and nervous systems. It keeps them in a state of sensitivity, open to the fluctuations of the vital force, which becomes evermore functional. This functionality does not lead to the obsession of bodily preservation since the body is no longer a thought construct. This absence of body mentalisation leaves it bathed in its own organic clarity.

"Rites purifying the body of all dualistic thoughts are awareness free of duality, the libation water is the play of the knowable, and the flowers, the nourishing essence of our own essence." MAHEŚVARĀNANDA, MAHĀRTHAMAÑJARĪ 45

Quietude (Santoṣa)

The same savour of tranquillity can be recognised throughout the diversity of our desires and experiences. At the heart of all our agitation is a call for appeasement. The object becomes merely a mirror of our own quietude and so loses its hold. There is thus a disinterest for objectivity and for the thirst of experience.

"The condition of 'I' is the resorption of the object in the subject, also referred to as rest (viśrānti)... because it is the end of all desire."
ABHINAVAGUPTA, ĪŚVARAPRATYABHIJÑĀVIMARŚINĪ, JÑĀNĀDHIKĀRA I, 1

Brilliance (Tapas)

Practising an art awakens a natural discipline which too becomes functional. We will be naturally and spontaneously inclined towards that which the embodiment needs. The rhythms of the day and night will become clear from an organic point of view. Our diet will follow these rhythms. We will eat food that does not overload the body unnecessarily and which is in accordance with the season and the requirements of the moment. This is all part of a certain asceticism, to abandon that which is not necessary in order to give ourself to practice. Our passion for the art becomes the heart of our activities, which themselves are organised around it. Forget the fairground entertainers who for thousands of years have been selling off their enlightenment techniques and improvement gymnastics into the market of desperation. This asceticism is of no interest to us. On the contrary, drawn like mystics to a fast of the heart, we will become established in the brilliance offered by our daily life, exactly as it is, leaving aside all hope of illuminating it with frills.

"The reality of Consciousness shines forth with its own brilliance. That being the case, what is the use of methods to reveal it? If it did not shine forth thus, the universe, deprived of light, would not reveal itself as it would be unconscious." ABHINAVAGUPTA, TANTRĀLOKA II, 10

Recognition (Svādhyāya)

The tranquillity felt whilst practising is the reflection of our own Presence. It becomes the background to all activities and situations. The desire for experience only exists so we tire of objectivity. There cannot be any situation that is more favourable, more rewarding or more impoverishing than another. The worldliness of experience resides in the fact that it is categorised and separated from its source, and used for our projections and fantasies. All situations bring us back to the essence of practice: a return to the Self (svādhyāya).

"The Fourth state must be expanded like oil so that it pervades the other three: waking, dreaming and deep sleep." VASUGUPTA, ŚIVASŪTRA III, 20

Abandonment (Īśvarapraṇidhāna)

Contemplation of embodiment weakens the idea of the body as a separate entity. This sensation of our own vacuity is transposed muscularly, organically, sensorially and cerebrally. It also occurs in privileged instants during the day: before sleep sets in when the day's events no longer have a protagonist and seem as though they unfolded spontaneously, during moments of surprise or urgency where there is no place for a doer. All action is without instigator. There is nothing to abandon and no-one to abandon it.

"He who abides in his own essence must surrender the conceptions of attributes belonging to previously grasped objectivity. This is abandonment." TRIŚIROBHAIRAVATANTRA, QUOTED BY JAYARATHA IN HIS COMMENTARY ON TANTRĀLOKA V, VERSES 130-131

Wearing Your Own Culture and Environment Like a Baggy Suit

When the environment becomes the extension of bodily sensibility, it is no longer stigmatised by socio-cultural criteria. The social landscape to which we belong is merely a system of conventions conditioned by geography, climate, language and history. It has no value in itself. We may feel restricted when there is total identification with a system, which becomes the unique point of view, or by a desire for exoticism, of belonging to another culture. The yoga practitioner rids himself of all 'Indianisation' and sees the uselessness of trying to replace one conditioning by another. These conditionings can be of some value in their context, but when out of place, they create conflicts. The space felt whilst practising, where the bodily clothing has found its ease, is transposed into social clothing, the environment and situations. Situations are no longer narrowed by a commentary. We are thus able to perceive our social suit, with its seams of fear, devoid of sense. It is seen and respected for what it is, and thus becomes baggy. This enables us to be at ease in all social circles, whilst not belonging to any.

"It is said that the perfect man has no rules, which does not mean there are no rules, but that his rule is that of the absence of rules, which constitutes the supreme rule."
SHITAO (THE MONK 'BITTER PUMPKIN') ON PAINTING

When Your House Is Burning, Warm Your Hands

"I've burned my own house down, the torch is in my hand. Now I'll burn down the house of anyone who wants to follow me." KABĪR

See how everything can collapse in the instant, even our vision of the world to which we are so attached. The toys of our childhood and the hopes of our accumulated projects have no importance whatsoever now. It will be the same in a few years when we look back at our current situation. All that we call our feelings, our experiences, our relationships, even the most intimate, will sooner or later abandon us. Our beloved is pain or indifference to another. When faced with a gut-wrenching situation or whilst drifting between two ports with no means of rescue, it is good to contemplate on the remnants and ruins of our world, to see our house burn.

No Practitioner, No Practice, No Process

In the Ucchaṣma Bhairava Tantra (quoted in the Śivasūtra, Swami Lakshman Joo, Page 16), it is said that: *"independent supreme God Consciousness exists beyond our individual state, in the same way our shadow exists."* Although we may try to join with it, catch up with it, or overtake it, this is impossible to do. This absence of state cannot be achieved by a means or by another state. It has already been achieved. Fundamentally, there is neither a process nor an entity activating a process.

"This light is not the power of the Great Goddess because it is not founded on anyone other than oneself, neither is it founded on the possessor of this energy, God.
It cannot be meditated upon because there is no subject to meditate, neither is it the meditator since it cannot be meditated upon.
It is not the worshipped because there is no worshipper, neither is it the worshipper since there is nothing to be worshipped."
ABHINAVAGUPTA, TANTRĀLOKA II, 24-25-26

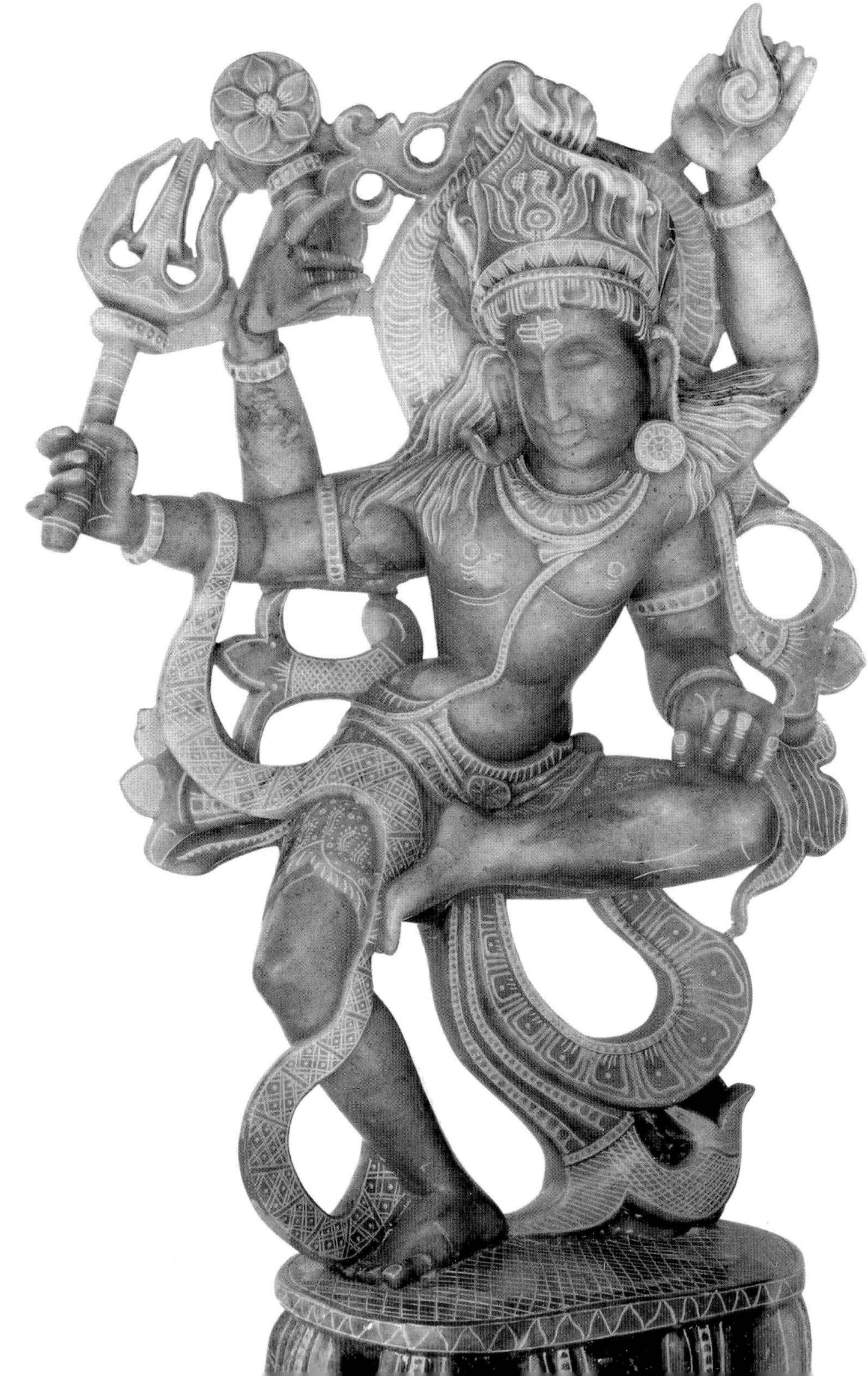

ACT

II

Contemplation of the body of Bhairava, "the dancer who plays and shines like lightning across a thick cloud-covered sky."

Abhinavagupta, Tantrāloka I, 3

• Earth (Pṛthivī Tattva)

Principal prāṇa: Apāna

क Phoneme: KA

Subtle element (tanmātra):
Odour (gandha), phoneme CA च

Organ of action (karmendriya):
Evacuation (pāyu), phoneme ṬHA ठ

Organ of perception (jñānendriya):
Smell (gandha), phoneme TA त

Energetic expression:
Mūlādhāra Cakra - vortex of foundation

Localised breath colouration: Apānavāyu

Ādhāra:
Located below the sex organ
and above the anus, embracing the mouth
of suṣumṇā, face down.

Bījamantra: LAṂ

Bīja vehicle: the elephant Airāvata

Number of petals:
Four, scarlet in colour, blossoming
with the golden coloured letters
VAṂ ŚAṂ ṢAṂ SAṂ
वँ शँ षँ सँ

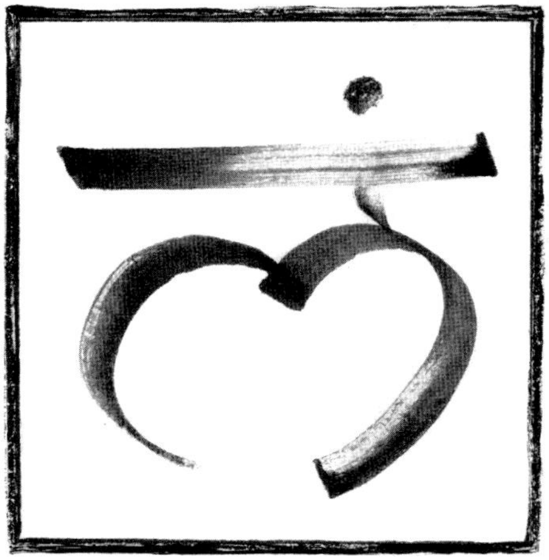

Deity:
Brahmā, red in colour, taking the form of a child
with four faces wearing a black antelope skin,
holding the staff, the flask, the rudrākṣa
and making the gesture that dissipates all fears.

Śakti:
Ḍākinī, red in colour, with red eyes,
frightening for the paśu, in her right hands she holds
the lance and the khaṭvāṅga (bone topped with a
human skull). Her canine teeth are menacing.
She is the death of her enemies.

Localisation:
Bhūrloka - physical world, of becoming.
Annamayakośa - body of food.

Yantra:
Square, bright yellow in colour, as sharp as lightning
containing the audible seed of the Earth.

"The imperishable fundamental nature (dharma) of all levels of manifestation (tattva grāma) is the Self, which constitutes the very heart of their own nature."
ABHINAVAGUPTA, TANTRĀLOKA I, 82-86A

• Water (Jala Tattva)

Principal prāṇa: Prāṇa

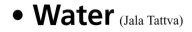

ख Phoneme: KHA

Subtle element (tanmātra):
Savour (rasa), phoneme CHA छ

Organ of action (karmendriya):
Procreation (upastha), phoneme ṬA ट

Organ of perception (jñānendriya):
Taste (rasana), phoneme THA थ

Energetic expression:
Svādhiṣṭhāna Cakra - vortex of settling into oneself

Localised breath colouration: Apānavāyu

Ādhāra:
Base of the genital organ

Bījamantra: VAṂ

Bīja vehicle: makara (mythical mount with the body of a crocodile or dolphin, the head of a lion, the trunk of an elephant and the tail of a swan, fish or peacock)

Number of petals:
Six, vermilion in colour, blossoming with the letters
BAṂ BHAṂ MAṂ YAṂ RAṂ LAṂ
बँ भँ मँ यँ रँ ळँ that have the sheen of lightning

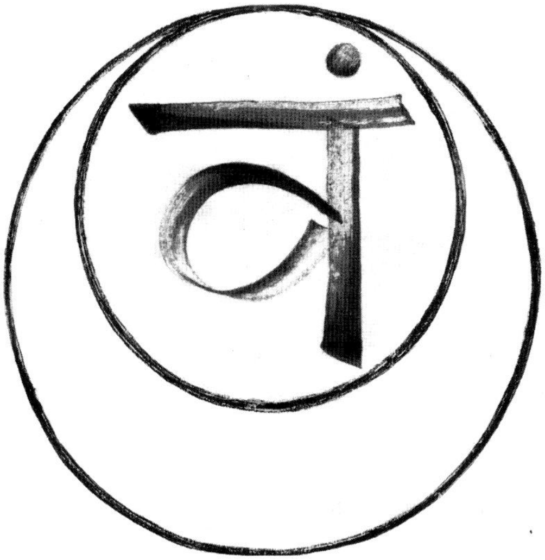

Deity:
Viṣṇu, standing on Garuḍa. He appears as a teenager with four arms, holding a conch, a disc, a club and a lotus. He is dressed in yellow and is wearing the knot of eternity or the knot of the infinite (śrīvasta) and the priceless jewel (kaustubha).

Śakti:
Rākiṇī, dark in colour, with four arms holding the lance, the lotus, the ḍamaru and shears. She has three eyes, curved tusks and is abominable in appearance. She likes white rice and blood.

Localisation:
Bhuvarloka - world of vibratory expansion through form. Prāṇamayakośa - subtle body.

Yantra:
White half moon.

• Fire (Tejas Tattva)

Principal prāṇa: Samāna

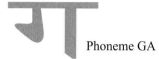

ग Phoneme GA

Subtle element (tanmātra):
Form (rūpa), phoneme JA ज

Organ of action (karmendriya):
Foot, movement (pāda), phoneme ḌA ड

Organ of perception (jñānendriya):
Sight (cakṣu), phoneme DA द

Energetic expression:
Maṇipūra Cakra - vortex of adamantine clarity

Localised breath colouration: Samānavāyu

Ādhāra: Root of the navel

Bījamantra: RAṂ

Bīja vehicle: a ram

Number of petals:
Ten, the colour of a rain-filled cloud,
blossoming with the luminous blue letters
ḌAṂ ḌHAṂ ṆAṂ TAṂ THAṂ
DAṂ DHAṂ NAṂ PAṂ PHAṂ
डँ ढँ णँ तँ थँ दँ धँ नँ पँ फँ

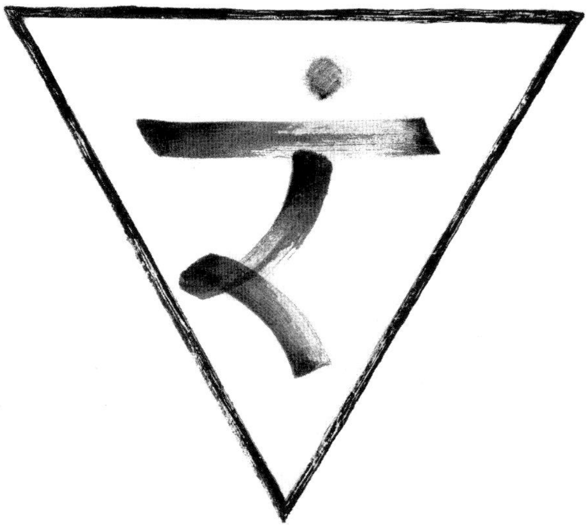

Deity:
Rudra, red in colour, astride a bull, with two arms:
one that gives grace, the other that removes fear.
He has the appearance of an old man with a body whitened by ashes and wearing light-coloured ornaments.

Śakti:
Lākinī, dark blue in colour, with three faces, whose gaze encompasses the Earth, atmosphere and heavens.

Localisation:
Svarloka - celestial world, place of immortality.
Manomayakośa - mental body.

Yantra:
Red triangle.

• Air (Vāyu Tattva)

Principal prāṇa: Udāna

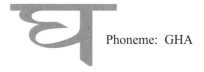

घ Phoneme: GHA

Subtle element (tanmātra):
Contact (sparśa), phoneme JHA झ

Organ of action (karmendriya):
Hand, grasp (pāṇi), phoneme ḌHA ढ

Organ of perception (jñānendriya):
Skin, organ of touch (tvak), phoneme DHA ध

Energetic expression:
Anāhata Cakra - vortex of non-emitted sound

Localised breath colouration: Prāṇavāyu

Ādhāra: The heart

Bījamantra: YAṂ

Bīja vehicle: speckled antelope

Number of petals:
Twelve, red in colour, blossoming with the vermilion red letters KAṂ KHAṂ GAṂ GHAṂ ṄAṂ CAṂ CHAṂ JAṂ JHAṂ ÑAṂ ṬAṂ ṬHAṂ
कँ खँ गँ घँ ङँ चँ छँ जँ झँ ञँ टँ ठँ

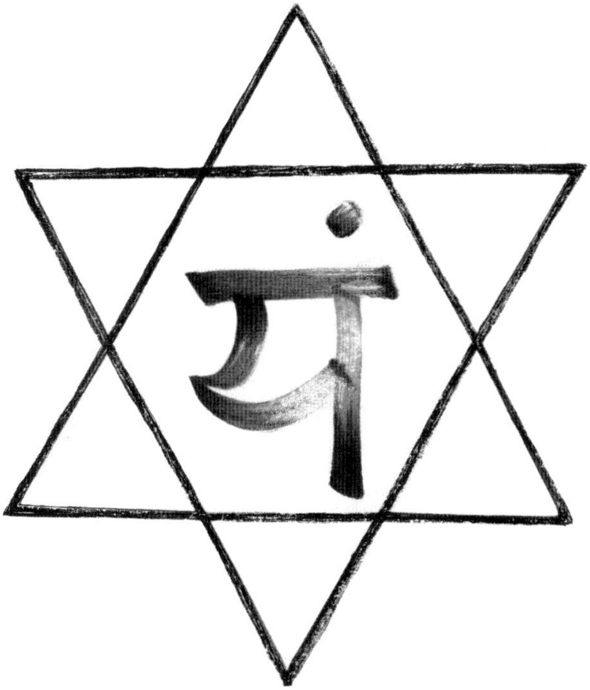

Deity:
Īśāna, with three eyes and two arms, performing the mudrā of the gift of grace and the appeasement of fear.

Śakti:
Kākinī, glistening yellow in colour and dressed in yellow. She has four arms and brandishes a noose and a skull. She wears a garland of bones.

Localisation:
Maharloka - world of vast Consciousness.
Vijñānamayakośa - body of intelligence.

Yantra:
Smoke coloured hexagon.

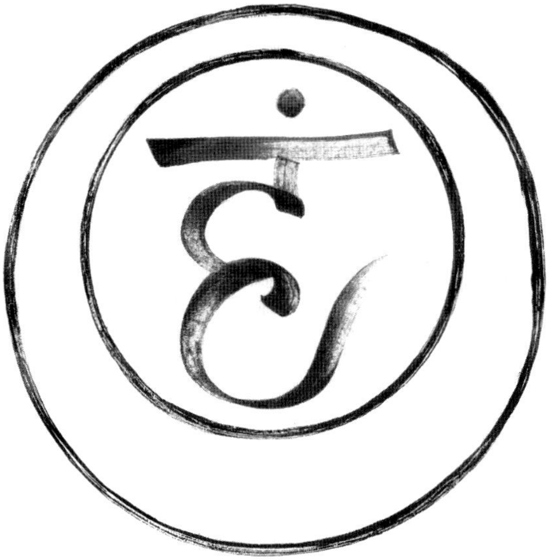

• Ether (Ākāśa Tattva)

Principal prāṇa: Vyāna

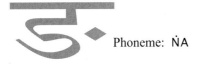

ङः Phoneme: ṄA

Subtle element (tanmātra):
Sound (śabda), phoneme ÑA ञ

Organ of action (karmendriya):
Speech (vāk), phoneme ṆA ण

Organ of perception (jñānendriya):
Hearing (śrotra), phoneme NA न

Energetic expression:
Viśuddha Cakra - vortex of purity

Localised breath colouration: Udānavāyu

Ādhāra: The throat

Bījamantra: HAṂ

Bīja vehicle: the white elephant

Number of petals:
Sixteen, dark grey in colour, blossoming with the sixteen red coloured vowels from A to Visarga
AṂ ĀṂ IṂ ĪṂ UṂ ŪṂ ṚṂ ṜṂ
ḶṂ ḸṂ EṂ AIṂ OṂ AUṂ AṂ AḤAṂ
अँ आँ इँ ईँ उँ ऊँ ऋँ ॠँ ऌँ ॡँ एँ ऐँ ओँ औँ अं अः

Deity:
Five-headed Sadāśiva, each with three eyes, which represent the five organs of perception and the five elements in their purest form, seated on a royal throne (mahāsiṃhāsana) carried by a bull. Half his body shines golden, the other half white. He holds the trident, the axe, the sword, the vajra, the fire, the king of serpents, the bell, the goad and the noose, and is performing abhayamudrā. He wears a tiger's skin and his body has been rubbed with the ashes of cosmic dissolution. A garland of serpents adorns his neck and chest. The diadem of the half-moon sits on his enormous chignon of matted hair (jaṭā).
It faces downwards, a flow of nectar pouring from it.

Śakti:
Sākinī, white in colour, and dressed in yellow.
She has three heads, each with three eyes. Her four arms hold the noose, the goad, the bow and the arrow.

Localisation:
Janaloka - world of humans, world of creative enjoyment.
Ānandamayakośa - body of bliss.

Yantra:
Full moon white coloured circle.

• Beyond the Elements

(Mahā Tattva) : **Giver of Breath**

It contains the seed of all the other elements.

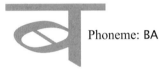

ब Phoneme: BA

Energetic expression:
Ājñā Cakra - vortex of command authority

Breath colouration: Udānavāyu

Ādhāra: the point between the eyebrows

Bījamantra: OṂ

Bīja vehicle: Nāda

Number of petals:
Two, white in colour,
blossoming with the letters
HAṂ हँ to KṢAṂ क्षँ

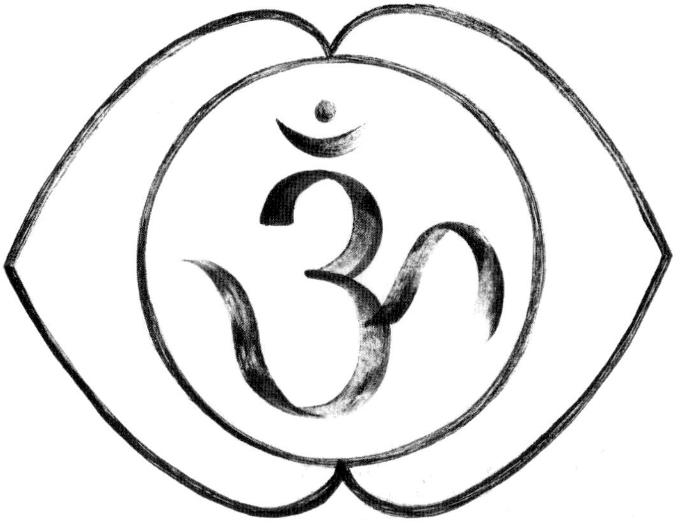

Deity:
The Liṅgam or Ardhanārīśvara. The masculine side of the deity has very pale blue coloured skin, and bears a trident. The feminine side has pink skin, is dressed in a red sari and bears a pink lotus.

Śakti:
Hākinī. She has four arms and six heads. Her skin is pale pink. She wears a red sari. She is sat on a pink lotus with her left leg bent and her right leg hanging. In her hands she holds Śiva's ḍamaru (small drum), a skull and a rosary. The ḍamaru represents the initial vibration or pulse (spanda) from which time-space emerges. The skull symbolises the end of all conceptualisation. The mālā is the spontaneous reciting of the ahaṃ mantra that resonates at the heart of all creation. Her right hand holds no object but performs the abhayamudrā, which seals the universe in an absence of fear.

Localisation:
Tapasloka - world of unfragmented energy.

Yantra:
White circle with two luminescent petals.
A liṅga sits in the centre of the circle.

Hymn to the Circle of Deities in the Body
(Dehasthadevatācakrastotra)

Abhinavagupta

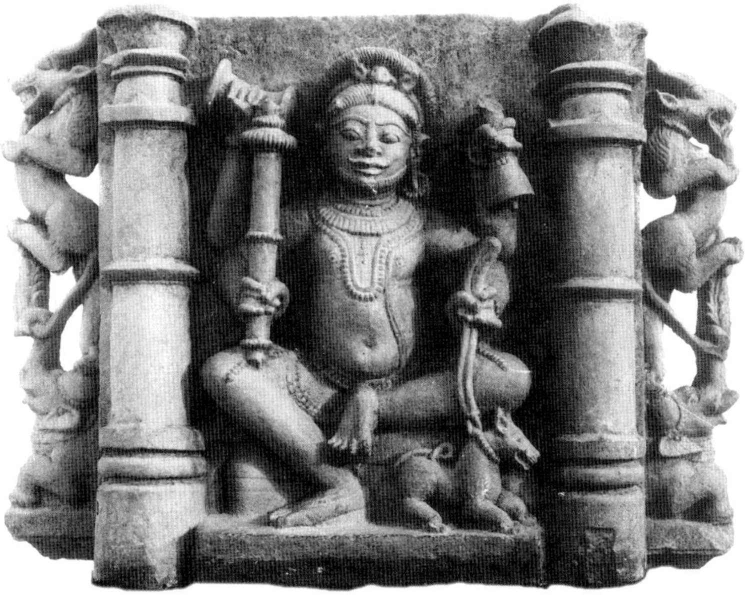

Bhairava
10th century (Kahjuraho, Madhya Pradesh)

I offer my respects to Gaṇapati, who expresses himself in the inhaled breath, and who is worshiped at the start of a multitude of treatises, likes to satisfy desires, and who is venerated by an infinity of intentions.

I praise Vaṭuka whom we refer to as exhaled breath, who obliterates the sorrow of men. His feet, identical to a lotus, are worshiped by the lineage of Siddha, the family of Yoginī and the best of Heroes.

I praise Ānanda Bhairava, fullness of Consciousness. The divinities of the senses worship him relentlessly in the lotus of the heart by offering him the pleasures of perceived objects.

I praise continually the Sadguru, whose form is devotion. By the power of his light the universe is revealed, which for his devotees is the expression of Śiva.

I praise Ānanda Bhairavī, pure Presence, who relentlessly amuses herself by provoking the creation, maintenance and disappearance of the universe.

I continually bow before Bhairavī, who is the embodiment of intelligence. She dwells on the eastern petal where she offers the flowers of certitude to Bhairava.

I praise Śāmbavī, the Mother who dwells on the south-eastern petal, whose form is the ego, and who venerates Bhairava with the flowers of egoism.

I eternally praise the damsel Kumārī, who is the embodiment of thought. Dwelling on the southern petal, she worships Bhairava with the flowers of doubt.

I bow eternally to Vaiṣṇavī, who is the embodiment of vibration. She dwells on the south-western petal and venerates Bhairava with the flowers of Sound.

I offer my respects to Vārāhī, who becomes the skin. She dwells on the western petal and enchants Bhairava with the flowers of the sense of touch that captivate the heart.

I praise Indrāṇī, who becomes vision. She lays on the north-western petal, where she worships Bhairava with magnificently coloured flowers.

I pay tribute to Cāmuṇḍā, who becomes the tongue. She lays on the northern petal, where she continually venerates Bhairava with varied dishes and their six flavours.

I continually bow before Mahālakṣmī, who becomes the nose. She dwells on the north-eastern petal, where she worships Bhairava with an infinite number of sweet fragrances.

I praise constantly the Self, the Lord of the body, dispenser of perfection, who is worshiped in the six darśana and who is the source of the thirty-six principles of the real.

I thus celebrate the wheel of deities in my body that continually surge up and quiver, the quintessence of experience, constantly present.

a = अ

ā = आ

i = इ

ī = ई

u = उ

ū = ऊ

ṛ = ऋ

ṝ = ॠ

ḷ = ऌ

ḹ = ॡ

e = ए

ai = ऐ

o = ओ

au = औ

aṃ = अं

aḥ = अः

Mātṛkā Yantra (The Wheel of Sonic Energies)

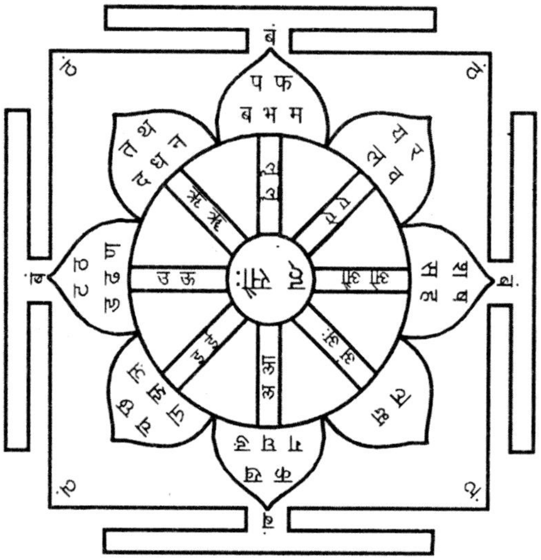

"The awakening of the wheel of sonic mothers takes place for the yogi." Vasugupta, Śivasūtra II, 7

The mātṛkā yantra is drawn using saffron (kesara) when worshipping Śakti, with sandalwood (candana) when worshipping Viṣṇu, or with ashes (bhasma) when worshipping Śiva. It is the first of ten saṃskāra (janana saṃskāra) that imbues the mantra with power.

One of the rituals of consecration is to place the phonemes in the different regions of the body (mātṛkā nyāsa).

Kālī is shown wearing a garland of fifty-one skulls, symbolising the phonemes of the Sanskrit alphabet (mātṛkā) and which make up the goddess' body of vibration.

"These fifteen are called vowels (svara) because they are of sound by nature... they shine of their own accord (svayam rājantaḥ) as does Consciousness. They contain the sun and the moon."
Abhinavagupta, Parātrīśikālaguvṛitti 5-9a

"At the confluence of expansion and contraction shines the absolute (anuttara: **a***), beatitude (ānanda:* **ā***), the energy of will (icchā:* **i***), maintenance (īśāna:* **ī***), opening (unmeṣa:* **u***), and resorption (ūnatā:* **ū***)."*
Abhinavagupta, Parātrīśikālaguvṛitti 5-9a

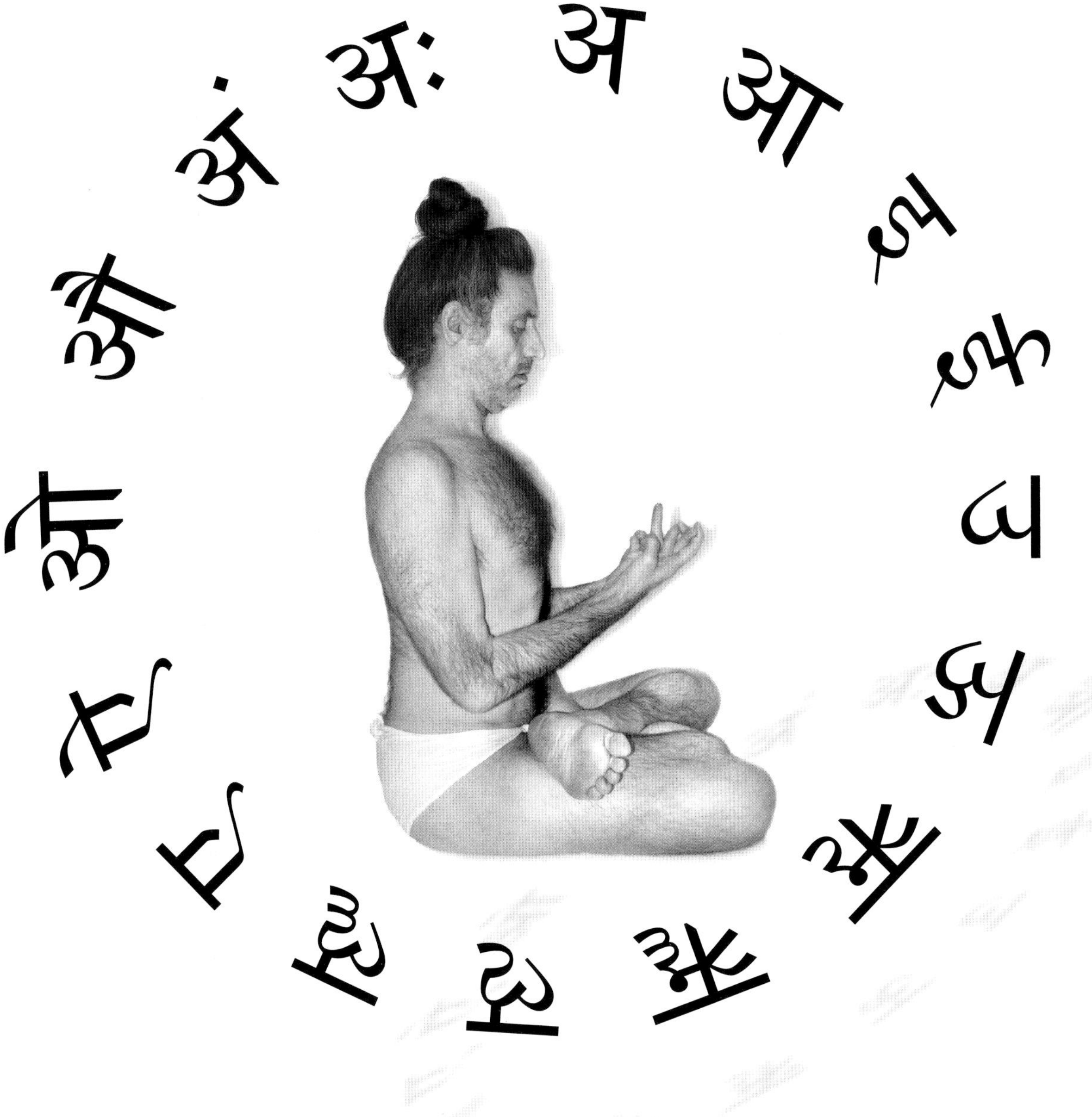

"Salutations to the wealth of touch (sparśalakṣmī), the supreme goddess who performs the Vow which is perpetually intent on the Yoni. This Vow is the manifestation of our innate vibration (svaghūrma), once drunk the supreme nectar of the juice of each state of being." Kubjikā Tantra 1/3

Emanation of the Semantics of

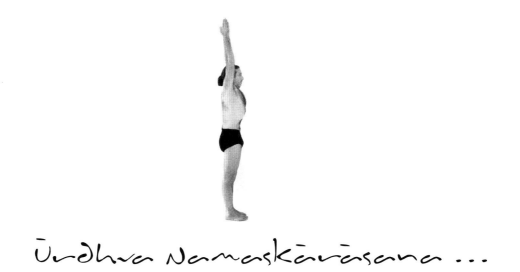

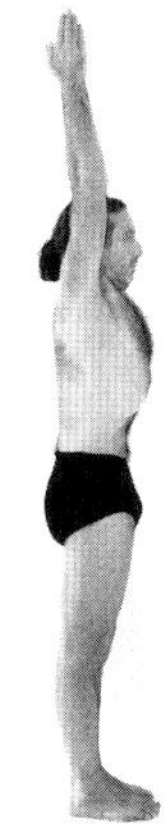

Ūrdhva Namaskārāsana ...

Āsana (Vyākaraṇāsanaparāmarśa)

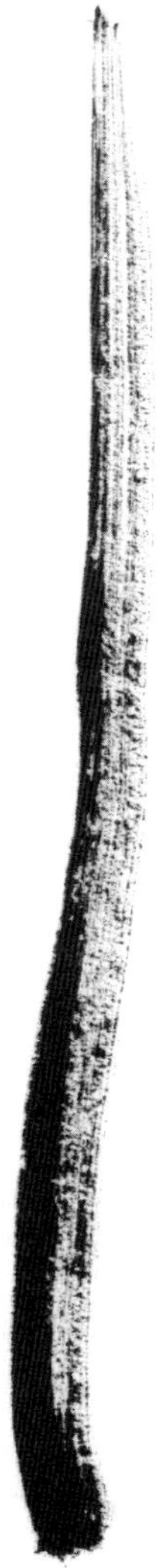

Contemplating Bodily Vacuity

> *If one meditates firmly on the void above (brahmarandhra), the void below (mūlādhāra) and the void in the heart, thus being free from all thoughts, then there arises simultaneously the thought-free state."*
>
> VIJÑĀNA BHAIRAVA* 45

Implicit Order

• Samasthiti, Ūrdhva Namaskārāsana

Sama means equilibrium, evenness. This word has many declensions rich in meaning:
• *Samavāya indicates reunion, meeting, contact, the relationship between the parts and the whole. "Samavāya is the perpetual reunion of the earth and the other elements, and of their qualities..."* CARAKASAMHITĀ I, 150
• Samabuddhi or samacittatva (mental evenness), Samadarśana (unified vision), samadhāna or samādhi. According to the Yogasūtra of Patañjali, *"That meditation having the manifestation of Truth, as if devoid of its own form, is called Samādhi."* YOGASŪTRA III, 3
• Samādhi, for which the Nirukta gives this definition: *"When the mind is established in the understanding of the Self, that understanding is called Samādhi."*
• Samāna, referred to as 'even breath', is one of the five breaths (vāyu) and participates in the union of apānavāyu and prāṇavāyu.
• Samarasa is the unique essence of all things.
• Samasaṃsthāna is the state of equanimity of psychophysical fluctuations. In Vācaspati Miśra's Yoga Bhāṣya (II.46), it is described physically as being Baddhakoṇāsana.
Sthiti comes from the root STHĀ, which means 'to be standing'. One of the literal meanings of this term is the action of standing in a steady and stable manner. It is also used to denote the continuum of existence. In cosmology, it comes after the emanation phase (sṛṣṭi). Whatever has the quality of stability is called sthiti, like the Earth. According to the Vaijayanti Kośa, sthiti means continuation (maryādā) and maintenance (dhāraṇā), but also installation (niveśa) and disposition (racanā).
All these nuances are found in the term Samasthiti, which is the art of verticality, wherein all notions of differentiation are lost in the feeling of unity. It is therefore not merely the act of standing, which would be an activity, but being or being held in and by the cosmic dharma (brahmādaṇḍa).
In Ūrdhva Namaskārāsana, we intensify the unfolding of the firmament of the root and its binding (mūlabandha), and of the firmament of the abdomen and its binding (uḍḍiyānabandha), in order to savour the unfolding of the space within the skull (internal jālandharabandha).

* SEE ADDITIONAL NOTES ON PAGE 379

Establishing the Earth: Standing Āsana

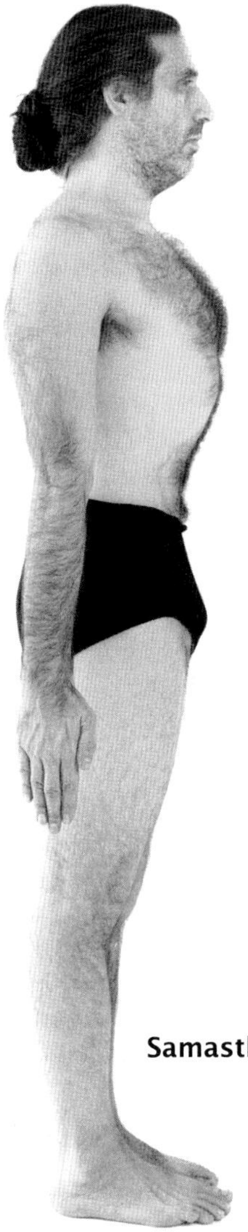

Samasthiti

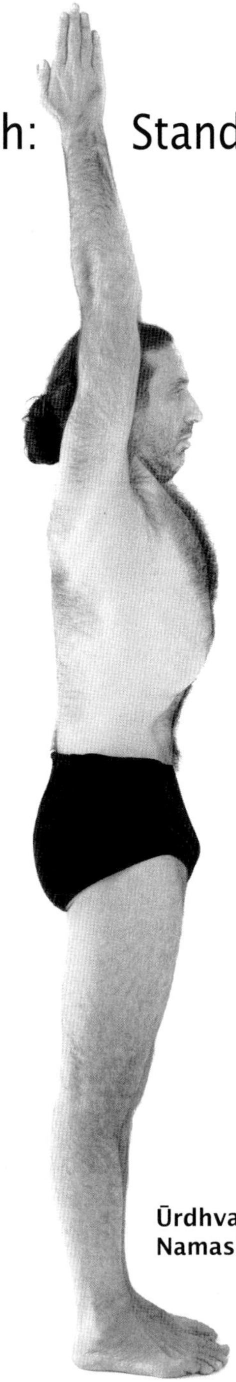

Ūrdhva Namaskārāsana

क

ka

earth (pṛthivī)

ACCORDING TO JAYARATHA, CONSONANTS DO NOT EXIST BY THEMSELVES. THEY ARE MERELY AN EXTERNAL MANIFESTATION OF VOWELS. WITHOUT VOWELS, AND ESPECIALLY THE A (ANUTTARA, THE UNSURPASSABLE), THEY CANNOT BE PRONOUNCED. THE ENTIRE MANIFESTATION, WHICH IS NOTHING MORE THAN THE EXPRESSION OF PHONEMATIC EMANATION, IS ONLY MADE POSSIBLE BY THE SEED OF THE ABSOLUTE.

THE GUTTURALS FROM KA TO ṄA STEM FROM THE CONDENSATION OF THE PHONEME A (ANUTTARA).

Divine Geometry, Wrathful Heroes and Nectar

• Utthita Trikoṇāsana: The Triad

The triangle symbolises the three divine energies (śakti) of will (icchā), knowledge (jñāna) and activity (kriyā). They unfold the knowing subject (pramātṛ), experience (pramāṇa) and the known object (prameya). These three energies, which in the absolute are one and the same, are the source of all manifestation. The Śiva Trikoṇa manifests the energy of knowledge (jñānaśakti). The Śakti Trikoṇa manifests the energy of activity (kriyāśakti). Fundamentally, there is no difference between them: Śakti Trikoṇa is localisation, the support (ādhāra), and Śiva Trikoṇa that which is placed (ādheya) on the support.

• Utthita Pārśvakoṇāsana: Junction and Dissolution

Pārśva means side or flank. Awakening the body's banks, the expression of Iḍā and Piṅgalā, is of utmost importance in āsana. An āsana should never be broached from the centre. This always denotes effort, whether muscular or mental. Activity does not belong to the centre, hence the reason why the central nāḍī is also called the cremation channel (śmaśāna nāḍī), where all differentiation is burnt and consumed. In this āsana, the meeting of the stretched flank with the thigh is part of the art of junction (saṃdhi). At the instant of junction, space-time boundaries disappear.

"Contemplate the vacuity in one's own body encompassing all directions simultaneously. Free from differentiation, everything is merely Void."

Vijñāna Bhairava 43

ख

Kha

water (jala)

> *"Unfolding of beatitude is worship.*
> *One should worship the Trikoṇa*
> *with sweet fragrances*
> *such as incense and flowers*
> *that delight the heart."*
>
> TRIKATANTRASĀRA

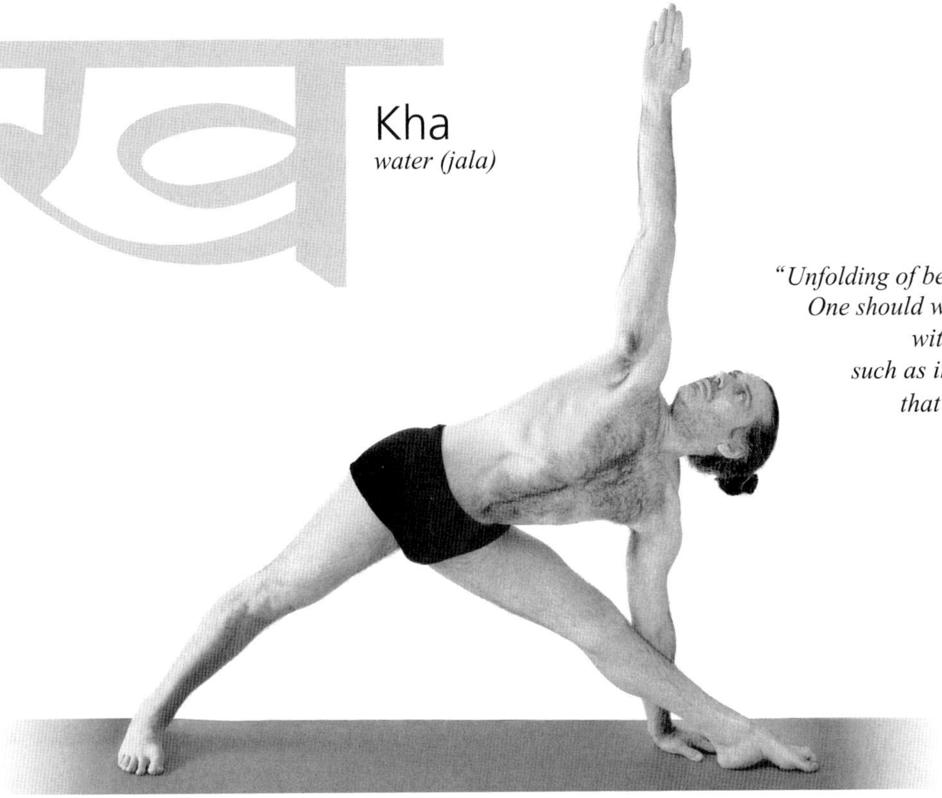

Utthita Trikoṇāsana

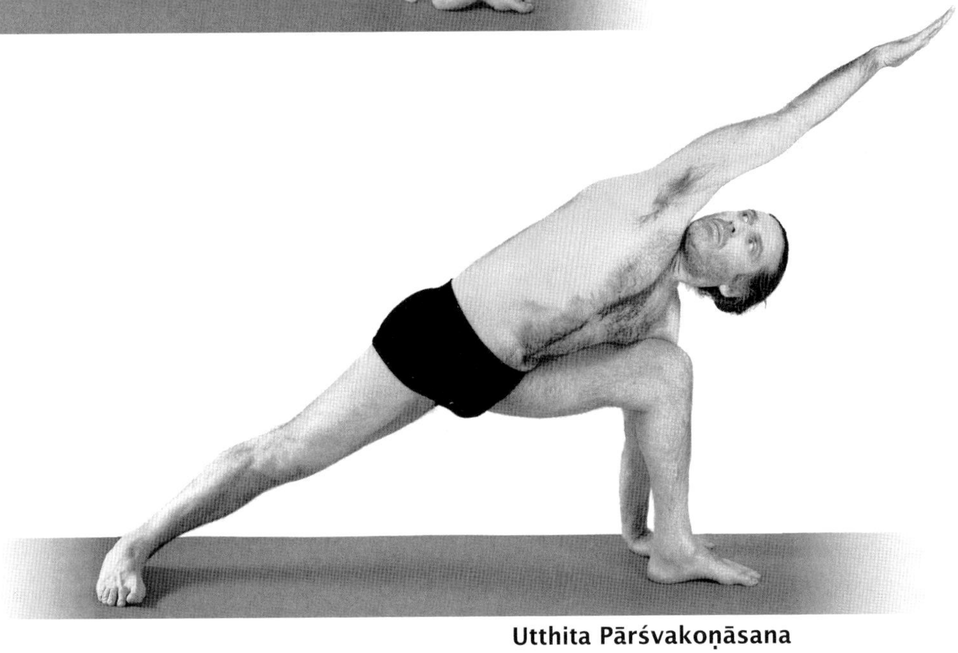

Utthita Pārśvakoṇāsana

• Ardha Candrāsana: The Soma Chalice

The half moon is the chalice of soma, the nectar of immortality. Candra is Soma (Sa + Umā), the perpetual union of Sa (Śiva) and Umā (Pārvatī). According to its etymology, soma is that which 'lives in Umā' (Umā saha), and represents the energy of will (icchāśakti). In its transcending aspect, the moon represents undifferentiated energy (akula) underlying the diversity of phenomena, of the knowable (pramāṇa), when the object (prameya) merges into the subject (pramātṛ).

It is also the semi-circle with the bindu that represents the last nasal sound (anunāsika) of the AUM, corresponding to the rising breath in Suṣumṇā, whose source is in the heart (phoneme A), crosses the throat (U), and then resonates in the palate (M) before hitting the centre of the eyebrows.

According to Abhinavagupta:
"It is by the grace of the full moon of the inhaled breath (apāna)
that one can grasp the essence of the Self as all things."
TANTRASĀRA V

"Either sitting on a seat or lying
on a bed one should meditate
on the body as being supportless.
When the mind becomes empty and
supportless, within a moment one
is liberated from mental dispositions."

VIJÑĀNA BHAIRAVA 82

*"If one contemplates in a thoughtfree way
on any point in the body as mere void
even for a moment, then, being free
from thoughts one attains the nature
of the Thoughtfree."*

Vijñāna Bhairava 46

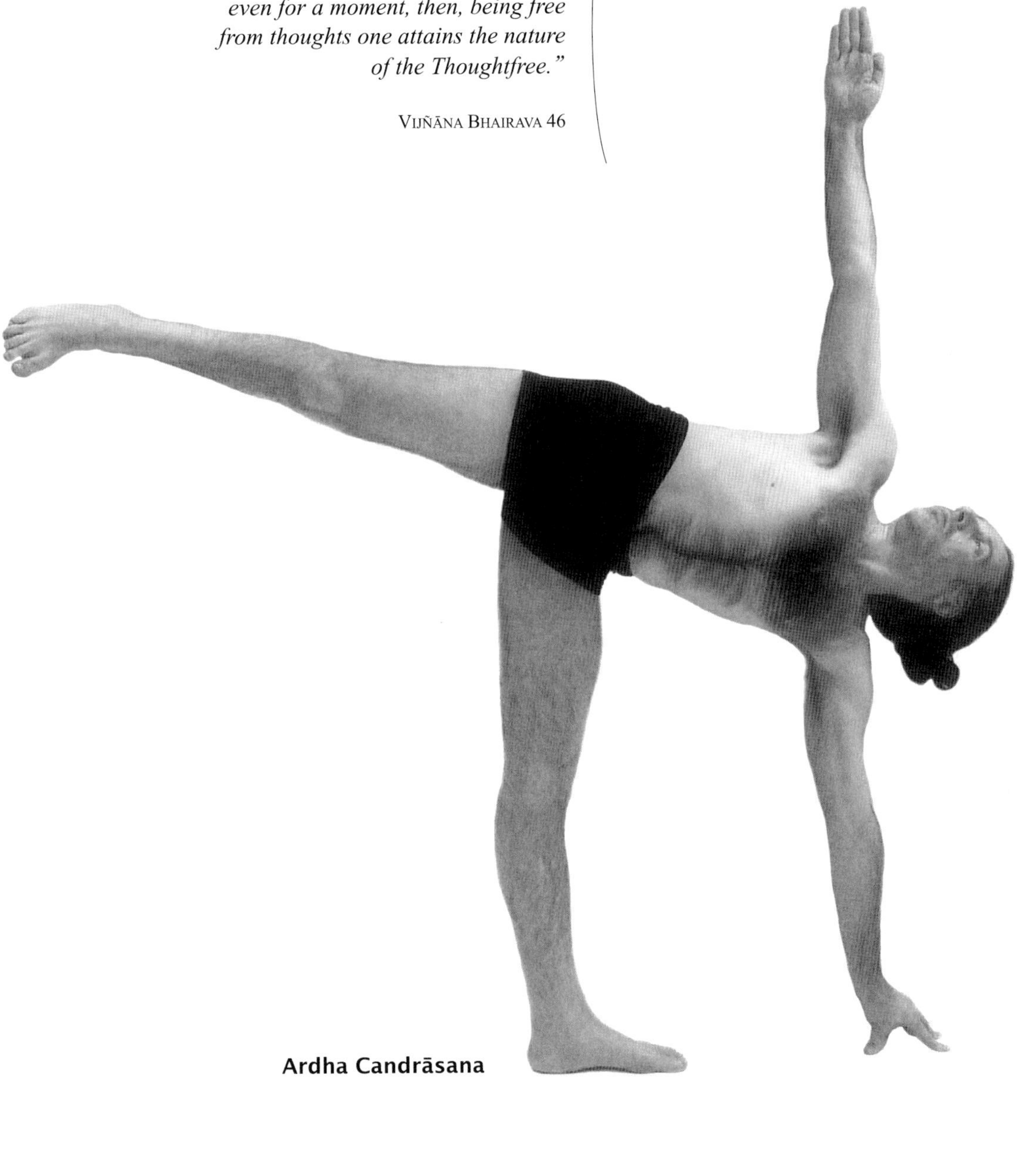

Ardha Candrāsana

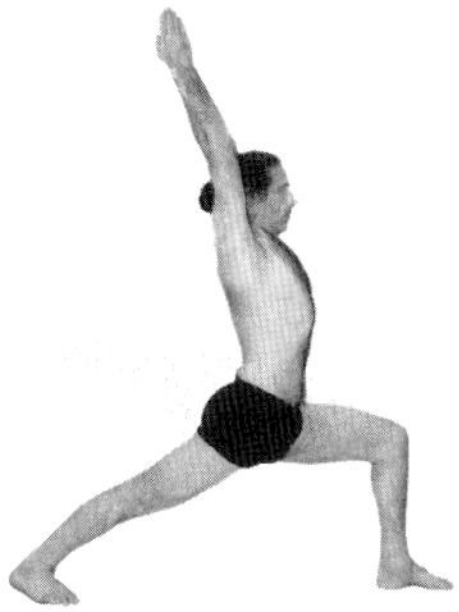

Virabhadrāsana 1 ...

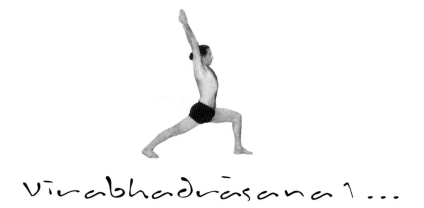

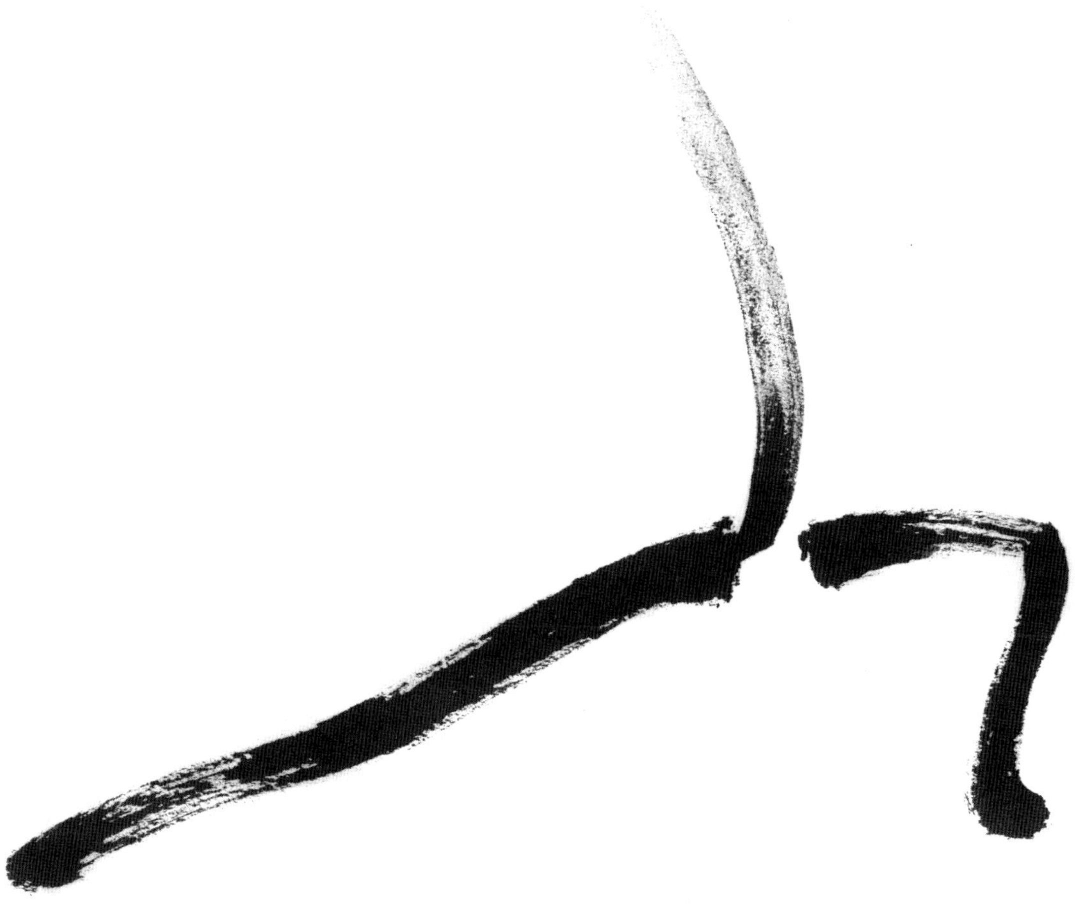

"O gazelle-eyed Goddess, if one contemplates on all the elements constituting the body as pervaded by void, then one's contemplation of the Void will become firm."

VIJÑĀNA BHAIRAVA 47

• Vīrabhadrāsana 1, 2, 3: The Hero of Auspicious Anger

According to the Dhātupāṭha, the nature of VĪR, the root of vīra (hero, warrior), and which denotes unfragmented energy, is found in the action of being everywhere in totality. Abhinavagupta defines heroic energy as: *"Whatever the hero accomplishes in thought, word or deed, through any activity requiring boldness and heroism apt to reveal such essence."*
TANTRĀLOKA XXIX, 5-6

Dakṣa had organised a very important sacrifice, known as Bṛhaspatisavana, to rid himself of the affront and humiliation bestowed upon him by Śiva. At a previous sacrifice performed by the Prajāpati, and to which Brahmā, Viṣṇu and Śiva had all been invited, when Dakṣa had entered into the hall of the temple, Śiva, his son-in-law, didn't deign to stand to welcome him. This had made Dakṣa wild with anger. He thus organised this great ritual where the gods, deva and other great dignitaries had all been invited, apart from Śiva. Pārvatī had gone to the sacrifice but her father didn't even look at her. Seeing that her husband had not been invited, she threw herself into the sacrificial fire.
It is said that Vīrabhadra was born from Śiva's wrath when he learnt of his wife's death. He threw a lock of his matted hair to the ground and it was from this that one of Śiva's most terrible guardians was born. Hence, even at the height of anger, in the extreme tension of a closed, knotted (symbolised by the matted hair) situation, by remaining in contact with the source of the event the unfragmented and radiant upsurge that is the true nature of the hero is able to gush forth.

This is what Śiva said to him:
"O my dear Vīrabhadra, listen carefully to what I am about to say. By carrying out my orders quickly, you will fill me with joy. Dakṣa, Brahmā's wicked son, has seen to the preparations for performing a sacrifice. He does not like me. He is ignorant and pretentious. O, best of the gaṇa, destroy his sacrifice and all that surrounds it, and then quickly return to me. Even if you encounter gandharva, yakṣa or any other entities, reduce them to ashes as quickly as you can. Do the same with Viṣṇu, Brahmā, Indra and Yama, pin them to the ground with your raging efforts. If anyone has defied the instructions of the venerable Dadhīci, reduce them too to ashes. Deva, politicians and other courtiers may try to seduce you and calm your anger. Burn them without hesitation. Once you have effortlessly destroyed the sacrifice, those performing it and their wives, in a playful and joyful mood, you may then quench your thirst."
ŚIVAPURĀṆA, RUDRASAṂHITĀ XXXII, 46-58

ग

Ga

fire (tejas)

"The jay's wings are alike on both sides. Why therefore would one define a yogi as introverted or extroverted?"

MAHEŚVARĀNANDA,
MAHĀRTHAMAÑJARĪ 60

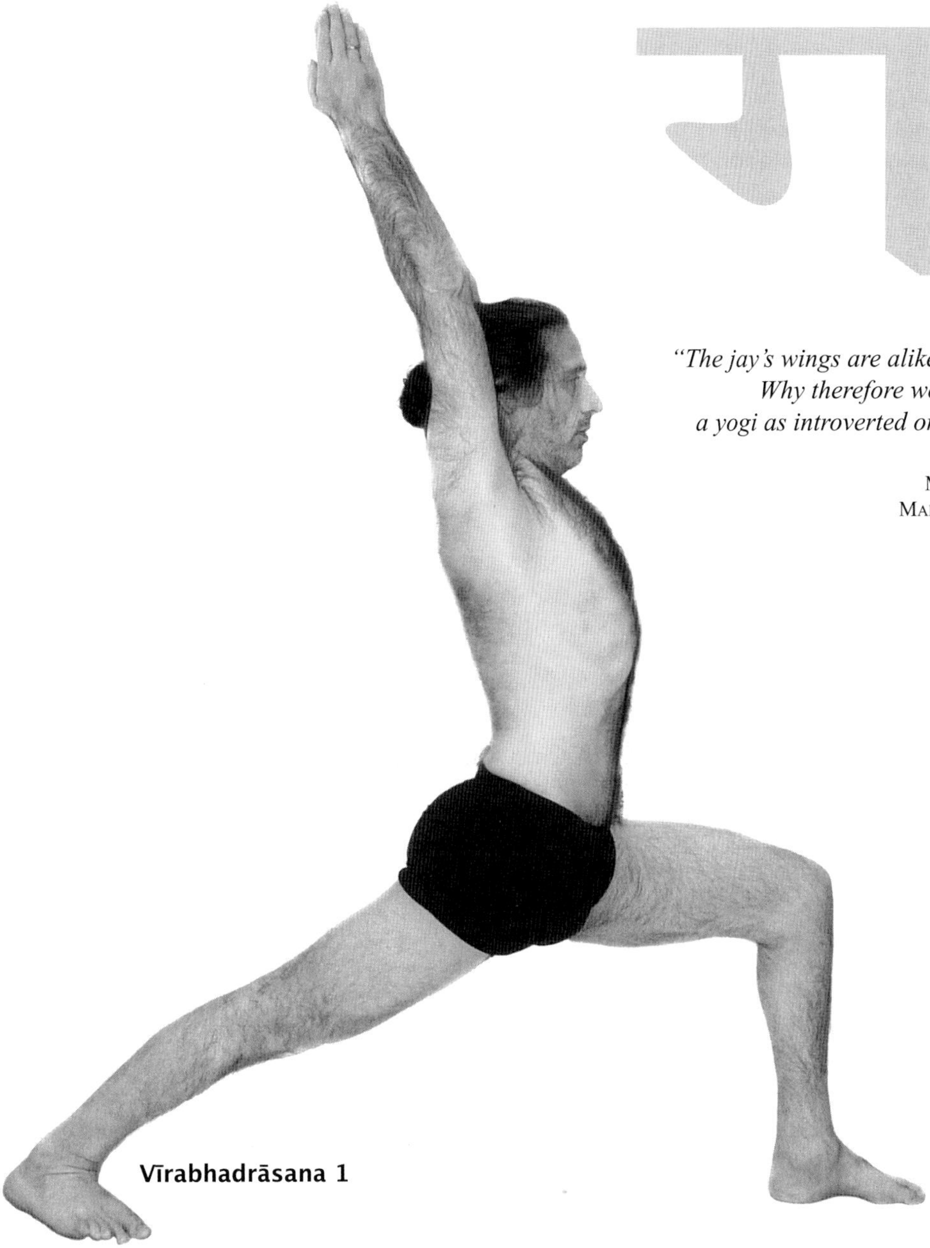

Vīrabhadrāsana 1

Dakṣa describes Śiva in the following terms:
"The sura, asura, brāhmaṇa and other sages all bow before me. How is it that this beggar, who is always surrounded by goblins and spirits, only does as he likes and sees fit to ignore me completely. He makes fun of rites, religious practices and all social conventions. Heretics, evil people and those who behave arrogantly before a brāhmaṇa are all of the same kind. And what's more, this beggar, who is my son-in-law, spends most of his time absorbed in himself or in lovers' games. Hear my malediction. Let Śiva, who has chosen to reside in cremation grounds, who is not noble by birth, be banished from the sacrifices. This untouchable is not to get his share. All you śaivites shall be excluded from vedic rites. You shall be rejected by those who follow the veda, and by the sages. You shall become marginalised as heretics and banished from society. You shall be devoted to drink and lust. Matted hair, ashes and bones will be your ornaments."
ŚIVAPURĀṆA, RUDRASAṂHITĀ XXVI, 14-18, 26-27

Dakṣa's sacrifice is that made to the divinities of fear and separation. We worship them and beg them for continuity, immortality, power, success, affective recognition and the like. This is the reason Śiva frightens Dakṣa so much, because he represents the end of all identities, of all affiliations, of all psychological banners, of all lifebuoys.

The gesture of Vīrabhadra reminds us of Christ chasing away the traders at the temple and shouting:
"Do not turn my Father's house into a place of trade."

Vīrabhadrāsana 1, 2, 3 represent the symbolic mudrā, in one's own body, of the destruction of Dakṣa's sacrifice.

"One should meditate on the body
as only enclosed by the skin
with nothing inside.
Meditating in this way, one attains
the One who is not an object
of meditation (i.e. Śiva)."

VIJÑĀNA BHAIRAVA 48

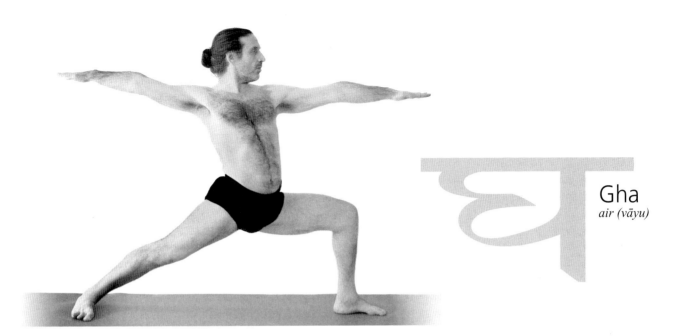

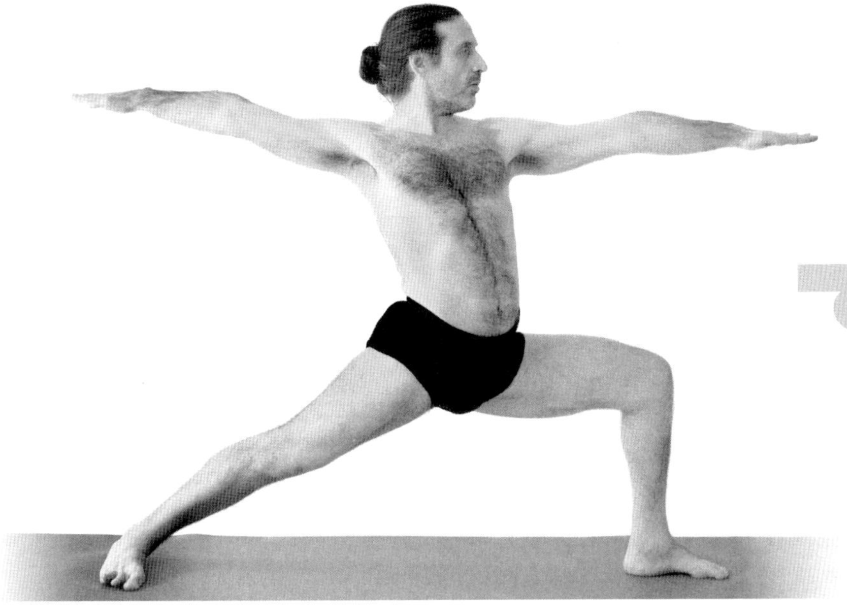

Vīrabhadrāsana 2

घ

Gha
air (vāyu)

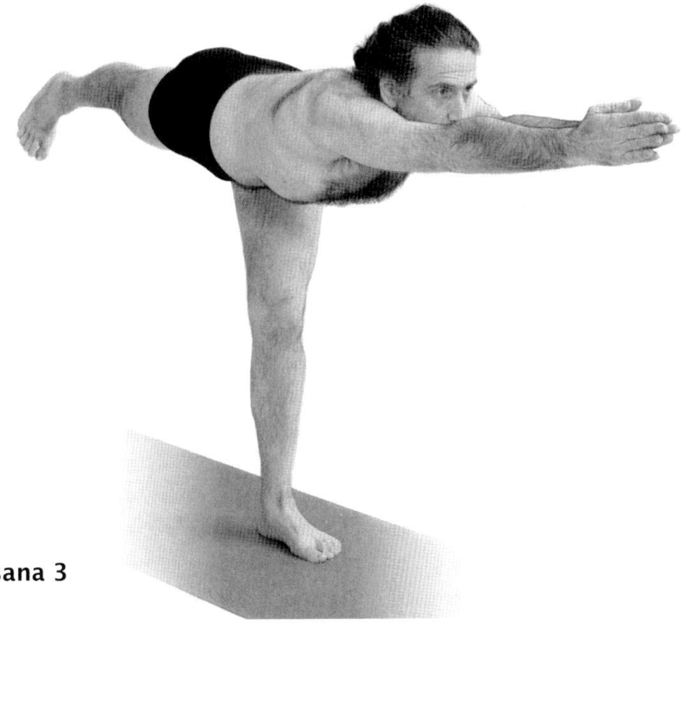

Vīrabhadrāsana 3

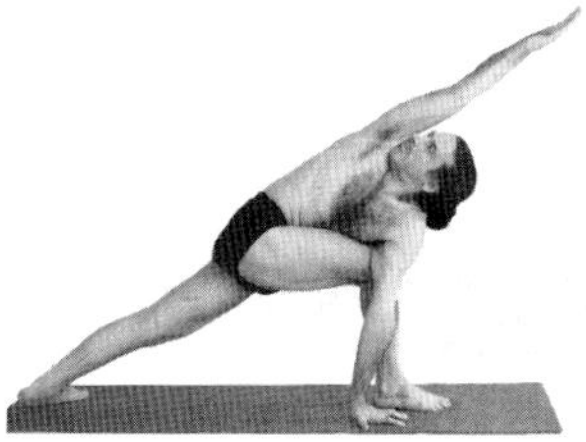

Parivṛtta Pārśvakoṇāsana ...

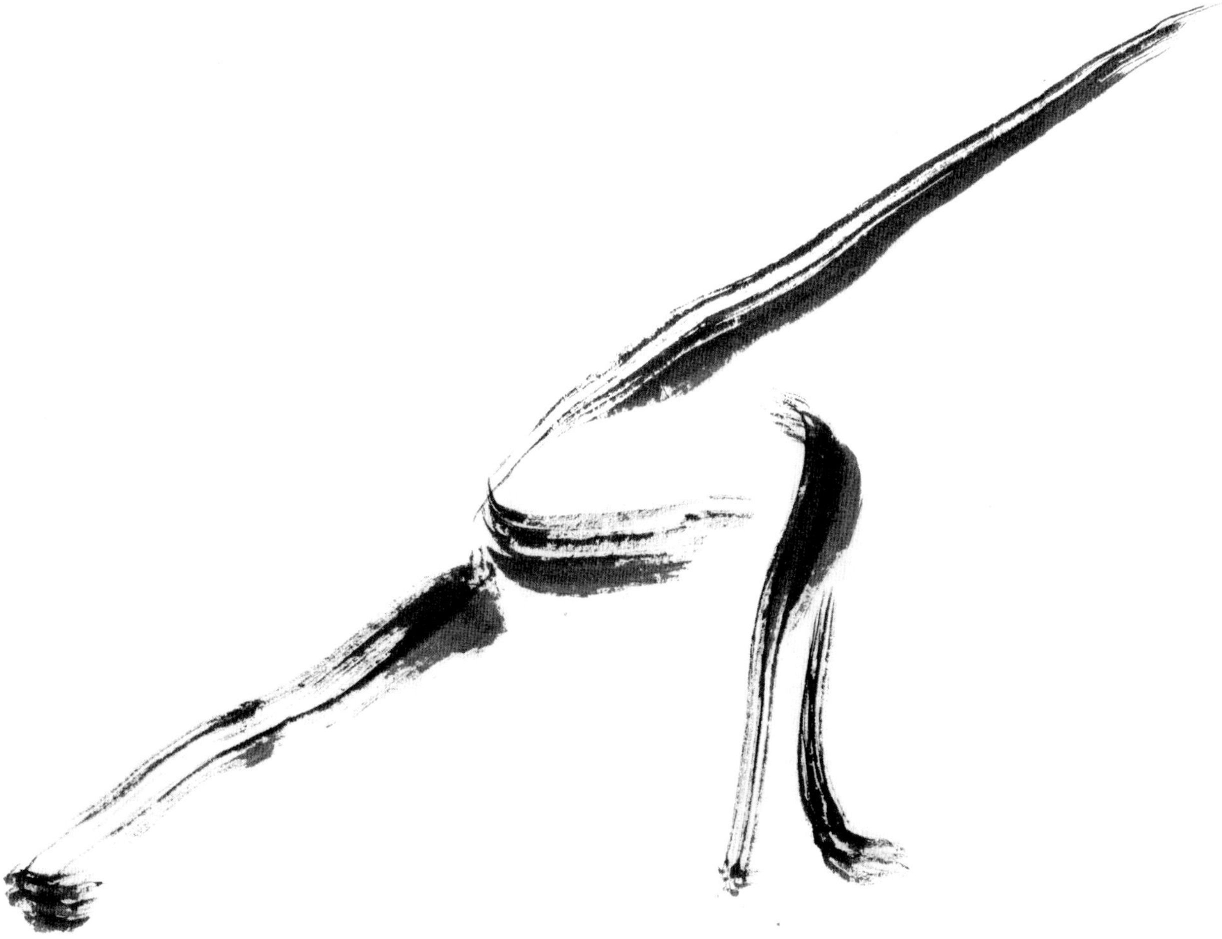

Contemplating the Vacuity of the Senses

If one merges one's senses in the space of the heart with an undistracted mind, then, O Blessed One, one attains supreme blessedness."
VIJÑĀNA BHAIRAVA 49

"The delight experienced at the time of sexual union when the female energy is exited and when the absorption into her is completed, is similar to the spiritual bliss and that bliss is said to be that of the Self."
VIJÑĀNA BHAIRAVA 69

Circumambulation and Churning (Parikrama, Manthāna)

- **Parivṛtta Trikoṇāsana: The Dance of Triangles**
- **Parivṛtta Pārśvakoṇāsana: The Great Churning**
- **Parivṛtta Ardha Candrāsana: From the Chalice to the Bindu**

Parivṛtta means revolved, turned round or back. This circumambulation is a reminder it is done from and around a centre. The universe itself is nothing other than the blossoming of this centre, of Viṣṇu's mythical navel (nābhi, from the root NAH - 'bandhane' to attach, to group together), the potentiality of all expressions of phenomenal emanation. All the contours and detours of our existence are merely its expression.

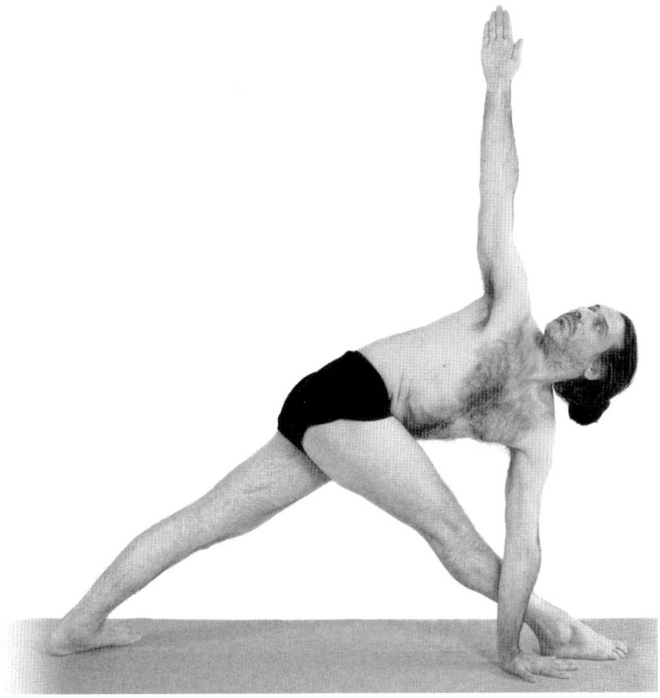

Parivṛtta Trikoṇāsana

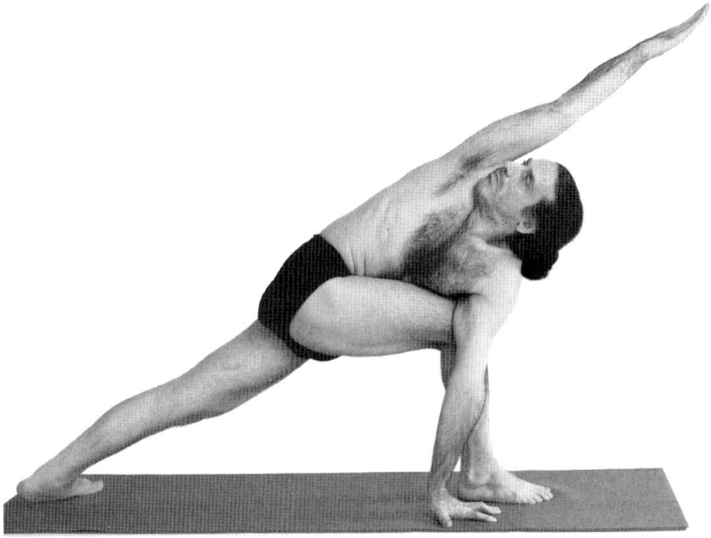

Parivṛtta Pārśvakoṇāsana

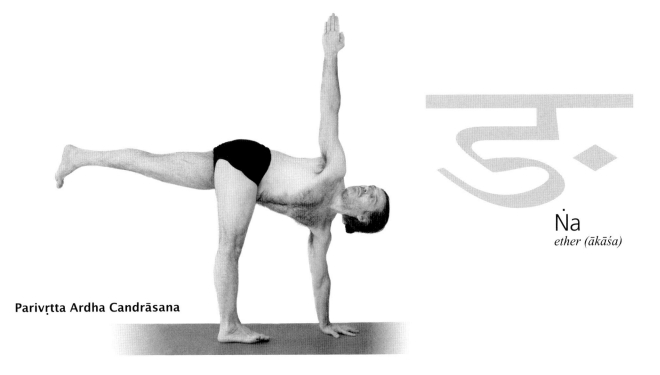

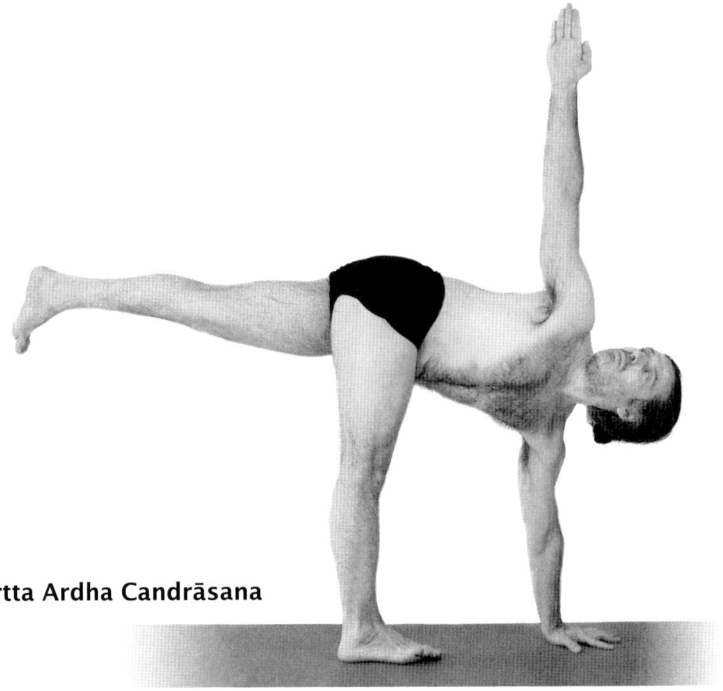

Parivṛtta Ardha Candrāsana

ङ

Ṅa

ether (ākāśa)

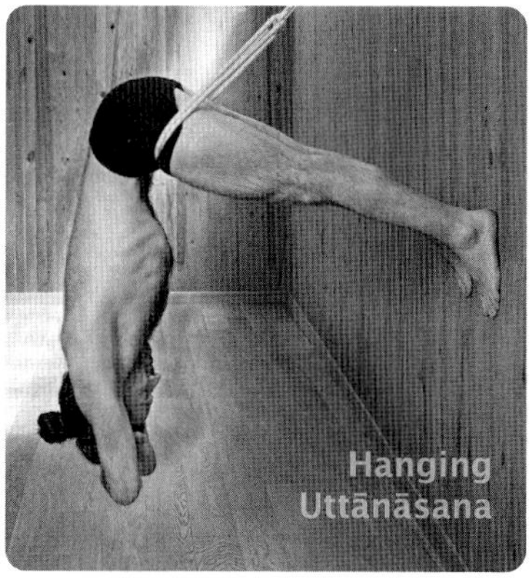

"O Goddess, even in the absence of a woman a flood of delight can be experienced by merely remembering with intensity the bliss of kisses and intimate embraces."
VIJÑĀNA BHAIRAVA 70

"When one is filled with joy arising from the pleasure of eating and drinking, one should meditate on the state of fullness. Then the great bliss will arise."
VIJÑĀNA BHAIRAVA 72

On Surging of the Sap

• Uttānāsana: The Vital Upsurge
• Pārśvottānāsana: On the Brightness of the Flanks
• Prasārita Pādottānāsana: The Feet in the Horizon

'Ut' indicates a will of intensity, of power, and the verb TAN means to extend, to stretch, to spread out and expansion. This energy of will (icchāśakti) is nothing other than the expression of the primordial vibration, the vital upsurge, spreading in itself, awakening a myriad of forms. There is no form that is not an expression of this will. Uttānāsana becomes the organic reflection of this surge that spreads without obstacle from the feet to the centre of the head. Pārśvottānāsana and Prasārita Pādottānāsana are declensions of this intensity. In Pārśvottānāsana, the sides of the chest and the flanks (pārśva) are explored. In yogic practices, the sides are activated and lose their identity in the silence of the centre. Prasārita means expanded, spread out. Pāda is the foot, but can also signify 'word' or 'vibration' in its aspect of ultimate reality and essence. In this āsana, the feet (pāda), which are the base or root, and which symbolically represent the ultimate reality (in Marathi, pāda also means the beginning of the instant, that which precedes manifestation) become the source of expansion (uttāna).

As it is said in the Kāmikāgama:
"Like a mirror or the water's surface, God reflects all forms yet has no form.
From Him, all things, mobile or immobile, are fully penetrated (vyāpta)."
ABHINAVAGUPTA, TANTRĀLOKA I, 66

च

Ca

smell (gandha)

THE PALATALS
FROM CA TO ÑA EMANATE
FROM THE VOWEL I
AND THE ENERGY OF WILL
(ICCHĀŚAKTI) SLOWLY
EMERGING OUTWARDS.

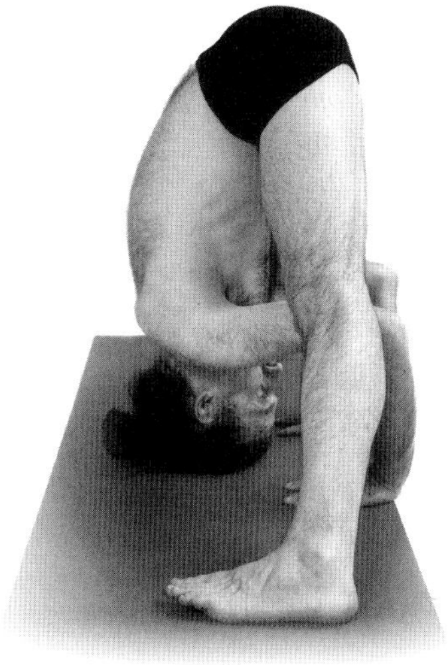

Prasārita Pādottānāsana

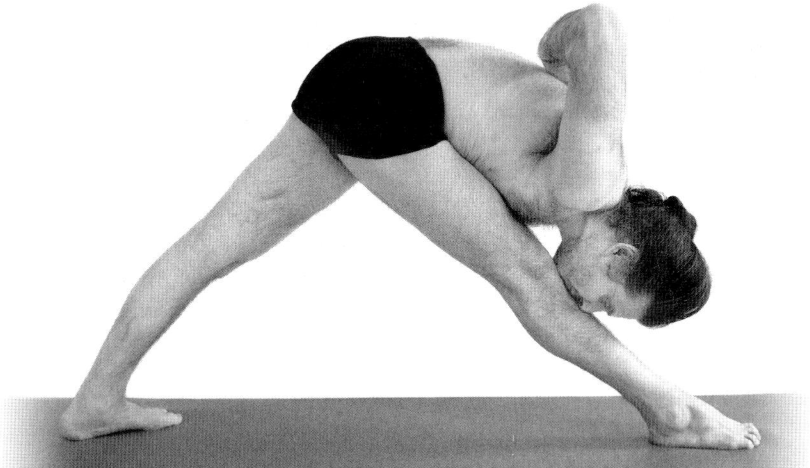

Pārśvottānāsana

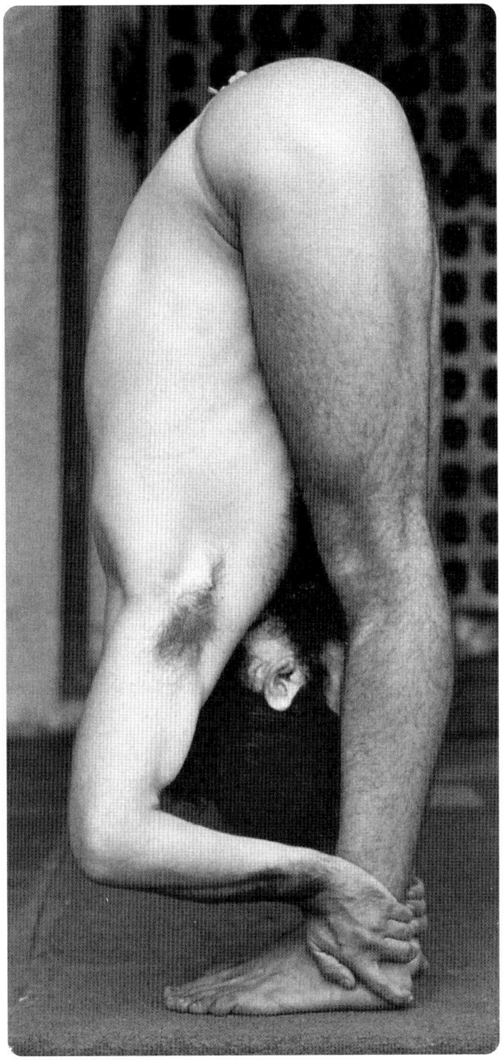

Uttānāsana

Awakening and Rooting of the Feet

• Pādāṅguṣṭhāsana, Uttitha Hasta Pādāṅguṣṭhāsana: The Semaphore of the Big Toes

Ādhāra, from the root DHRI, literally means that which holds or contains, but also means support. The term lakṣya, object of contemplation, is also used.

The first place of contemplation or ādhāra, as described by Gorakṣanātha, are the big toes. The awakening of the big toes, and especially of their roots, unfolds the various sections of the feet and legs, and in particular will be felt by the lifting of the knees and thighs. In this āsana, a 'luminous' length is given to the inner legs, from the heels to the groins, and from the groins to the heels. The vital point, referred to as kṣipra, located between the big toe and the second toe, is stimulated.

"First is the ādhāra of the pādāṅguṣṭha. There, in the big toe, one should meditate upon the light.
This makes the vision steady."
GORAKṢANĀTHA, SIDDHASIDDHĀNTAPADDHATI II, 10

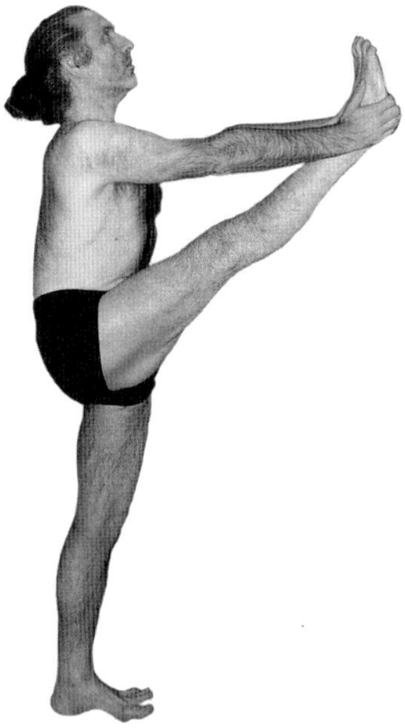

"Whenever the universal Consciousness of the all-pervading Lord is revealed through any of the sense organs, since their nature is the same, then by absorption into pure Consciousness the fullness of the Self will be attained."
VIJÑĀNA BHAIRAVA 117

"Immerse yourself in the joy of listening to music or songs, or other pleasures that delight the senses. Let this resonate within you as your own nature."
VIJÑĀNA BHAIRAVA 73

"O gazelle-eyed goddess, by applying a trick of tickling under the armpits there arises suddenly great bliss by which Reality is revealed."
VIJÑĀNA BHAIRAVA 66

छ

Cha

taste (rasa)

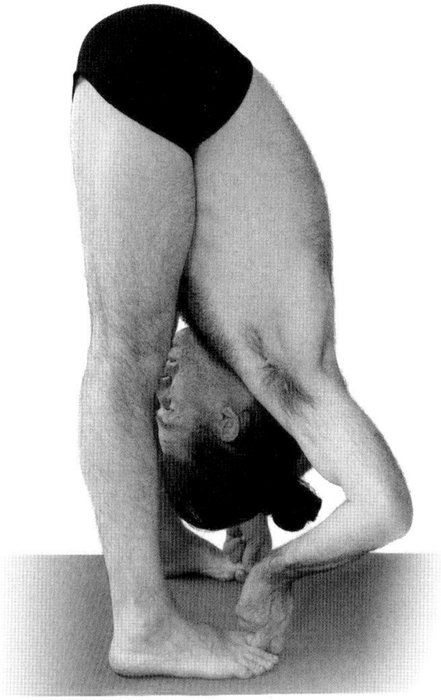

Pādāṅguṣṭhāsana

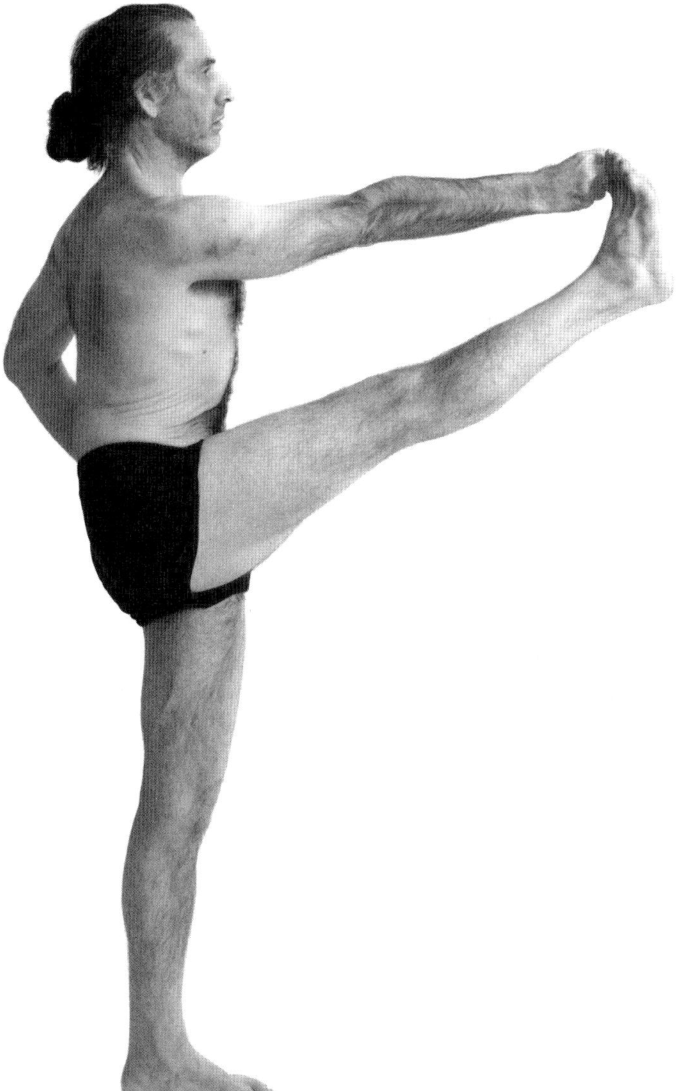

Uttitha Hasta Pādāṅguṣṭhāsana

Contemplating the Vacuity of the Mind

> *If one's mind is absorbed at the dvādaśānta,*
> *the body is void in all parts with firm intellect,*
> *then the firmly established Reality is revealed."*
> VIJÑĀNA BHAIRAVA 50

• Pādahastāsana: Spreading and Humility

In this āsana, the feet (pāda), which are the base or root, and which symbolically represent the ultimate reality, become the source of expansion (uttāna) of the back of the legs, and are placed on the hands (hasta), the etymology of which in Sanskrit means: 'that which unfolds outwards'. Here, the binding of the extremities awakens the back of the legs, especially the calves and back of the knees. This āsana seals and fills the extremities by the feeling of power it creates in the feet, particularly the heels, but also by the spreading of the hands that are cleansed of their desire to grasp and to grip because of the weight of the feet and the contact of the back of the hands with the ground.

• Ardha Baddha Padmottānāsana: Budding of the Root

In this āsana, the intensity of spreading (uttānāsana) is combined with half Padmāsana, which tones the lower abdomen. The cleansing of this region prepares the blossoming of the lotus, symbolising the vertical thrust of the region between the anus and the genitals, and which is achieved by the binding of the root (mūlabandha). The bind (baddha) is the passageway to a functional relationship with the vital energy, and no longer its exploitation by our psychological projections.

"The functions of the body are his worship." VASUGUPTA, ŚIVASŪTRA III, 26

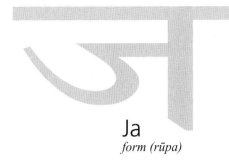

*"If one fixes one's mind on dvādaśānta**
every moment, in any way and
wherever one is, then the fluctuations
of the mind will dissolve and within days
one will experience an extraordinary state."

VIJÑĀNA BHAIRAVA 51

ज

Ja

form (rūpa)

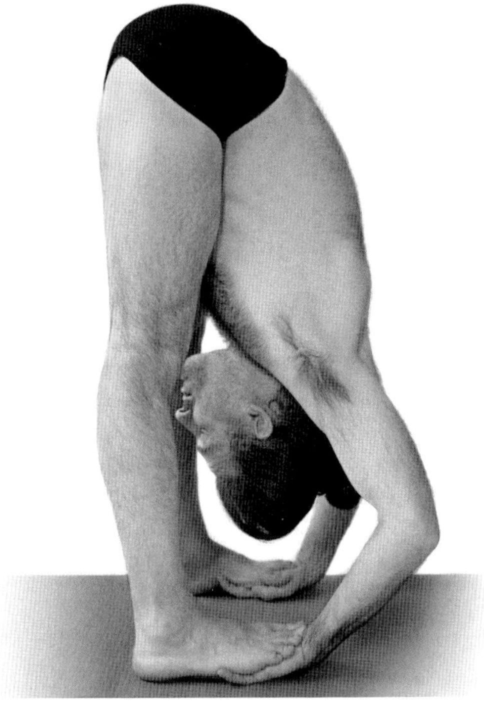

Pādahastāsana

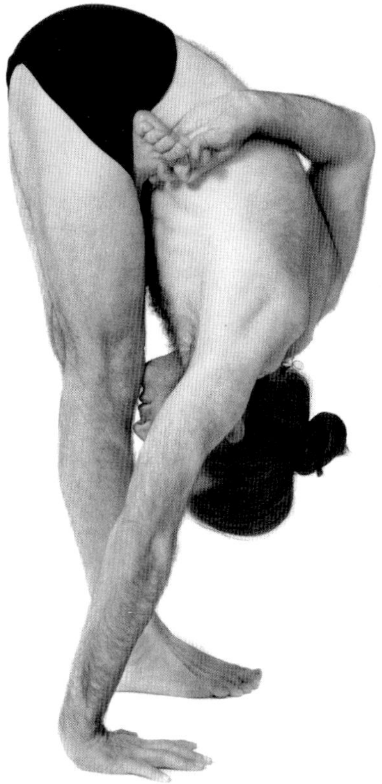

Ardha Baddha Padmottānāsana

* *Dvādaśānta:*
1 ūrdhva dvādaśānta, the space above, 12 fingers above the head (brahmarandhra)
2 bāhya dvādaśānta, the space outside, 12 fingers in front of the nose
3 āntara dvādaśānta, the space inside the heart

• Siṃhāsana: The Roar of the Unknown

Hiraṇyakaśipu, an asura god, obtained powers from Brahmā that made him almost immortal. He could be neither killed by beast nor by man, neither by day nor by night, neither inside nor outside a house and not even by weapons. Hiraṇyakaśipu personifies the ignorance that makes us live within reassuring concepts. Despite his almost complete immunity, he was constantly in conflict with the gods and didn't cease to torment them. The gods here symbolise situations, which were never in harmony with his desires. He also tyrannised his son who was a Viṣṇu devotee. One day, wanting to prove the stupidity of his son's belief in the omnipresence of Viṣṇu, he kicked a pillar in an excess of rage. Viṣṇu leapt out of the pillar in the form of a man-lion (Narasiṃha), who was neither beast nor man. He attacked Hiraṇyakaśipu at twilight, which was neither by day nor by night, and whilst he stood at the threshold, which was neither inside nor outside. Narasiṃha then tore out his entrails using his claws, which were not weapons.

How far can our insatiable desire for security go?
All the ramparts we build to make ourselves invulnerable
are never sufficient to protect us from our own fears.
Despite all of our fortresses, there is always a breach
into which the roaring of the unknown rushes.

*"Whether one is seated on a moving vehicle
or whether one moves one's body slowly,
one attains a peaceful state.
Then, O Goddess, one realises
the divine flood of Consciousness."*

Vijñāna Bhairava 83

Oneiric Lands and Mythical Creatures: Āsana of Initiation into Lucid Dreams

Siṃhāsana

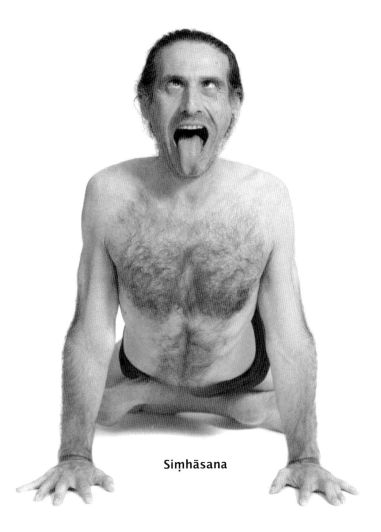

• Vātāyanāsana: Roaming of the Divine Horse

In the Vedic period, the end of the year, especially the month of December, was considered as very auspicious and was chosen for the start of a very special sacrifice: that of the horse. It was thought that at this time the earth prepared itself to receive the seed of the Sun God. It was in this season that a horse was left free to roam as it pleased for one year before sacrificing it.

The horse symbolises the sun and by extension, the radiant Self and the senses. In the Ṛgveda, it is said that the sage sees the horse's head as a solar disc crossing the sky.

When left to roam free, the senses are abandoned since nothing can be found in exteriority.

> *"If you want to control a bull,*
> *give him a big field."*
> CHAN PROVERB

The senses then become simple observers and are no longer a means to grasp and appropriate the world.

The horse's head is often identified with that of Viṣṇu in his solar disc form. Viṣṇu incarnated himself in the form of a man with a horse's head (Hayagrīva) in order to kill a demon (Rākṣasa). As for the fiercely beautiful goddess with a horse's head, Itarala (see photo page 66), she had a lion as a throne and is seated in the āsana referred to as that of 'royal ease' (rājalīlāsana).

Indra killed the asura (agitation of the senses) with a weapon made from the bones of a horse's head given to him by the sage Dadhīci.

The senses are therefore said to be white (śveta) as they no longer colour things. This realisation gave the name to an Upaniṣad that bears witness to the understanding of the sage who composed it. The Upaniṣad of the immaculate white horse: Śvetāśvataropaniṣad.

"Wherever the mind goes, whether outside or within, there itself is the state of Śiva. Since He is all pervading, where else could the mind go?"

VIJÑĀNA BHAIRAVA 116

"Wherever the mind finds satisfaction, let it be fixed there, for there itself the nature of supreme bliss will become manifest."

VIJÑĀNA BHAIRAVA 74

Jha

touch (sparśa)

झ

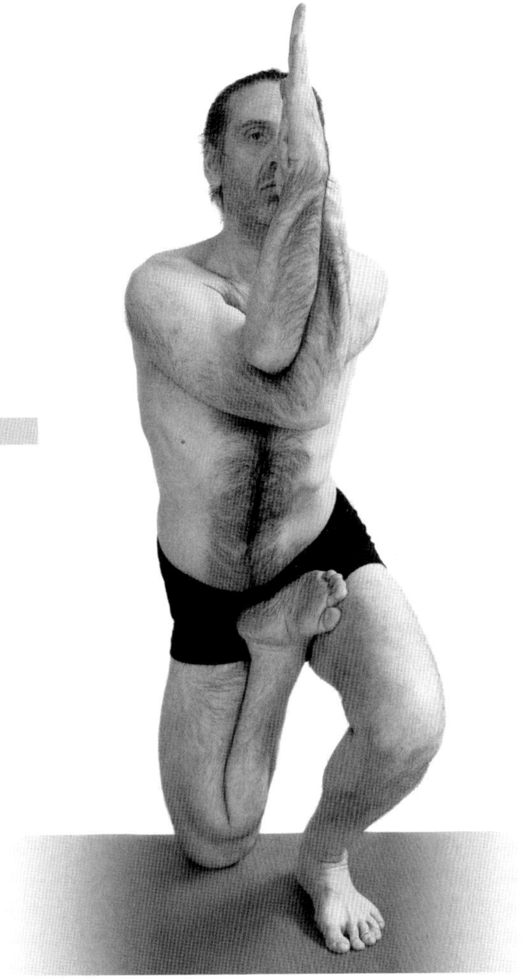

Vātāyanāsana

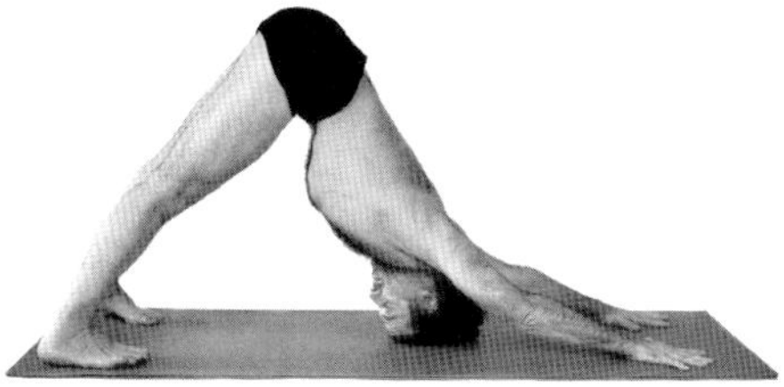

Adho mukha śvānāsana …

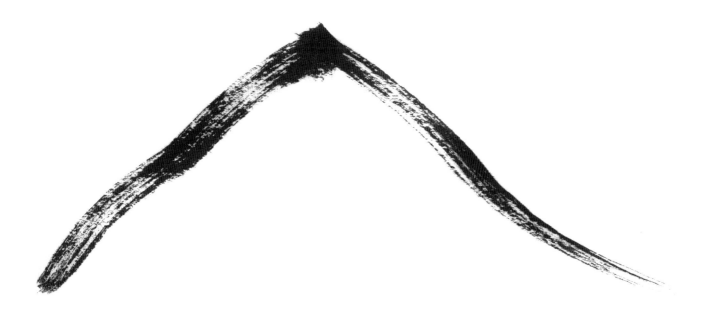

Contemplating the Source of Spontaneous Arising

> *Energy and its source are one.*
> *Existence (Śakti) is thus the essence (Śiva)."*
> Vijñāna Bhairava 18

• Adho Mukha Śvānāsana, Ūrdhva Mukha Śvānāsana: Dogs Howling to the Absolute

Kāla Bhairava (He who makes time tremble), the dark form of Śiva, is accompanied by a black dog. When he uses the dog as his vehicle, Śiva is referred to as the 'Master of Dogs' (śvapati), He who uses a dog as a horse. Rudra is also known as the 'Lord of Dogs' (śvaneśa). The absolute in its most stripped and inaccessible form is associated with an animal that is impure in the eyes of the Hindu tradition. Thought, which by nature is discursive, should become silent otherwise it is like a pack of enraged dogs. This can only happen when thought recognises its source, for which the pure and impure are only mental categories. It then becomes a vehicle.

To discourage half-hearted seekers, Dattātreya was followed by four very aggressive dogs. They represent the four Veda, accumulated knowledge and the conceptions we have of the world and of ourselves. All of this must come to an end in order he who is dressed in space (digambara) and who has abandoned himself (Avadhūta, another name of Dattātreya) can be recognised.

A story about Śaṅkarācārya tells how he had carried out his morning ablutions and was on his way to a temple. On a narrow path he found himself face to face with an untouchable who was carrying a jug of liqueur and followed by four dogs barking incessantly. Fearing he would be sullied by the presence of an untouchable and his dogs, and that he would be bitten, he asked the stranger to step aside in no uncertain terms. The stranger did not move and replied that there was only the unique reality of the Self and nobody to be sullied or not sullied. Śaṅkarācārya bowed at the stranger's feet and worshiped him, reciting verses from the Mānīśāpañcaka. The untouchable revealed his true identity and was no other than Śiva, and the dogs were recognised as the four Veda. For Eknāth and Tukārām, the dog is the symbol itself of devotion (bhakti).

In this āsana, the diaphragm finds its space and elasticity and can once again become a bridge between the gross and subtle bodies, and is no longer a barrier of tension.

ञ

Ña

sound (śabda)

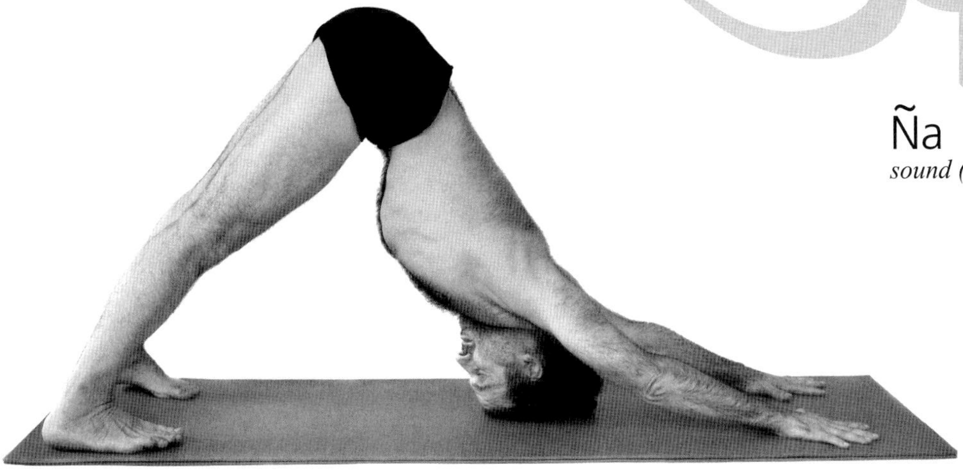

Adho Mukha Śvānāsana

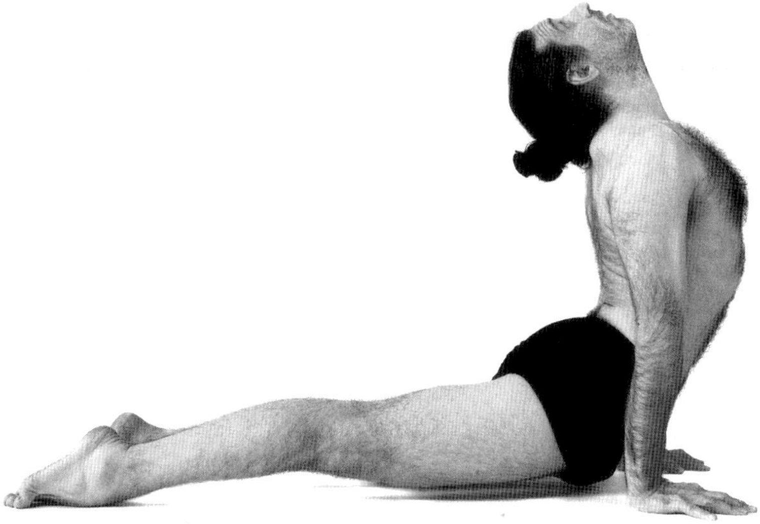

Ūrdhva Mukha Śvānāsana

• Vīrāsana: The Quiet Hero

The organs of action (arms and legs) are conditioned to ensure survival. In sitting āsana, the legs are reposed in different ways and learn to become quiet and free from the desire for movement linked to defence, aggression or escape.

According to a sermon by Master Eckhart:
"The gospel says that Christ was sitting in the temple and was teaching. The fact he was sitting signifies being at rest. Because he who is sitting is in a more ready state to accomplish those things that are pure than he who moves or is standing. Sitting signifies rest; standing, work; and moving, instability. This is the reason the soul must be seated in humility under the crushing weight of all creatures. This is why it finds true peace. The light of this peace comes from silence, whilst within the soul is seated and dwells... It is the reason Masters, those who must teach the Sciences, are seated. Because he who is lying down has an unrefined mind, that is to say unrefined blood that rises to the brain and obscures intelligence. But when man is seated, the unrefined blood falls and a light mind hurries upwards towards the brain. Thus the memory is enlightened."
MASTER ECKHART, SERMON 90

It is interesting to note that the phoneme RA and bījamantra RAM are the seed of fire. Jayaratha says the sound RA shines with an instantaneous brilliance, like the lightning flash that symbolises the verticality of breath beyond inhalation and exhalation.

Here, as in other sitting āsana, the three major joints of the lower body are cleansed: ankles, knees and hips, leaving the pelvis completely free of all extensions and able to bring to maturity the churning of breath in its different modalities (pañcavāyu).

"At the moment Energy quivers,
be aware that you are not separate from it.
Energy (Śakti) is known as the mouth
of Śiva or the gateway that leads to Him."

VIJÑĀNA BHAIRAVA 20

Installing the Throne and Surrendering of Weapons: Sitting Āsana

The cerebrals from Ṭa to Ṇa
are also connected
to the energy of will (icchāśakti)
which abides in itself.
This energy of will is connected
to a sudden illumination
that creates the phoneme Ṛ.

ट

Ṭa
procreation
(upastha)

"That is āsana (seat)
which is determined by
the agent through his autonomy,
for when the aspect of universality
is the main principle, then in the act
of sitting, the location and seat are
determined through autonomy only."

Abhinavagupta, Parātrīśikāvivaraṇa,
Jaideva Singh, Page 254

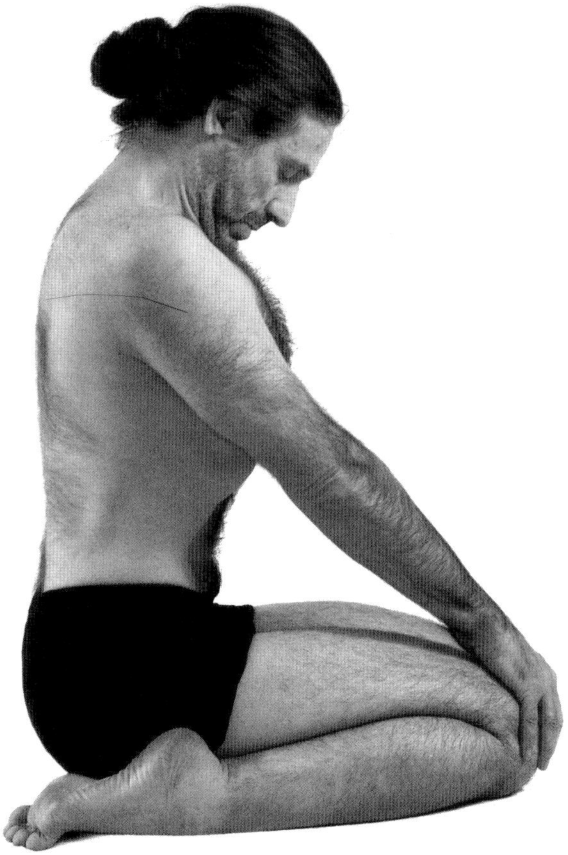

Vīrāsana

• Siddhāsana: Divine Drunkenness

In the Haṭhayogapradīpikā, it is said there is no āsana to equal Siddhāsana. Symbolically, Siddhāsana represents the essence itself of all āsana, which is to be seated as Presence or Consciousness, and, as Abhinavagupta says, *"shines with its own brilliance."* (TANTRĀLOKA II, 10).

It is the source of all activities but which activities cannot reach. It is described as making the unmanībhāva attitude, or absence of conceptualisation, and the three locks (mūlabandha, uḍḍiyānabandha and jālandharabandha) gush forth spontaneously, which puts an end to all identification with the psychosomatic continuum. Siddhāsana spreads the ink of the inner night where *"man must reside in the absence of images and ties. There lies the greatest of joys."* (SUSO). This night is known as Kevala Kumbhaka, when the modalities of inhalation and exhalation cease.

"When there is mastery of Siddhāsana and it is firmly established, without effort, by itself, then appears the suspension of the mind's functions, and the three bandha follow easily and spontaneously."
HAṬHAYOGAPRADĪPIKĀ I, 42

• Gomukhāsana: The Mouth of Abundance

One of the meanings of 'go' is cow. It is known and worshiped as Kāmadhenu, 'the cow that grants all desires.' The word 'dhenu' indicates the notion of stock and beverage, a sacred beverage, giving rise to the name of Sabardughā, the cow that provides not only milk as food and nectar, but also the milk of prosperity. Clouds are thus regarded as cows of the sky that spread the blessing of rain upon the earth. The cow is but food and a boon. This boon is a continuous flow, and this is the reason the river Sarasvatī is also visualised as the cosmic cow. This unreserved abundance that is asking to be milked, becomes the heart of sacrifice.
Another meaning of 'go' is senses. Mukha means face or mouth, as well as opening. What could be found at the mouth of the senses but this instant before their exteriorisation as diversity (indriya vṛtti), where, although vibrant (indriya śakti), they are still bathed in the blindness of the world?

"The first form of worship is the movement of all the senses when they reside in non-duality."
YOGINĪHṚDAYA, PŪJĀSAṂKETA III, PAGE 221

Gocarī is also one of three energies that pervade the universe and which are the expression of Khecarī:
"As Gocarī, she brings about a knowledge of objects and exists as the internal organ (antaḥkaraṇa)."
ABHINAVAGUPTA, PARĀTRĪŚIKĀVIVARAṆA, JAIDEVA SINGH, PAGE 38

The names of āsana refer to archetypal energies that are felt intuitively. Their literal representation is not needed.

"Just as parts of space are known by the
light of a lamp or the rays of the sun,
in the same way, O Dear one,
Śiva is known through Śakti."

VIJÑĀNA BHAIRAVA 21

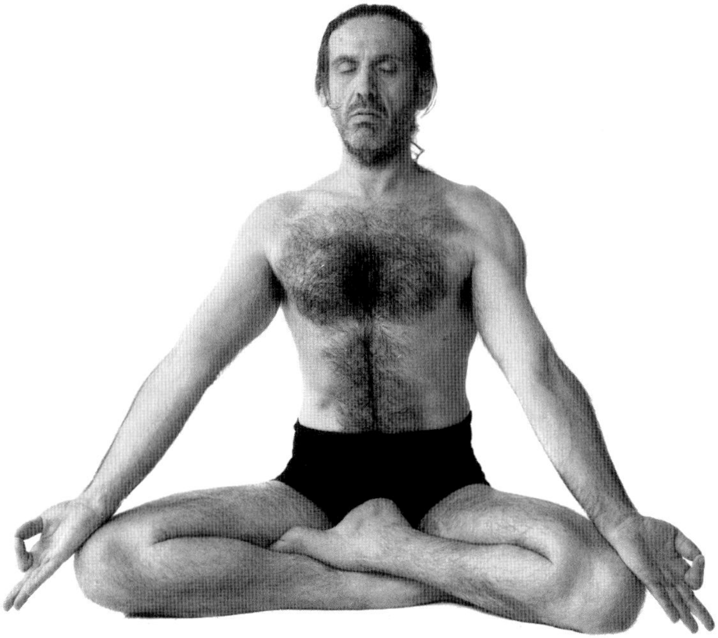

Siddhāsana

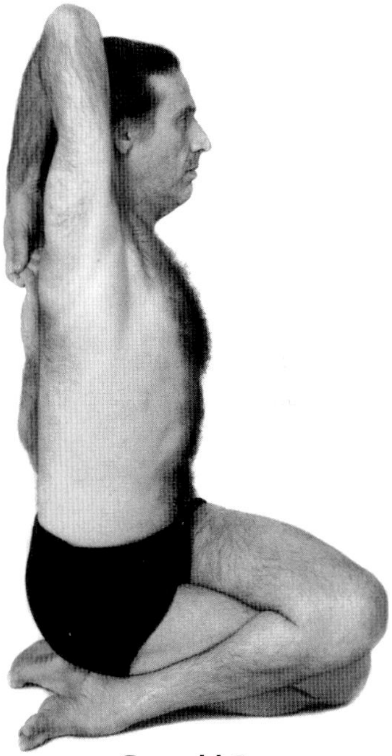

Gomukhāsana

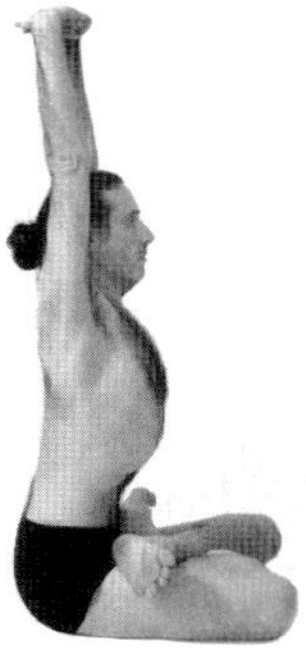

Parvatàsana ...

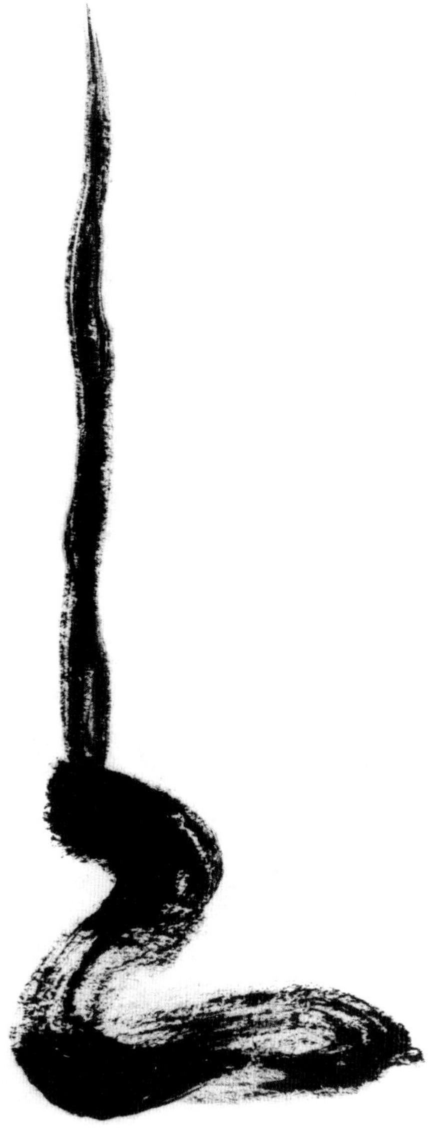

"If one observes a desire as it arises spontaneously, one should put an end to it immediately. It will merge at that point from whence it has sprung."
Vijñāna Bhairava 96

"Who am I when neither my will nor my knowledge has arisen? I am this in reality! Having become that, one should be merged in that and one's mind should be identified with that."
Vijñāna Bhairava 97

• Padmāsana, Baddha Padmāsana: The Sacrificial Altar

"Through the practice of this pose, the vital breaths of the practitioner are immediately balanced and flow harmoniously through the body." Śivasaṃhitā III, 90

The descent of the root of the thighs in this āsana creates an intense space between the pubis and the diaphragm, leaving the two lotuses of mūlabandha and uḍḍiyānabandha free to blossom.

"In Siddhāsana, the top part of the spine is more stretched than its other parts, while in Vīrāsana it is the lumbar area that is more stretched. Some of these postures may be more comfortable, but for accuracy and efficacy Padmāsana is the best of them all. In Padmāsana the thighs are lower than the groin, the lower abdomen is kept stretched, with maximum space between the pubis and the diaphragm, enabling the lungs to expand fully."
Śrī B.K.S. Iyengar, Light on Prāṇāyāma, Chapter 11, Paragraph 15

Padmāsana is therefore the royal āsana for practising prāṇāyāma. The different regions of the body, namely the arms, legs, trunk, neck and the head are balanced in silence. Padmāsana is used in the variations of Śīrṣāsana and Sarvāṅgāsana to cleanse and purify the apānic region located below the navel, which includes the pelvis and legs.

• Parvatāsana: The Mountain of the Depths

She is worshiped as the 'axis mundi' (Mount Meru) or as Kailāśā, the impenetrable abode of the gods. It is the place of all ascetism, where one meets one's own nakedness and death. This is where Arjuna went to accomplish terrible austerity so as to be fit to propitiate Śiva. One day after he had just killed a wild boar with an arrow and was getting ready to lift it onto his shoulders, another hunter, who was none other than Śiva, arrived and said it was he who had killed the boar. Arjuna, failing to recognise Śiva, refused to give in and started a fight with this stranger that lasted all night. It was only as the night was dying, after Arjuna had exhausted all his strategies and strength, and was forced to admit defeat, that Śiva revealed himself. The mountain is always a place of light and darkness: the blinding light of lofty heights and the darkness of the night of the soul we must cross. Despite all our efforts and desperate attempts to hold on to all our concepts and identifications, this mountain cannot be climbed. It is only by abandoning our hold that the goddess of the mountain (Pārvatī) reveals herself. Abandon is Pārvatī.

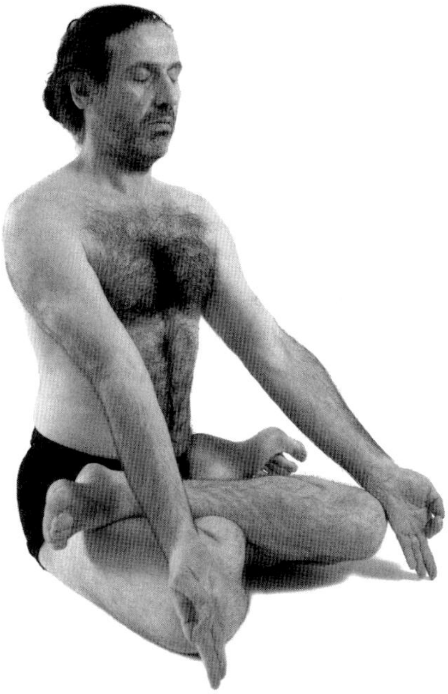

Padmāsana

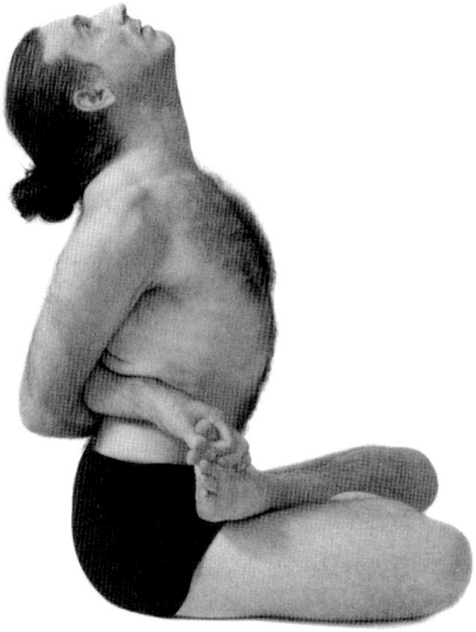

Baddha Padmāsana

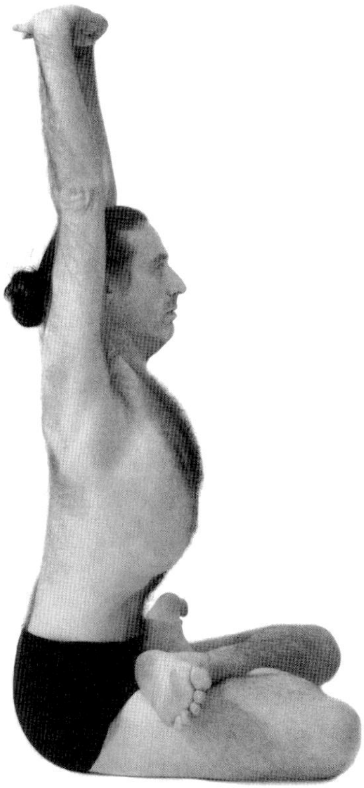

Parvatāsana

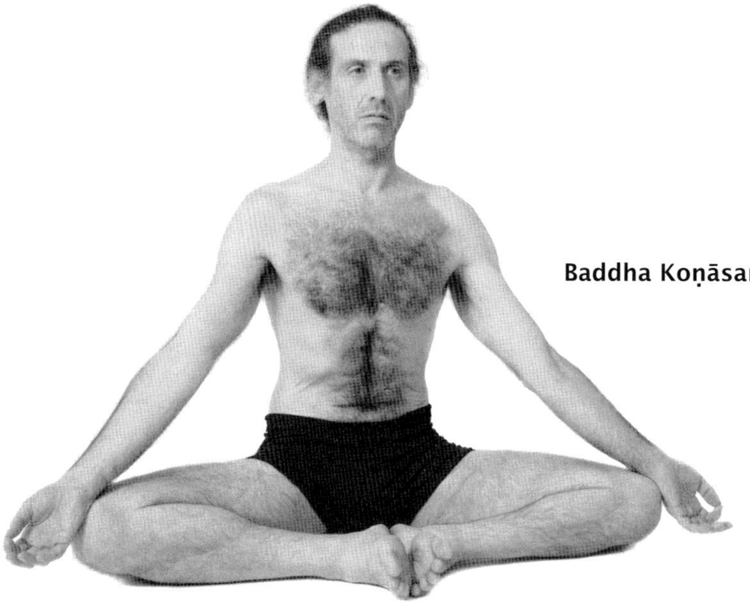

Baddha Koṇāsana

• Baddha Koṇāsana: The Celestial Cobbler

This is the pose Indian cobblers adopt whilst working. What is the work accomplished by this bound (baddha) angle (koṇa)? In baddha, the phoneme BA symbolises buddhi, which here means 'awakening to certainty'. What is this certainty? Whatever the aspect of manifestation, whether the experimenter, the experience or the object of experience, they are only the expression of a unique and same reality.

Even the triangular shape of the āsana suggests the three-current unfolding of spanda: the energy of will (icchāśakti), intuition (jñānaśakti) and action (kriyāśakti). This triangle also symbolises Māyā, as the principle of generation and emanation of the universe.

In the Haṭhayogapradīpikā, it is referred to as the beneficial āsana (Bhadrāsana) or Gorakṣāsana.

"The Siddha and the Yogi call it Gorakṣāsana. Sitting thus, the fatigue felt in āsana and bandha is dissipated."

HAṬHAYOGAPRADĪPIKĀ I, 53

• Mūla Bandhāsana: The Womb

"That Brahman which is the root of all existence, and on which the restraint of the mind is based is called the restraining root (mūlabandha), which should always be adopted since it is fit for the Rāja Yogi."

ŚAṄKARĀCĀRYA, APAROKṢĀNUBHŪTI 114

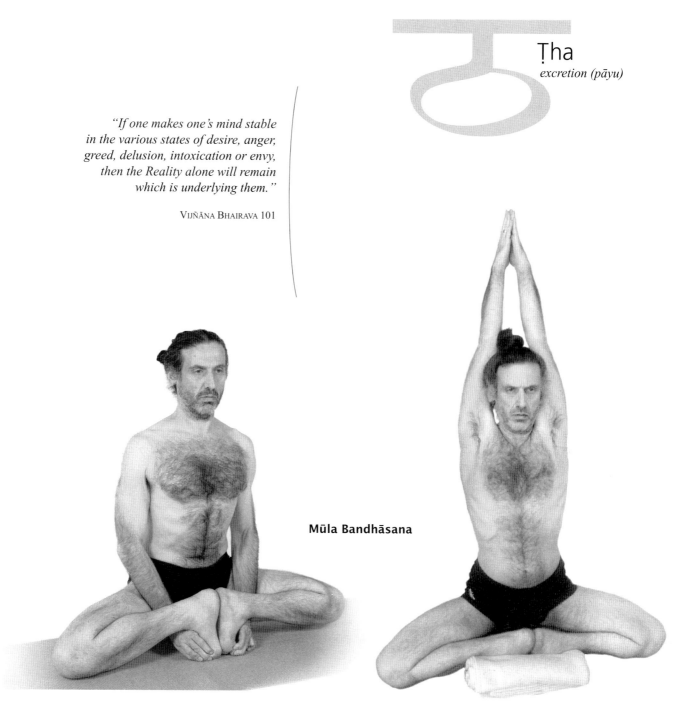

ठ

Ṭha

excretion (pāyu)

"If one makes one's mind stable in the various states of desire, anger, greed, delusion, intoxication or envy, then the Reality alone will remain which is underlying them."

Vijñāna Bhairava 101

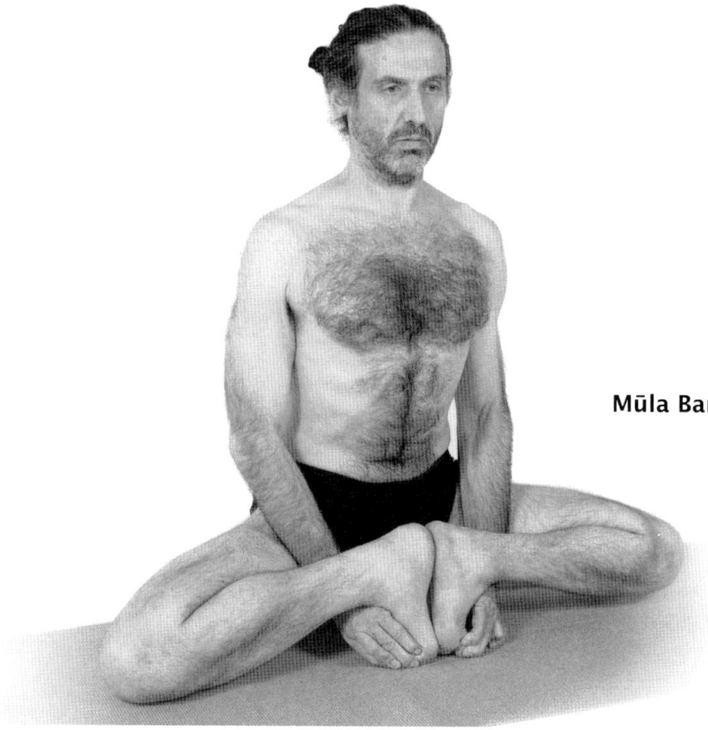

Mūla Bandhāsana

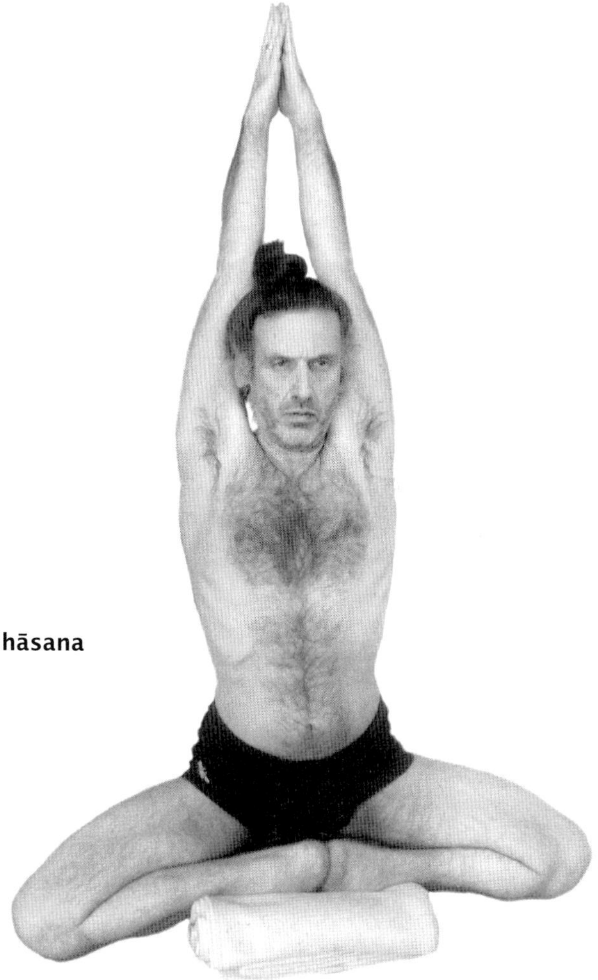

• Vāmadevāsana 2: He Who Cooks a Dog's Entrails

The semi-vowel 'VA' comes from the junction of the vowels 'U' (energy of awakening) and 'A' (the Without-Equal). According to the Tantrāloka, it causes emanation to rain down. 'VA' is the seed of water and of the god Varuṇa, who is the Lord of water and of the oceans.

During a terrible famine caused by a drought, Vāmadeva cooked the entrails of a dog in order to feed himself. It is said that Indra appeared before him as a sparrowhawk and gave him honey, which symbolises rain and food. When we abandon our references of what is considered acceptable or not acceptable, we are left with the entrails of each situation, which resonates with unfragmented energy.

"He is God (deva) because He plays without concern for what is to be sought and what is to be rejected."
Abhinavagupta, Tantrāloka I, 101

• Kandāsana: The White Gown of the Goddess

"Soft in texture and white in colour, it is described as having the form of an enveloping cloth."
Haṭhayogapradīpikā III, 113

The bulbous root, the source from which the seventy-two thousand nāḍī unfold, is the navel of exteriorisation of the body and world as objects of experience. This exteriorisation corresponds to the sleeping of the kuṇḍalinī śakti that is said to sleep above the bulb. According to the Yoginīhṛdaya, the sacred places of pilgrimage (pīṭha) are found in the bulb. These pīṭha are the various constellations of energetic mapping expressed in cakra and in the subtle and gross bodies. Kanda also represents the inclusive sphere (saṃpuṭa) of Śiva and Śakti.

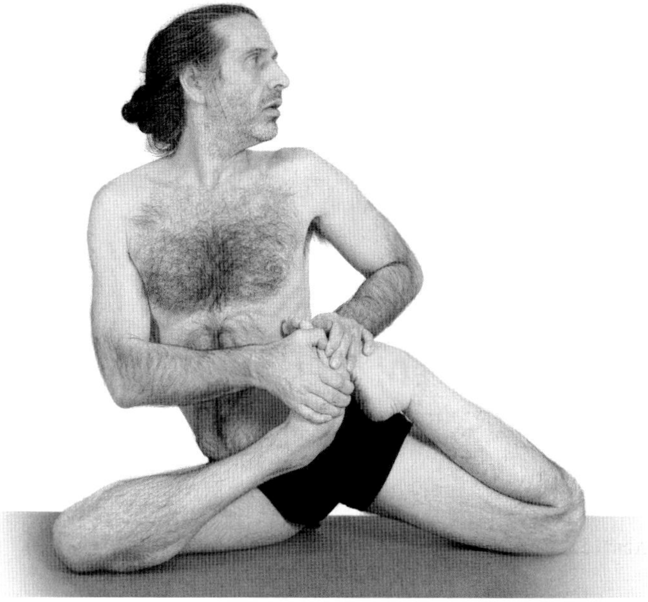

Vāmadevāsana 2

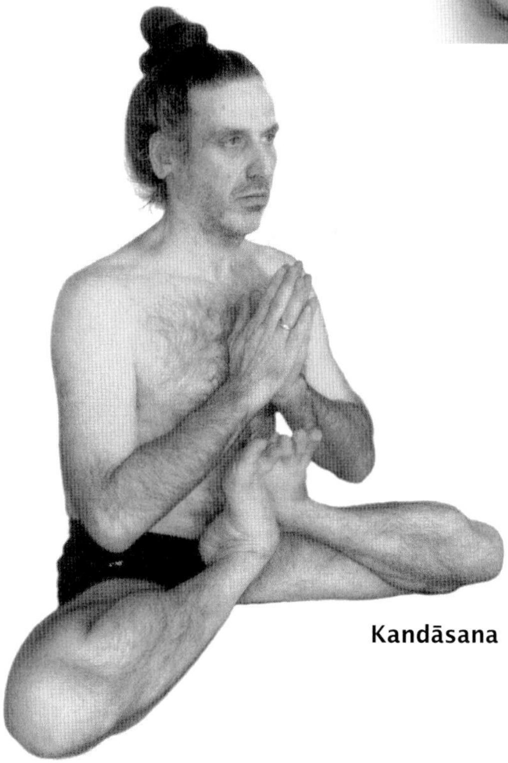

Kandāsana

"While making assertions like 'I am, this is mine', etc. the mind goes to that which is supportless. Inspired by this meditation one becomes peaceful."

Vijñāna Bhairava 131

• Yoga Daṇḍāsana 1 & 2, Adho Mukha Yoga Daṇḍāsana: The Armpit of the Real

In the Vijñāna Bhairava, it is said that by *"fixing the mind on the void under the armpits, it will merge in that void and attain peace."* (79)

Śiva is sometimes represented seated with a staff (daṇḍa) supporting his armpit.
The head rests on the hand and activities are able to nap.
The breathing naturally alternates between the right and left nostrils during the day.
But one nostril may become blocked thus preventing the breath from alternating regularly.
A staff was used to regulate the uneven flow of breath and to unblock the nostril.

The armpits are an important place of contemplation in āsana.
The opening of the armpits participates in pacifying the frontal brain and temporal regions.

Symbolically, in yoga, daṇḍa phenomenally represents the spine,
but also the vertical energy (udāna) that burns subject-object differentiation.

Yoga Daṇḍāsana 1

Yoga Daṇḍāsana 2

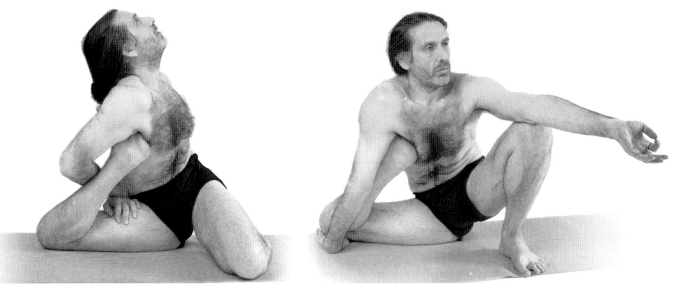

"All association with pleasure and pain occurs through the senses. Therefore detach yourself from the senses and abide within your own Self."

Vijñāna Bhairava 136

"Knowledge illumines everything in this world; and the Self is the one who illumines. Since they have the same nature, knowledge and the known should be contemplated as one."

Vijñāna Bhairava 137

ड

Ḍa

motion:
foot (pāda)

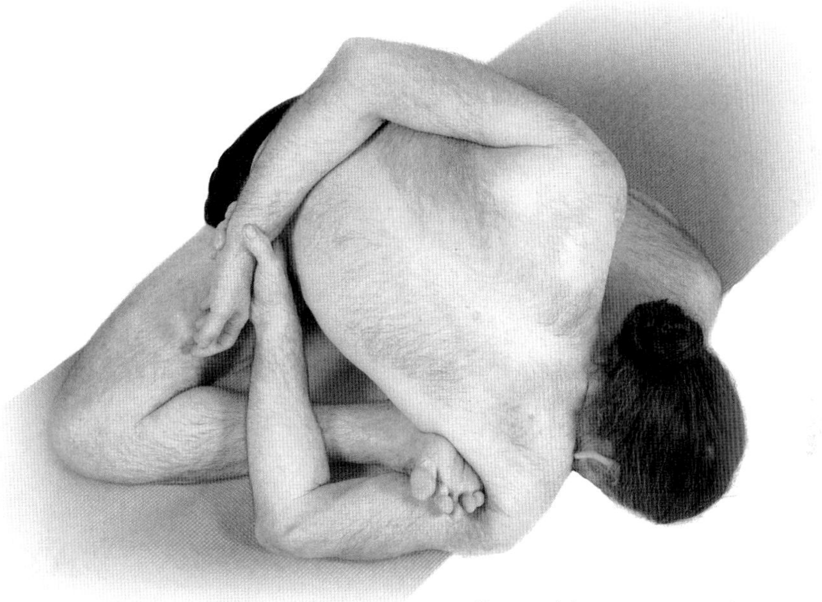

Adho Mukha Yoga Daṇḍāsana

Contemplating the Great Cremation

One should meditate on one's own fortress as if it were consumed by the Fire of Time, rising from the foot. At the end of this meditation the peaceful state will appear."

VIJÑĀNA BHAIRAVA 52

• Supta Vīrāsana: On the Silence of the Confluence

The action of lying down (supta) takes us back to the unobstructed spreading of the vital upsurge. Supta describes the mudrā of Ananta, the infinite, or Ādiśeṣa, the cosmic serpent that lies down, thus becoming the web and support of the world. In the far reaches of Pātāla is the last of the seven infernal regions, which are the backstage of the earth. In this land of darkness, inhabited by the nāga, bordering on nothingness, can be found the couch in which Viṣṇu falls asleep when the dissolution of the worlds takes place. This couch supports and wears creation like a crown. The gandharva, nāga and even the deva are unable to fully understand it. This is why it is referred to as Ananta (the infinite). The sage Garga obtained the secrets and mastery of astronomy by worshiping it.

Āsana are merely contemplation and worship of the embodiment's different constellations, and of the infinite in which they appear. In Supta Vīrāsana we can plunge into the depths of the abdominal cavity and make contact with the tides that support its physiology, in particular apānavāyu.

Lying Down in the Infinite:
Supine Āsana

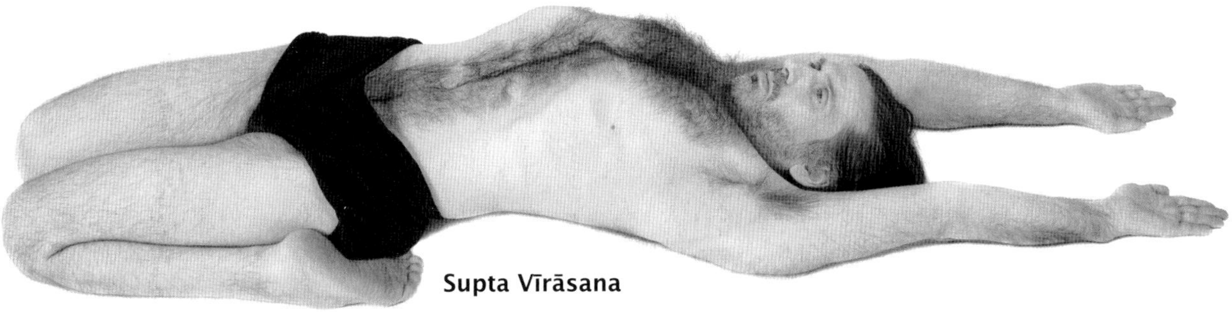

Supta Vīrāsana

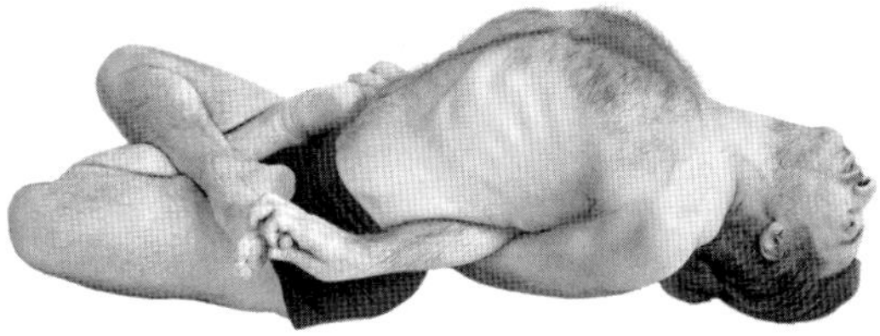

• Supta Vajrāsana: The Bones of Adamantine Reality

The sage Dadhīci took responsibility for the weapons entrusted to him by the gods. Although they assured him that they would return quickly, a thousand years had already passed. To keep the weapons from the envy and hate of the asura, Dadhīci absorbed them into his body. When the gods returned, not seeing the weapons, they demanded the sage return them immediately. He returned them in the form of his bones, thus causing his death. It is said that all weapons were created from his bones, including Indra's thunderbolt. We are entrusted with a natural brilliance, which, through its sharpness, can be considered as a weapon cutting into the flesh of our fears. At the heart of childhood flitting, the vision of reality perspires this brilliance, which one day disappears into the background, behind the waves of bodily chemistry. When the gods come to claim this brilliance, we will only be able to offer them the bones of our ordinariness, and we won't have any choice. At the end of our spatiotemporal contraction, only the spontaneous flash of primordial astonishment, often compared to a thunderbolt or diamond (vajra), will remain.

Supine variations of Padmāsana, and of course Supta Vajrāsana, are preparations for the different stages of Vajrolī (coming from vajra) Mudrā.

The deep organic suction and prāṇic churning in the pelvic and abdominal cavities cause the currents that maintain the coagulative descent of energy (apānavāyu) to be drawn-up beyond the modalities of inhalation and exhalation, of life and death.

"Meditating in this way by imagining
that the entire world has been burnt,
a person whose mind is undisturbed
will attain the highest human condition."

VIJÑĀNA BHAIRAVA 53

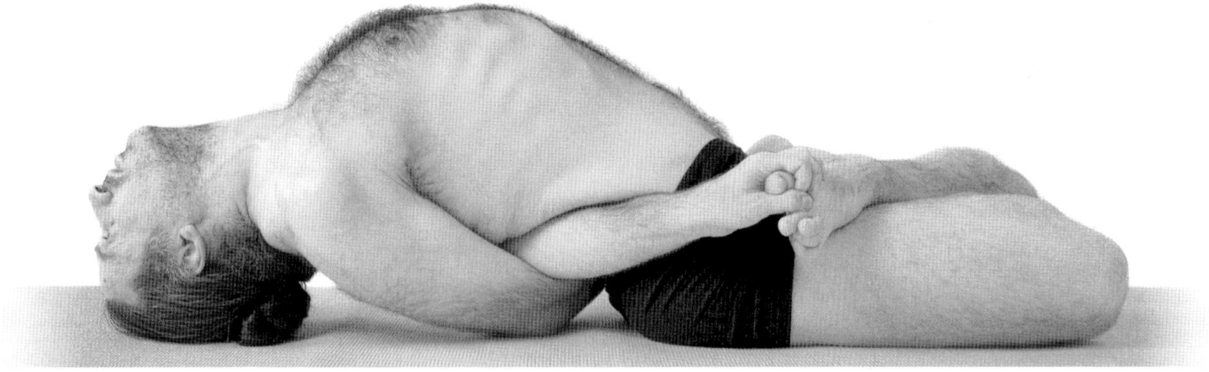

Supta Vajrāsana

Contemplating the In-Betweens

"Meditating on the knowledge of two things or states, one should rest in the middle. By abandoning both simultaneously, the Reality shines forth in the centre." VIJÑĀNA BHAIRAVA 61

• Bhujapīḍāsana, Tittibhāsana: Chrysalis and Flying Off

Āsana are archetypal energies that enable us to explore certain organisms, whether mineral, vegetal, animal, divine, cosmic, etc. The breath precedes the structure, which is organised according to a certain breathing pattern, a certain ambiance. In these āsana, the shape of the chrysalis and its associated breathing pattern, as well as the unfolding of the insect (tittibha) from its cocoon, can be intuited.

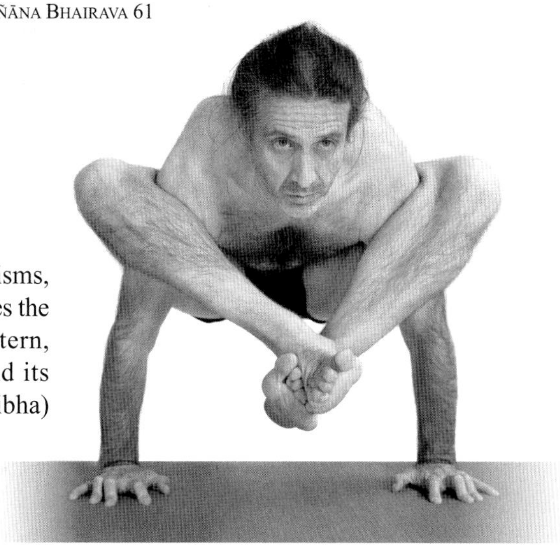

Bhujapīḍāsana

• Aṣṭāvakrāsana: The Laughter of the Cripple

A legend tells that Kahoda recited the Veda to his wife whilst she was carrying their child. It is said that the baby, whilst still in the womb of his mother, said to his father: *"It is thanks to you that I have learnt the Veda, but it is such a shame you distorted them by your poor pronunciation."* Cut to the quick, Kahoda cursed his son promising him that he would be born deformed in eight places. This is precisely what happened and the reason he was named Aṣṭāvakra. Years later, Aṣṭāvakra went to the king's palace to participate in a debate to which the greatest scholars had been invited. He had difficulty entering because the guards thought he was a beggar.

He challenged Bandi, the scholar of Mithila's court, who had conquered and humiliated his father: *"Take the lead from my verse and I will do the same from yours."* Bandi was unable to finish the thirteenth verse. *"It is said that the thirteenth day of the moon is ill-fated, thirteen is the number of continents on this earth..."* At this point Bandi stopped and Aṣṭāvakra completed the verse: *"For thirteen days the hirsute one hurried, thirteen syllables or more for the longer ones."* Aṣṭāvakra's laugh was like the sun that filled King Janaka's court with its rays and burned away the hypocrisy of the paṇḍita who had smirked upon seeing him. He said to the king that this farce made him laugh and he wondered how the king could hope to find the truth in the company of these charlatans: *"They cannot see beyond appearances and cannot feel the presence behind the body's clothes. If a pot is broken, does this affect the space inside the pot? If a pot has a flaw, does this deform the space inside it? Whatever you perceive, it is merely your own reflection. Does jewellery such as bracelets, necklaces and rings exist as something other than gold?"* AṢṬĀVAKRA GĪTĀ 139

The Absence of Gravities: Balancing Āsana

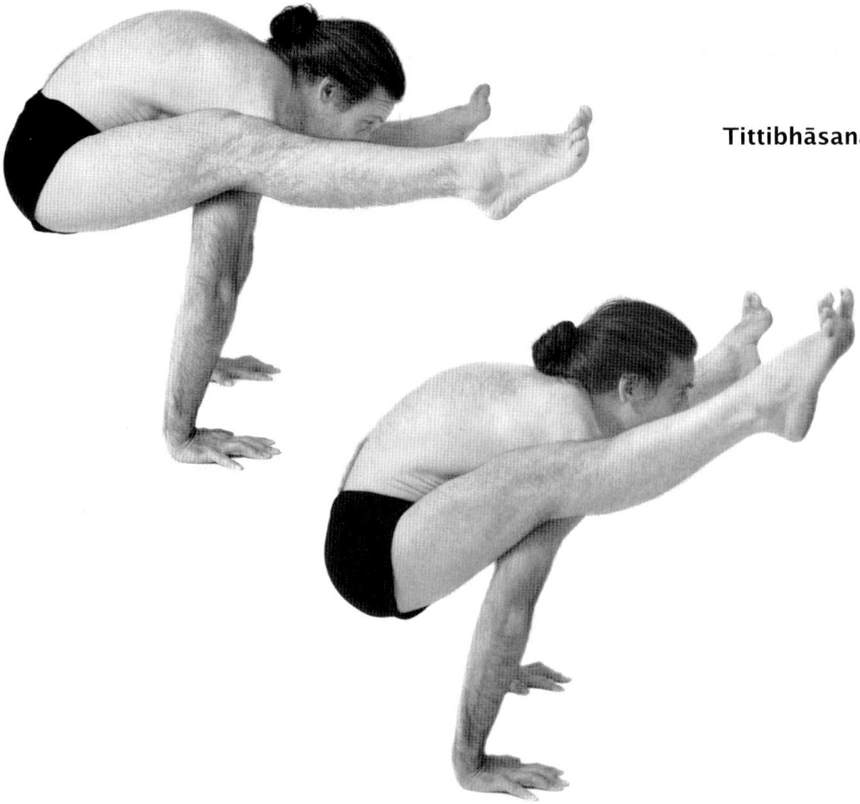

Tittibhāsana

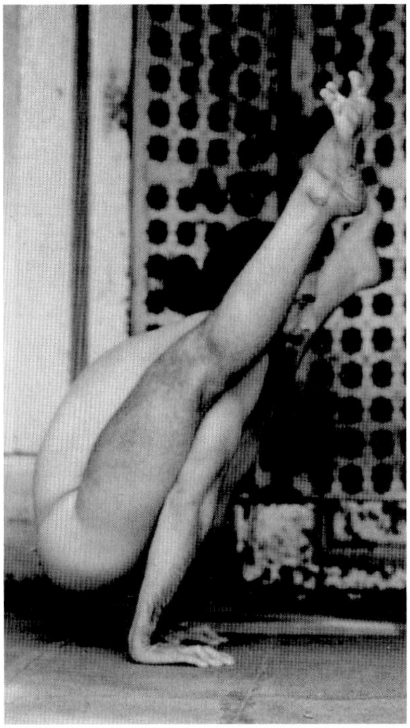

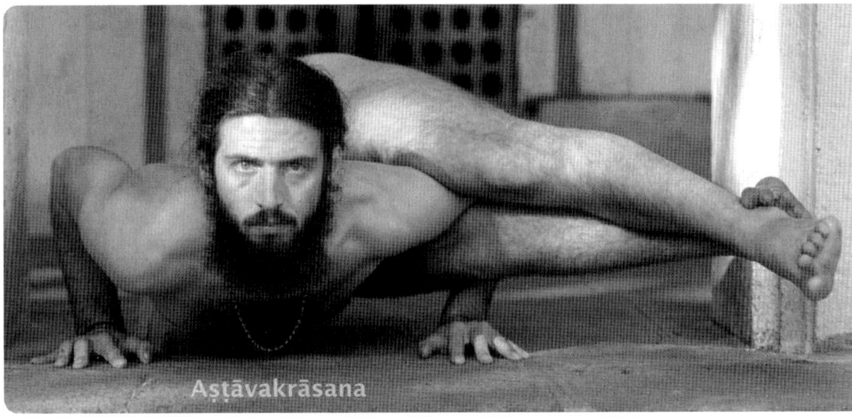

Aṣṭāvakrāsana

"One's mind should neither be engrossed in suffering nor in pleasure. O Bhairavī, you should know the middle state, then the Reality alone remains."

VIJÑĀNA BHAIRAVA 103

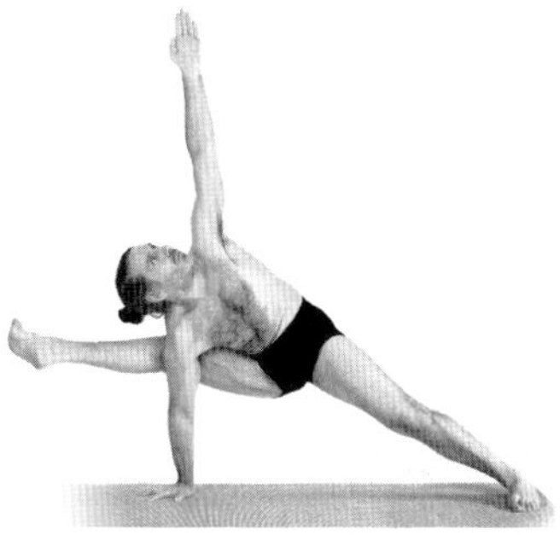

Viśvāmitrāsana ...

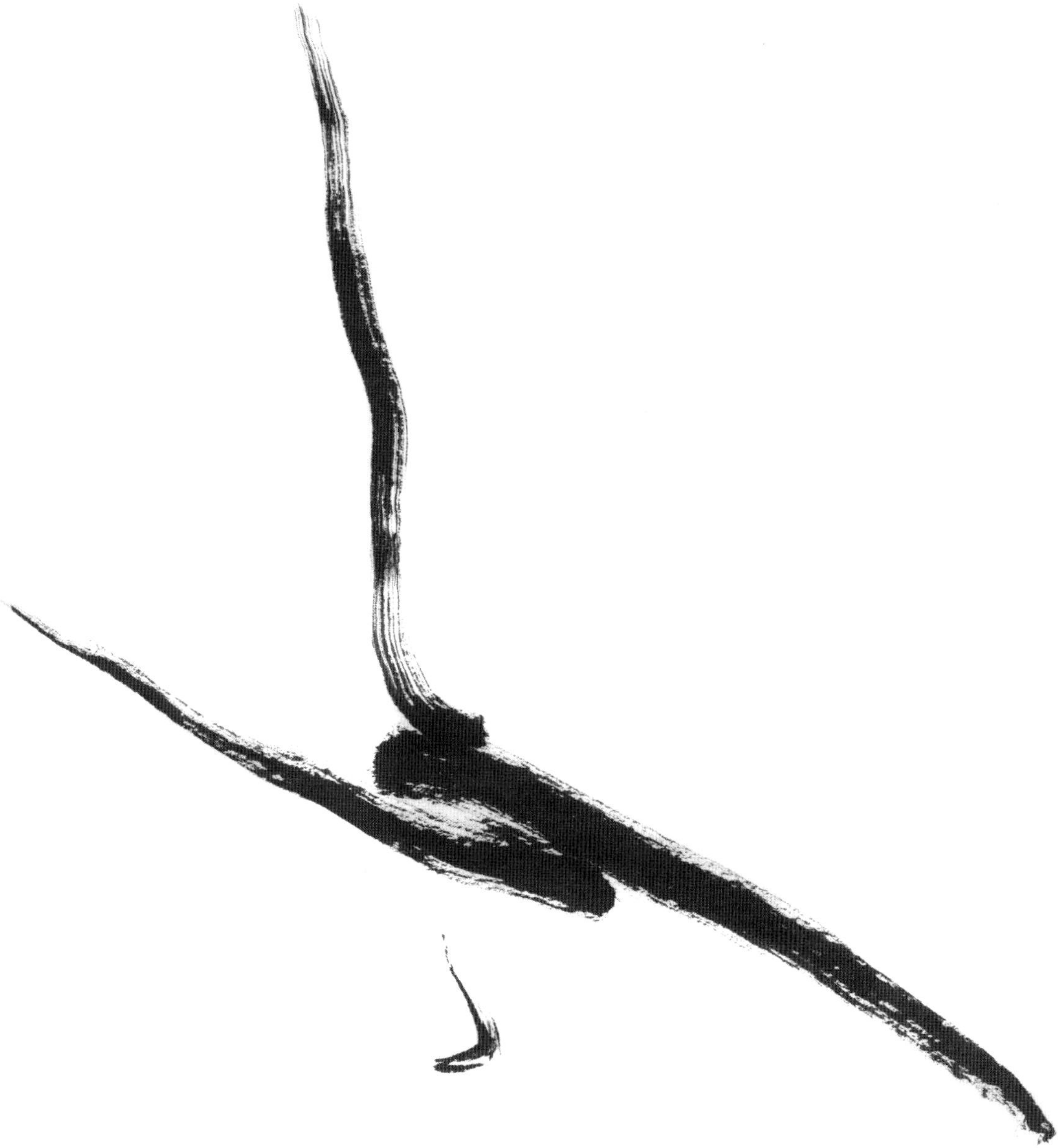

• Vasiṣṭhāsana, Kaśyapāsana, Viśvāmitrāsana: The Heavenly Lords

All three form part of the seven ṛṣi (saptaṛṣi), who are the seven stars of the Great Bear. The quarrels between Vasiṣṭha and Viśvāmitra are well known. Their long animosity started when Viśvāmitra wanted to forcefully take the cow Kāmadhenu, who granted all boons. It was after losing this battle that Viśvāmitra, ashamed of himself, relinquished his kingdom and became a hermit. Viśvāmitra was not a brāhmaṇa, but a king and a warrior. It was only after long austerities that he obtained the title of Brahmaṛṣi, a brāhmaṇa sage, but he was only satisfied when it was Vasiṣṭha who honoured him with the title of Brahmaṛṣi.

It was Vasiṣṭha who gave the meaning of his name: *"I am known as Vasiṣṭha because I am Vasumān. The Śruti says that Earth, Air, etc. are Vasu. The elements (vasu) are under my control and I have the power to reduce the body to an atom (anima)."*

The postural form of Kaśyapa, Lord of Creators (Prajāpati), when placed between the other two āsana, seems to regulate, or rather link the quiet strength of Vasiṣṭha and the warrior spirit of Viśvāmitra, who are no longer in conflict.

But let Vasiṣṭha and Viśvāmitra confront each other! Even the great sages are merely puppets in the vast and incomprehensible play of Consciousness.

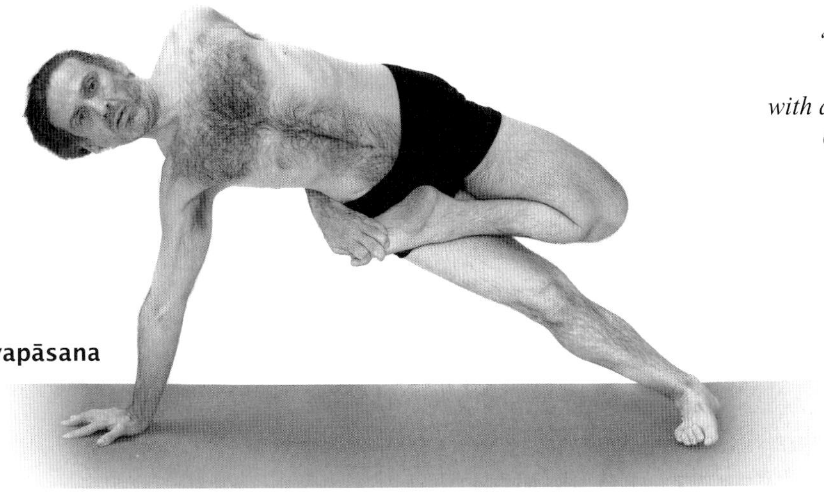

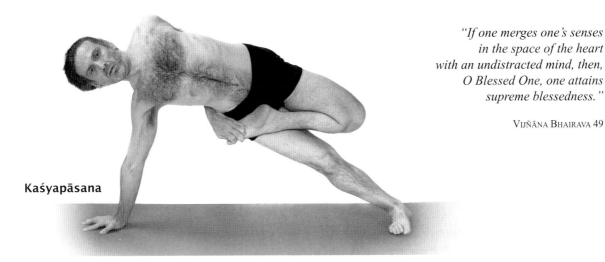

Kaśyapāsana

"If one merges one's senses
in the space of the heart
with an undistracted mind, then,
O Blessed One, one attains
supreme blessedness."

VIJÑĀNA BHAIRAVA 49

Ḍha

grasping: hand (pāṇi)

ढ

"After the sweet intoxicating nectar of bliss has made the heart quiver, the yogi longs for the acid flavour of worldly fury."

MAHEŚVARĀNANDA, MAHĀRTHAMAÑJARĪ 62

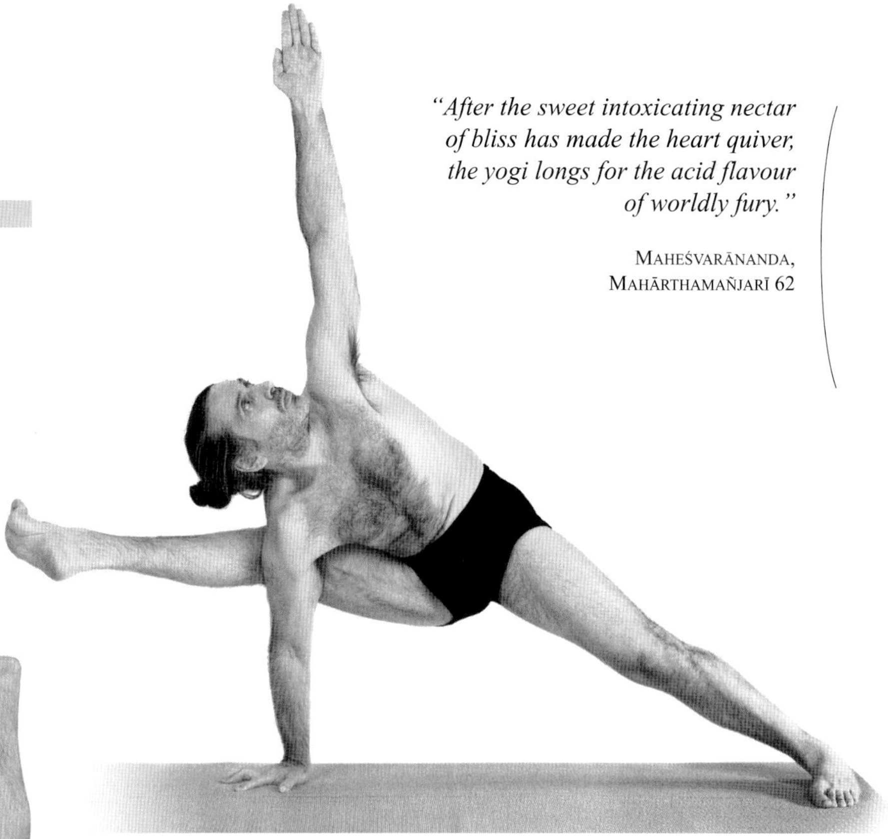

Viśvāmitrāsana

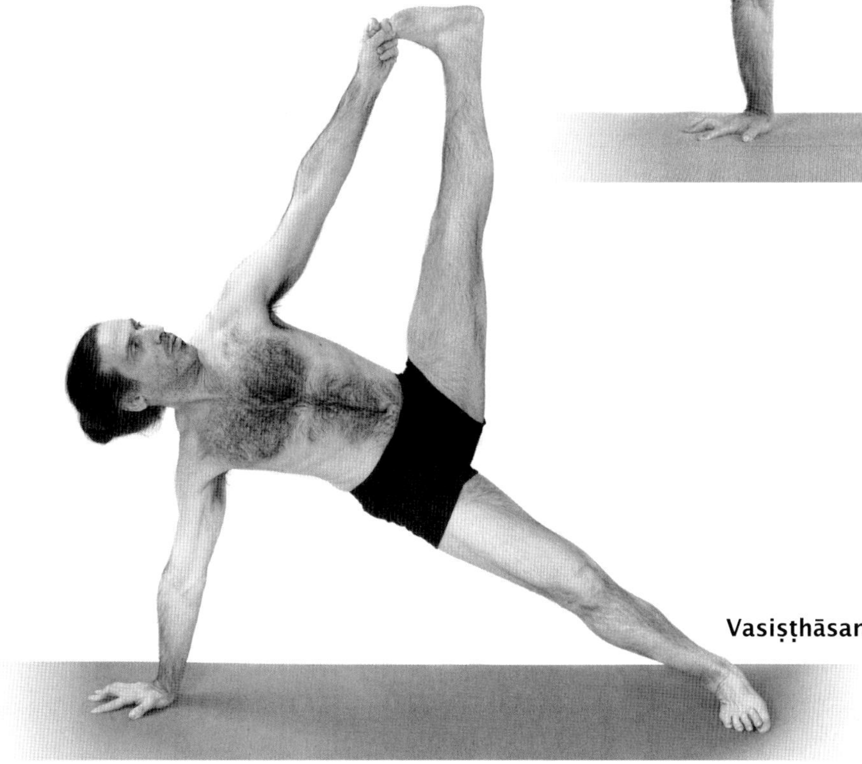

Vasiṣṭhāsana

• Bakāsana, Pārśva Bakāsana: The Crane's Questioning

In their exile, the Pāṇḍava tasted the kiss of death when, through thirst, they refused to reply to a genie's questions and they drank enchanted water from a lake.

The genie appeared before Yudhiṣṭhira as a crane. The great wader scrutinised Yudhiṣṭhira and after preening its long feathers said:
"Your brothers are under my power, I have sent them to the land of the dead. He who wishes to drink from this lake must first answer my questions. Answer or else drink and die."

"Ask your questions, I will answer them as best I can."

The last two of the thirteen questions asked were:
"What is the most wonderful thing in life? What is the way?"

"Day after day thousands of people die, yet we act as though we will live forever. That is what is most wonderful. The argument is futile. The scriptures differ. No sage possesses the whole Truth. The truths of Dharma are hidden from our eyes. Ignorance reigns over this world. What good men embrace in their daily life, that is the way!"

"Magnificently answered. Choose one of your brothers so he may live again."

"The dark-skinned Nakula."

"It is said that you dearly love Bhīma and Arjuna. Why do you prefer to save Nakula?"

"My father had two wives, Kuntī and Mādrī. Mādrī is as dear to me as Kuntī, my own mother. Nakula is Mādrī's son, let him live."

"Since you speak with such nobleness, all your brothers will live again. I am Dharma, your father."

"Just as you are about to go to sleep,
at the verge of wakefulness,
when the world has faded away
but sleep has not yet come,
there the supreme Goddess shines."

VIJÑĀNA BHAIRAVA 75

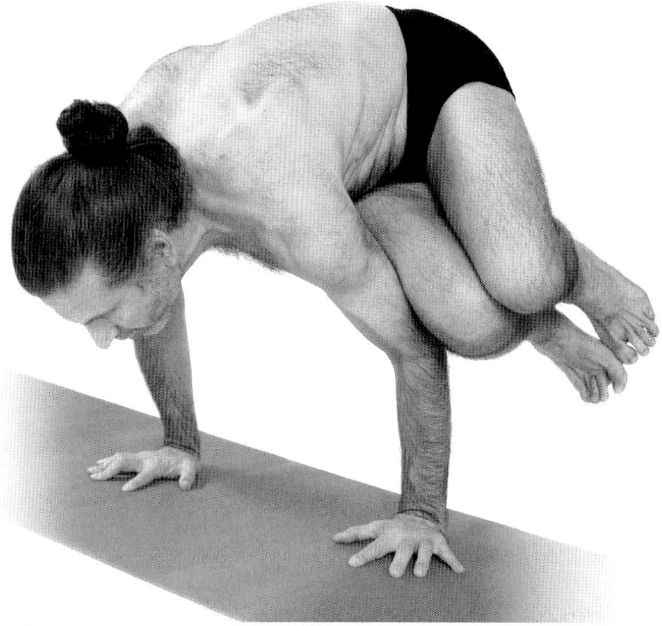

Pārśva Bakāsana

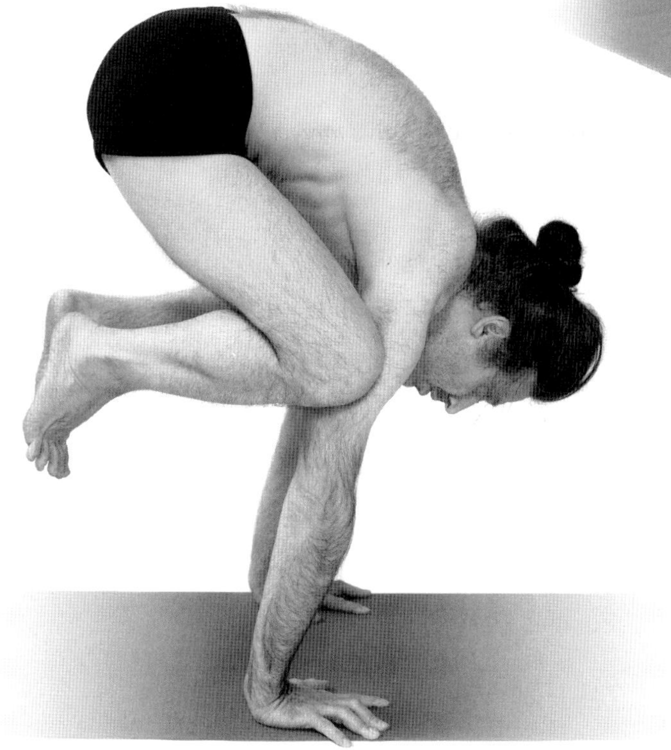

Bakāsana

Contemplating the Quiver at the Source of Situations

At the beginning and end of sneezing, in a state of fear or sorrow,
standing on top of an abyss or while fleeing from a battlefield,
at the moment of intense curiosity, at the beginning or end of hunger;
the illusion of separation ceases."
VIJÑĀNA BHAIRAVA 118

• Eka Pāda Kouṇḍinyāsana 1 & 2, Eka Pāda Gālavāsana: The Dance of the Legs

Kauṇḍinya, also known as Viṣṇu Gupta, or he who was saved from Śiva's anger by Viṣṇu, belongs to Vasiṣṭha's family and was a grammarian. Gālava was the son of Viśvāmitra. This is the story that is told about the origins of his name.

A terrible drought that had lasted for twelve years plunged the country into famine. Viśvāmitra had left his family to go and settle on the banks of the river Kauśikī where he could carry out his austerities. His wife, no longer able to support the crying of her starving children, decided to sell one of her sons at the market. She told herself: *"It is better to lose one child so the others may live."* She made a rope from darbha leaves and fixed it around the boy's neck (gāla) to take him to the market. Her tears and the boy's heartrending sobs caught the attention of a stranger by the name of Satyavrata. After having listened to her story, he consoled her and said that he would take care of her family until Viśvāmitra returned. She joyfully threw away the rope without further ado. From that day on, the boy was called Gālava.

All mythologies are acted out and reinvented not only in the body itself, but also in the body of situations. Who is able to say what makes wisdom blossom? Are there situations more favourable than others? Are not all situations the opportunity to return to the essential, like the sage Kauṇḍinya who offended Śiva or the sage Gālava who was to be sold at the market?

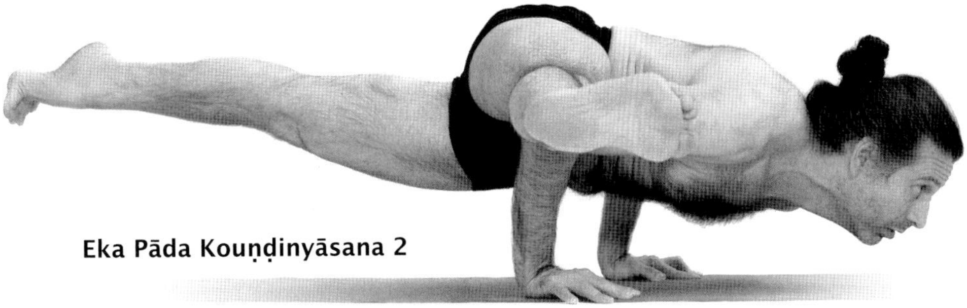

Eka Pāda Kouṇḍinyāsana 2

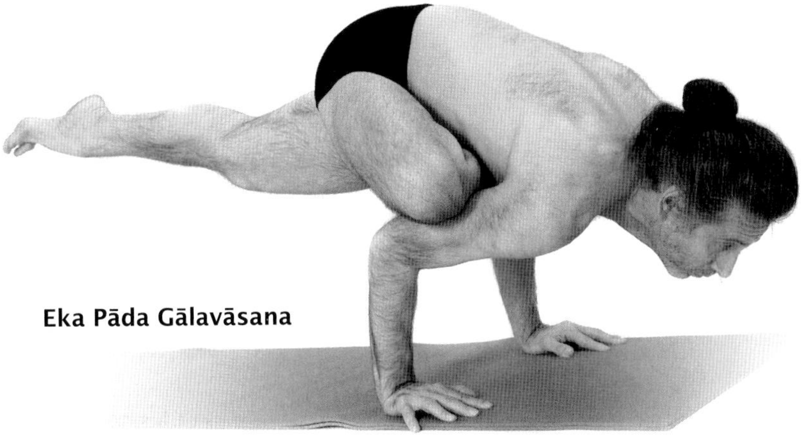

Eka Pāda Gālavāsana

ण

Ṇa
speech (vāk)

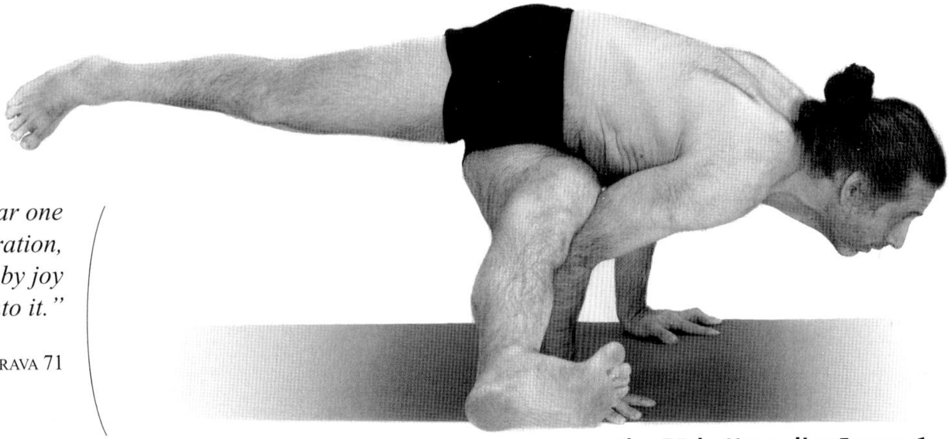

"When reunited with a dear one
after a long separation,
let yourself be overwhelmed by joy
and be absorbed into it."

VIJÑĀNA BHAIRAVA 71

Eka Pāda Kouṇḍinyāsana 1

Contemplating the Dissolution

• Ūrdhva Kukkuṭāsana, Gālavāsana, Pārśva Ūrdhva Kukkuṭāsana: The Cock's Crow

Nāgasena, the Buddhist sage, described to King Milinda the five attitudes of the cock that the practitioner must observe. The first is to go to bed early and completely abandon the day's activities. The second is to rise early and prepare one's living space for meditation. Being attentive to the emergence of the body and its functions and to the emergence of the world when coming out of deep sleep is the symbolic preparation of this space.
In the same way the cock continuously scratches away at the ground to find its food, the practitioner must continually scratch away at his activities whilst bearing in mind the question: 'who am I?' This is the third attitude.
In the same way the cock has eyes but cannot see at night, the practitioner lets the inclusivity of Consciousness envelop the world and becomes blind to differentiation. This is the fourth attitude.
In the same way the cock, albeit persecuted, does not leave its abode, the practitioner, whatever the situation, remains attentive to his own Presence. This is the fifth attitude.
The cock also represents desire and greed, agitation and perpetual projections from the past and into the future. Yet at the heart of desire, once it has been satisfied, the realisation of tranquillity shines forth. There is nowhere to go; everything is already perfect. It is the desire itself that enables us to go beyond (ūrdhva) it, to burn it away.

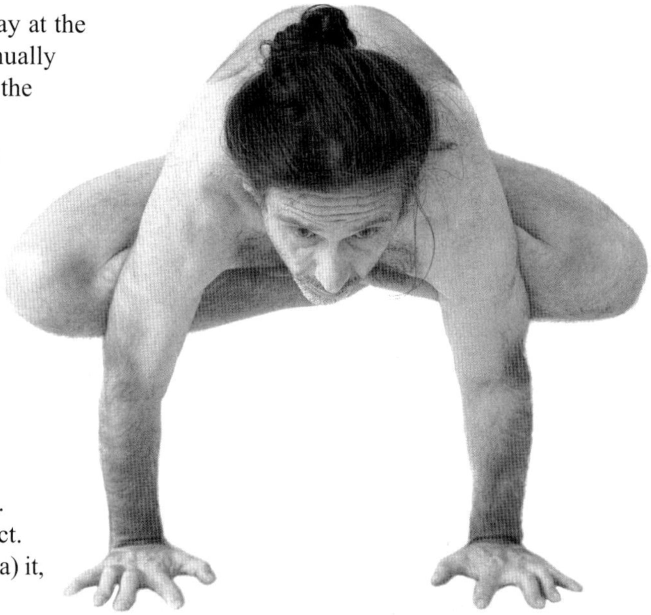

Ūrdhva Kukkuṭāsana

of the Universe

"If one meditates on the subtle and subtlest elements in one's own body or of the world as if they are merging one after another, then in the end the Supreme Goddess is revealed."

VIJÑĀNA BHAIRAVA 54

"Contemplate the universe and its constituent worlds dissolving into ever more subtle forms, until the mind merges with Consciousness."

VIJÑĀNA BHAIRAVA 56

THE DENTALS, FROM TA TO NA, ARE CONNECTED (LIKE THE CEREBRALS) TO THE ENERGY OF WILL (ICCHĀŚAKTI) WHICH ABIDES IN ITSELF, BUT WHICH IS CONNECTED TO STILLNESS, AND THIS BRINGS ABOUT THE PHONEME Ḷ.

त

Ta
organ of smelling: nose (ghrāṇa)

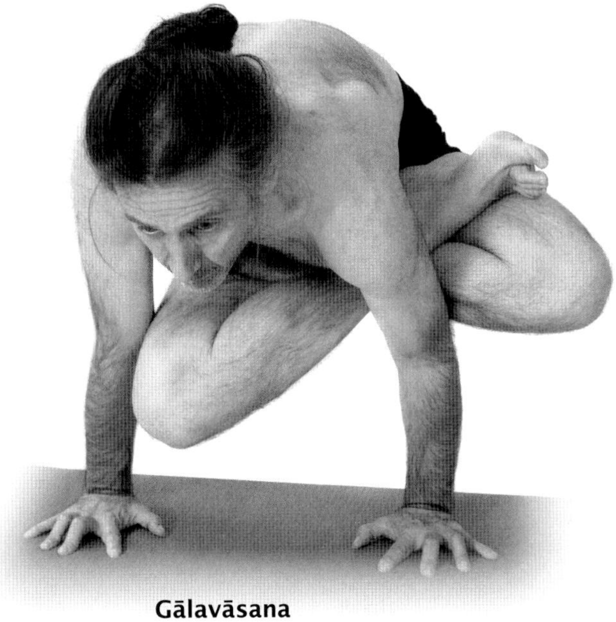

Gālavāsana

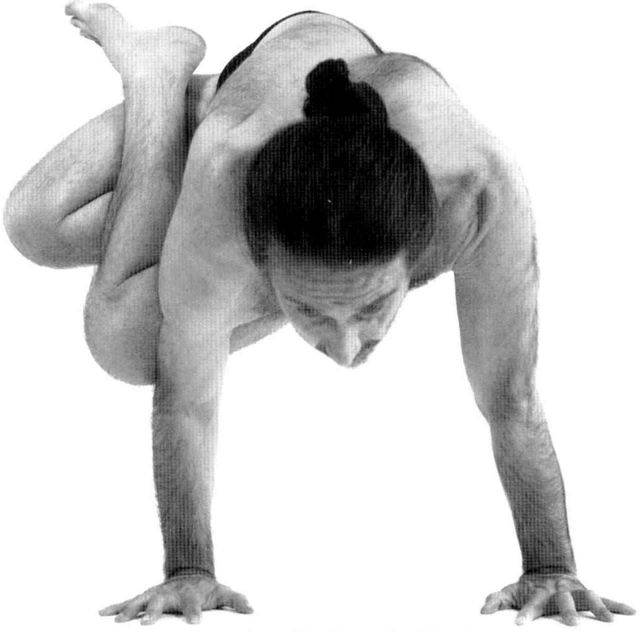

Pārśva Ūrdhva Kukkuṭāsana

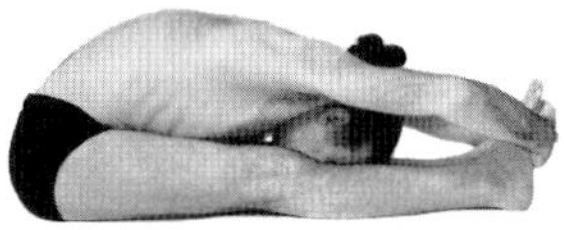

Paścimottānāsana ...

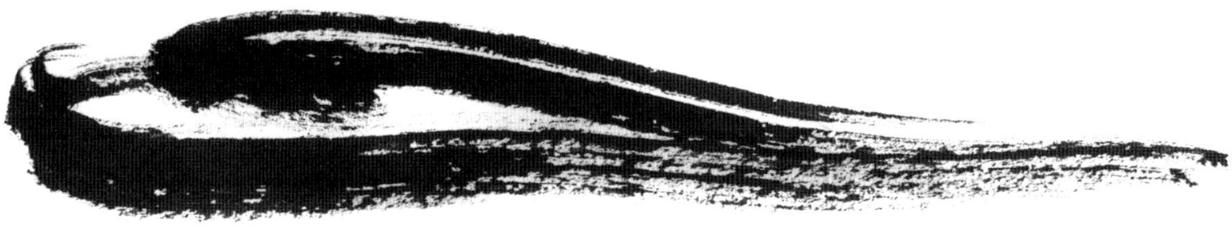

"O Great Goddess! Contemplate the vacuity of this entire universe.
Let the last traces of the mind die away,
and be the container of this space."

VIJÑĀNA BHAIRAVA 58

"Contemplate both your body and the universe
as being woven by the same web of Consciousness.
There is no separation, just the never-ending
awakening of Consciousness."

VIJÑĀNA BHAIRAVA 63

Ūrdhva Mukha Paścimottānāsana

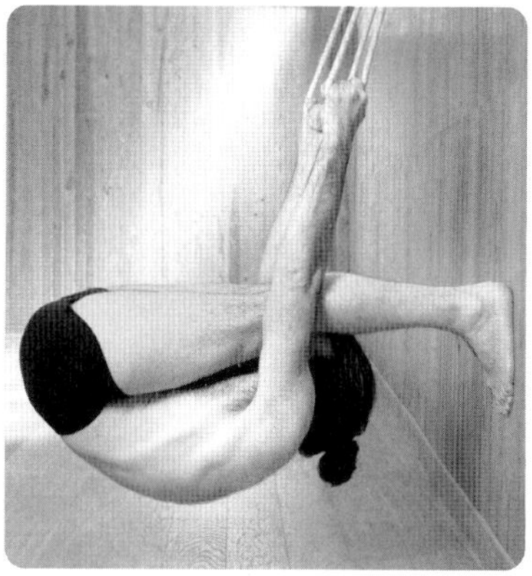

• Paścimottānāsana: The Western Transmission (Paścimāmnāya)

Kubjikā, the hunchbacked goddess, gives her breath to this vision that is intimately associated with the 'Mountain of the Moon', and hence its savour of interiorisation. Perhaps it was the goddess who whispered the three names of this āsana to the yogi? The spreading of the west (Paścimottānāsana), the terrible (Ugrāsana) and living in Brahman (Brahmacaryāsana).

These names refer to the different approaches and moods of the āsana. Paścimottānāsana explores the spreading of the rear side, the extension of the back and the flow of prāṇa by the posterior path (paścimavāyumārga). It unfolds the energy of activity (kriyāśakti). In resonance to this, Ugrāsana unfolds the anterior side of the trunk and the pelvic, abdominal and thoracic cavities. It unfolds the energy of knowledge (jñānaśakti). Brahmacaryāsana explores the root of the spine and its prāṇic extension (mūlabandha). It is linked to the energy of will (icchāśakti).

The Breath of Night: Forward Extension Āsana

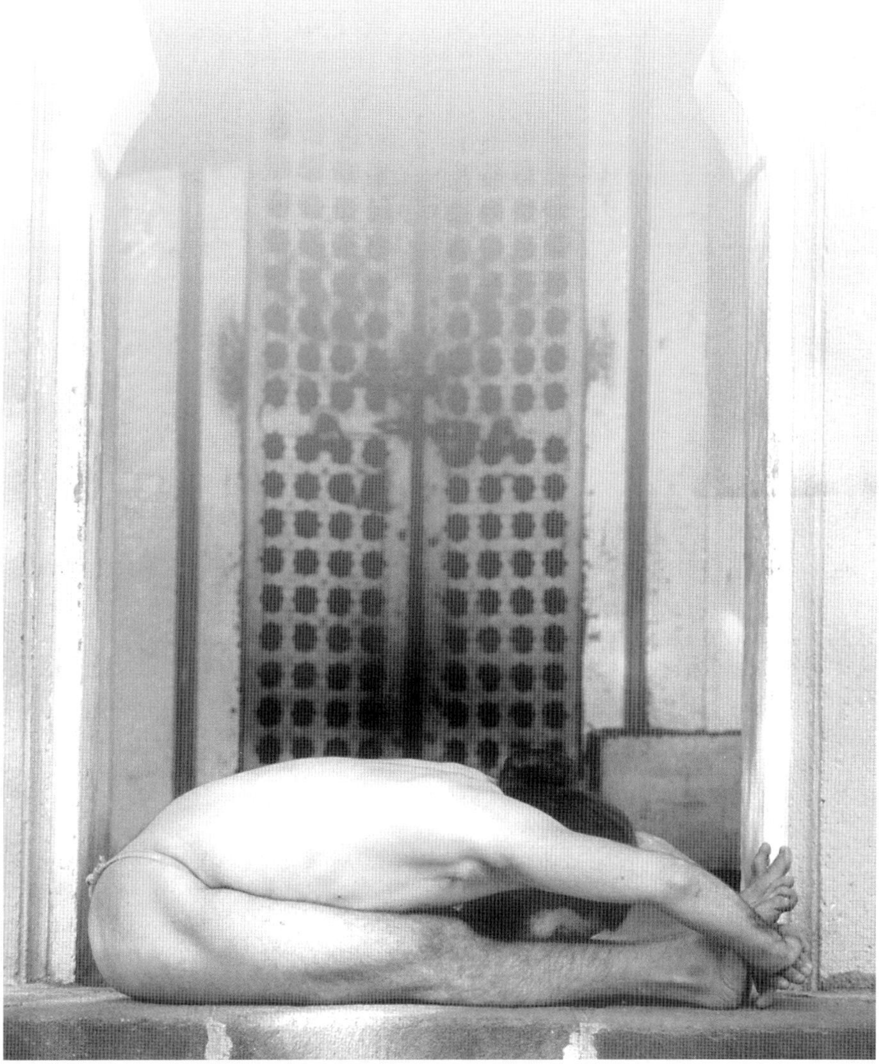

Paścimottānāsana

Contemplating Spontaneous Spatiality

"The yogi should contemplate simultaneously on the whole world or his own body as filled with the bliss of the self, then by his own blissful nectar he becomes united with the supreme bliss." Vijñāna Bhairava 65

"One should meditate one one's own Self in the form of the vast sky, unlimited in all directions, then the Power of Consciousness is free from any support and reveals her own nature." Vijñāna Bhairava 92

• Jānu Śīrṣāsana: The Head of the Knee or The Crowning

In forward extensions, abandoning the head towards the knee and beyond symbolises surrender and capitulation of all strategies. Frontal brain perception dies away and makes way for the humility of the earth. One is crowned by one's own vacuity. The knee of the bent leg unfolds concentric circles, like those around the knees of the glorified Christ in Christian iconography. In Yoga, the head is found at the source of sensation, which is in itself spaciousness.

• Parivṛtta Jānu Śīrṣāsana: On Returning to the Self

Here, the intensified rotation of the head of the knee unfolds the āsana. The back of the head is abandoned towards the knee. The face is swallowed up by the space of the posterior skull. Circumambulation is carried out from a centre. One can only turn around oneself.

Jānu Śīrṣāsana

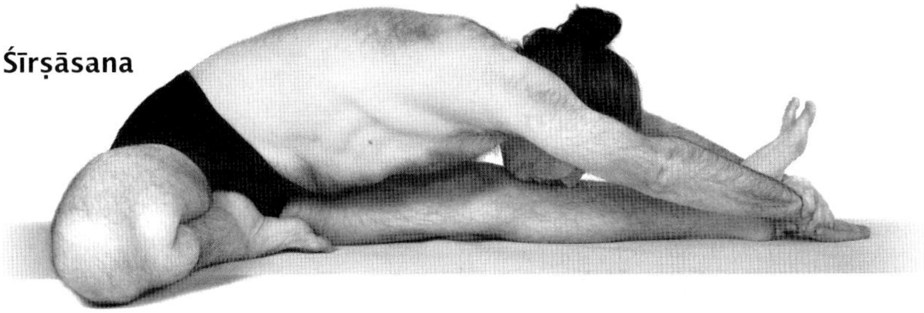

Jānu Śīrṣāsana in Mūla Bandhāsana

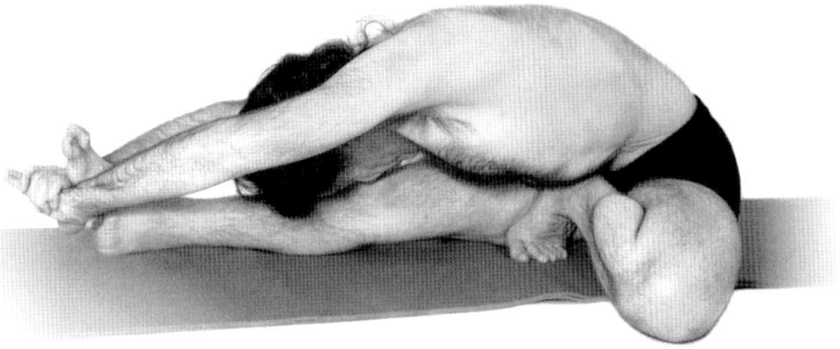

थ

Tha

organ of tasting: tongue (rasanā)

Jānu Śīrṣāsana in Yoga Daṇḍāsana

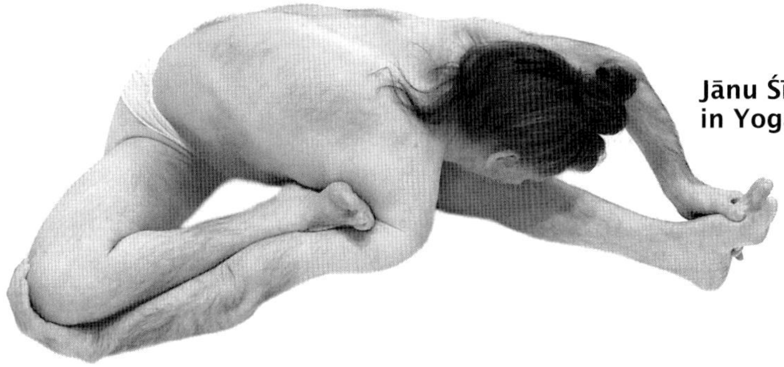

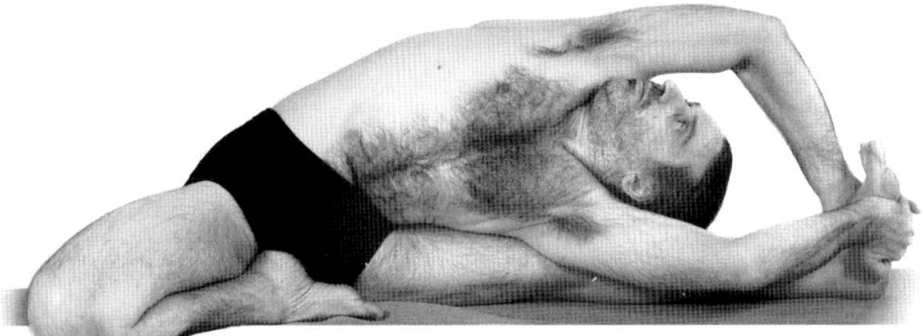

Parivṛtta Jānu Śīrṣāsana

• Ardha Baddha Padma Paścimottānāsana: Intensifying the Spreading of the West

The position of the foot in Padmāsana allows the thighbones to descend. The descent of the root of the thighs causes the lower back to spread. The foot in Padmāsana, and its binding, intensify the depth of the abdominal cavity and its cleansing. Here, the apānic and samānic regions are churned. The heel is in contact with the navel, thus facilitating contemplation of this place (ādhāra), the sixth in Gorakṣanātha's classification.

"Contemplation of the vibration as OṂ in this ādhāra leads to the dissolution of sound (nādalaya)."
GORAKṢANĀTHA, SIDDHASIDDHĀNTAPADDHATI II, 15

It is interesting to note the connection between the ādhāra of the navel (nābhyādhāra), the ādhāra of the throat (kaṇṭhādhāra) and the ādhāra of the middle of the eyebrows (bhrūmadhyādhāra). There is often much tension in the abdomen, especially in our societies where a flat tummy is extolled. This dictatorship is imposed much more on women than on men. When the abdomen is tense, the throat, eyes, space between the eyebrows and the face reflect this contraction.

Nābhyādhāra, located at the root of the navel, is also the place of the kandāsana bulb, the root of the nāḍī network.
"It is said that the bulb of the navel in the form of the lotus is the receptacle of all bodily currents (nāḍī)."
GORAKṢANĀTHA, AMARAUGHAŚĀSANA

This ādhāra is the place where praṇava (OṂ) is manifested in its subtle, still unified form.

"One should contemplate the entire sky which is the nature of Bhairava as if it is pervading one's head. Then one experiences everything as the form of Bhairava and one enters into the glory of His nature."

VIJÑĀNA BHAIRAVA 85

द

Da

organ of seeing: eye (cakṣu)

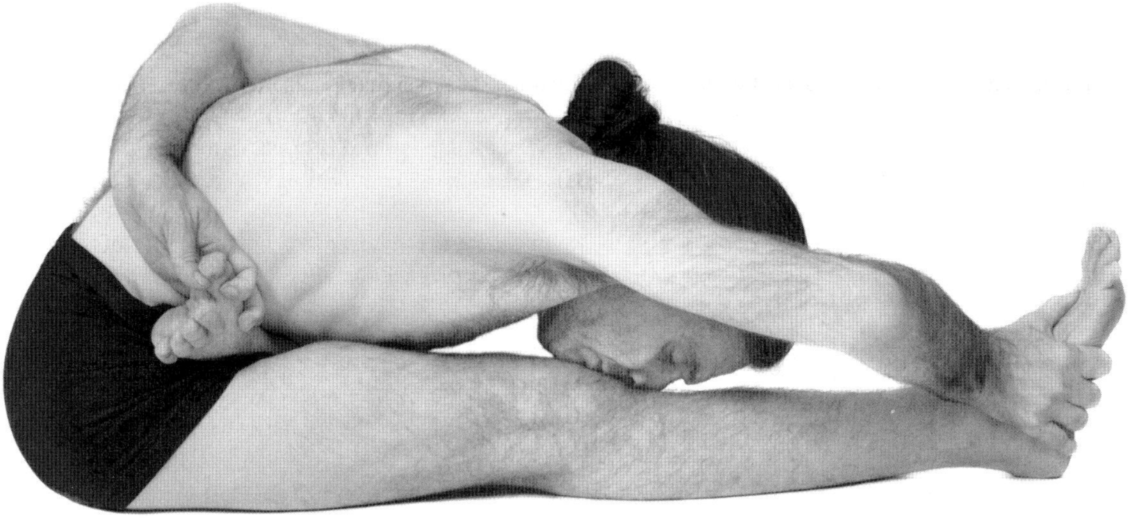

Ardha Baddha Padma Paścimottānāsana

• Krauncāsana: The Precipice

Although the trunk lifts up along the leg, it is the descent of the head of the thighbone into the hip socket and the space subsequently created that is explored, as well as the depth of the groin that opens like a precipice. Above this precipice, positioned high-up, beams the diaphragm, which entices towards it all movements of exteriorisation of the forehead and eyes, and their tendency to pull upwards.

• Marīcyāsana 1 & 2: The Son of the Creator

Marīci, son of the creator (Brahmā), lends his name to this current of poses that unfold both forward extensions and lateral extensions (Marīcyāsana 3, 4). Marīci is one of the sages that parented the world (prajāpati) through various lineages or families (gotra). It is said that Marīci was born from the mind of Brahmā. Correspondingly, the constellations that host these two āsana are the upper abdomen and lower abdomen, which are the organic mind where the alchemy of food assimilation and transmutation takes place.

"After accomplishing samyama on the umbilicus circle, the yogi knows the organisation of the body."
Vyāsa, Yogabhāṣya III, 29

This bodily organisation is expressed in the lineages (gotra) of the three humours (tridoṣa): wind, bile and phlegm; and the seven constituents (saptadhātu): skin, blood, flesh, ligaments, bones, marrow and sperm.

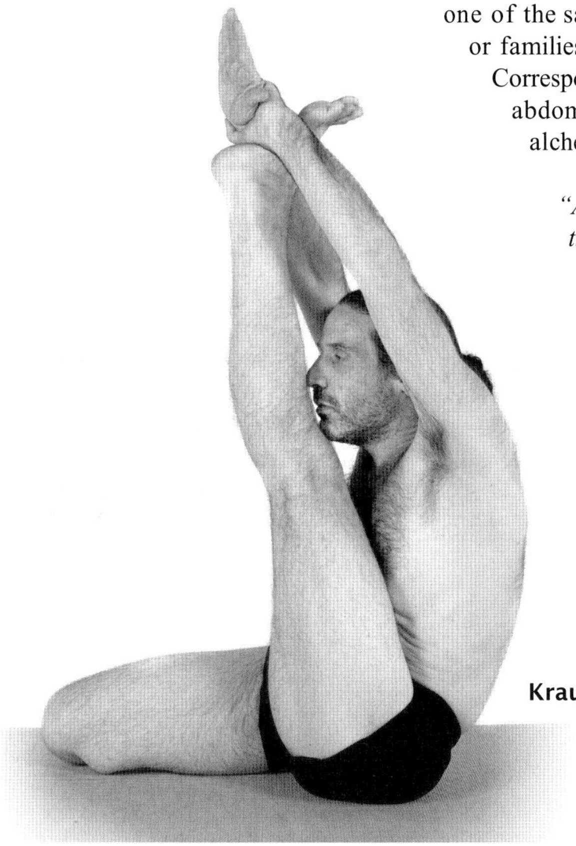

Krauncāsana

"If one contemplates the void of the external space which is eternal, supportless, empty, all-pervading and free from limitation, in this way one will be absorbed in non-space."

Vijñāna Bhairava 128

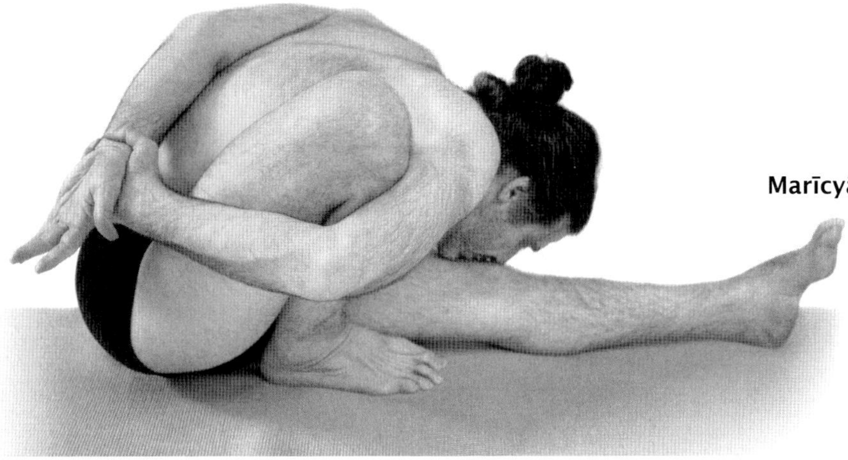

Marīcyāsana 1

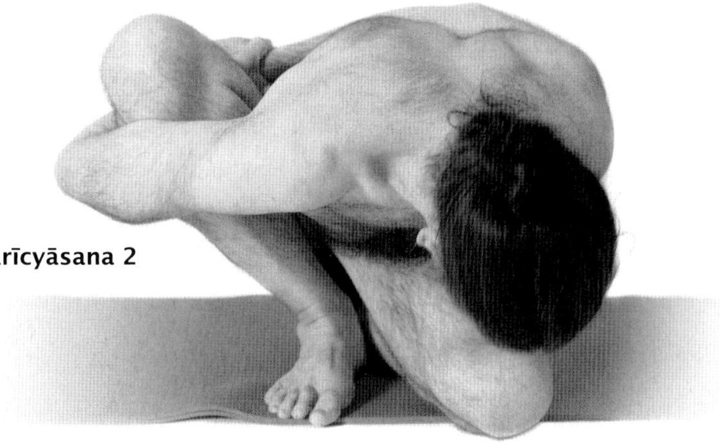

Marīcyāsana 2

Contemplating the Engulfment of the Object

> *Whatever the object of contemplation,*
> *be it an empty space or a wall, it echoes the contemplation itself,*
> *which is absorbed into the spatiality of your own nature."*
> Vijñāna Bhairava 33

• Kūrmāsana: On the Incarnations of Viṣṇu

After being cursed by Durvāsa, the gods were going to lose their immortality and have to get used to wrinkles and grey hair. Mahāviṣṇu advised them to churn the ocean of milk to extract the nectar of immortality from it. They would then be free from this curse. They asked the asura to help them. The mountain Mandara was used as a churning stick and the serpent Vāsuki as a rope. But having no support, the mountain sank into the ocean. Mahāviṣṇu took on the form of a tortoise and dived to the bottom of the ocean to support the mountain, which he lifted higher and higher.

In the maṇḍala of the body, Gorakṣanātha places the tortoise in the sole of the feet (Siddhasiddhāntapaddhati III, 2). The awakening and rooting of the feet in āsana act as a support for the bodily universe and unfold Bhairava's churning (Manthānabhairava).

The descent (avatāra) is merely the recognition of the presence of Consciousness as a background. Without this background, activities would not be possible. The ocean of milk is perpetually churned at the heart of our activities, whether pleasurable (deva) or painful (asura), by inhalation or exhalation (rope), thus putting the spine (stick) into motion. Behind the scenes of the world and its activities lie their web and their support (kūrma) through which they can be expressed.

"When a Yogi withdraws his senses like a tortoise withdraws its limbs, he surrenders worldliness. It can be said he no longer grasps sense objects and leaves them and the sense organs to rest in their source."

ABHINAVAGUPTA, GĪTĀRTHASAṂGRAHA II, 60

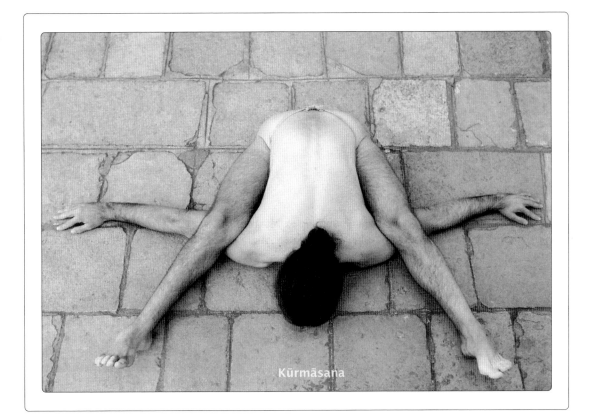

• Yoga Mudrāsana: The Seal of Non-Separation

For Kṣemarāja, mudrā can be defined in three ways: that which gives joy (muda), that which dissolves ties (mu), and that which seals the universe in Turiya (mudrayati iti) when *"the non-state of states, as Consciousness, takes upon itself the world's activity as resting within Itself."* This is the true nature of mudrā.

Yoga Mudrāsana represents the total inclusivity of Consciousness, to which nothing can be added or taken away. This realisation seals (mudrā) the universe as being Consciousness itself, where *"the entire mass of entities dissolves into the sky of Consciousness, like a little autumn cloud."*
Kṣemarāja, Pratyabhijñāhṛdaya 19

From a physiological viewpoint, the intestines are highly stimulated and cleansed of all congestion. This evacuation echoes the non-retention of psychological memory. Stimulation of the digestive fire (jaṭhara agni) lets us assimilate what we ingest. Symbolically, this power of digestion is the ability to burn and consume events characterised by subject-object polarity.

• Adho Mukha Baddha Koṇāsana: The Cobbler's Prostration

The deep descent of the thighs calls for the trunk to lengthen along the floor. Irrigation of the pelvis and abdomen cleanses this region of all congestion. The pelvis symbolises the earth, which is turned over and aerated, thus preparing it for the germination of mūlabandha.

Dha

organ of touching:
skin (tvak)

ध

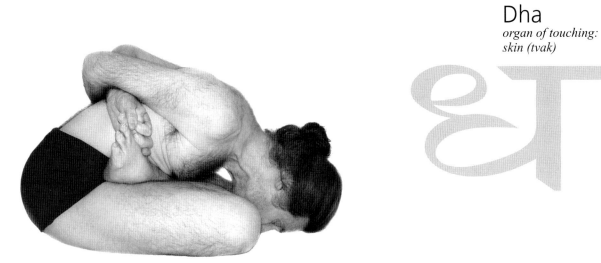

Yoga Mudrāsana

"Give your undivided attention to the sounds of musical instruments.
Listen to the vibration of each sound die away into space and silence.
In this way you will be absorbed into the sky of Consciousness."

VIJÑĀNA BHAIRAVA 41

"Contemplate a jar and the empty space inside it.
Leave aside the enclosing walls and feel the empty space in its entirety."

VIJÑĀNA BHAIRAVA 59

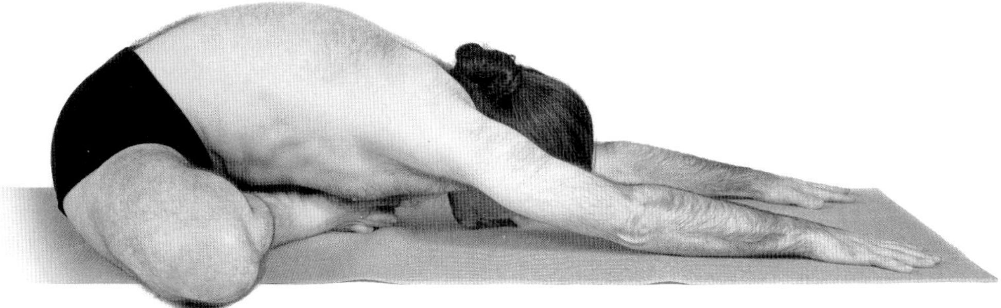

Adho Mukha Baddha Koṇāsana

• Eka Pāda Śīrṣāsana: Over and Beyond the Head

In emergency situations, the gaze becomes the vision beyond subject-object polarity. Here, Śiva beheads Brahmā.

• Skandāsana: The Lord of War

He is called Skanda or Subrahmaṇya, or Kārttikeya because he was fed by six mothers (kṛttikā). He looked at each in turn and so developed six faces. He killed the demon Tāraka to whom Śiva had granted a boon: only Śiva's own son would be able to kill him. Tāraka, intoxicated by his power, terrorised the world. This terror brought about the gushing forth of light that was incarnated by Skanda, the Lord of War. In each situation there is the germ of its own destruction and the return to tranquillity. The Lord of war is merely the momentary expression, according to circumstances, of the perpetually benevolent Śiva.

• Bhairavāsana: The Cry of the Absolute

He provides support (BHṚ) since he supports the worlds, but he also permits them to be born and fed (RU). And his cry (rava) then devours them.

"Rising from the heart, when frightened, is a cry prompted
by the awareness of time's inexorability.
Thus the fear of existence is revealed."
Abhinavagupta, Tantrāloka I, 97

The Art of Knotting: Binding Āsana

"Fix your eyes on a space filled with variegated light of the sun or of a lamp. Let the universe be filled with this light, the mirror of Your essential nature."

VIJÑĀNA BHAIRAVA 76

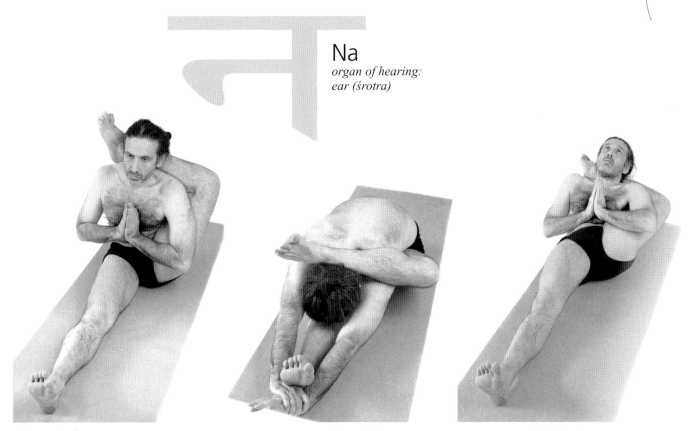

न

Na
organ of hearing: ear (śrotra)

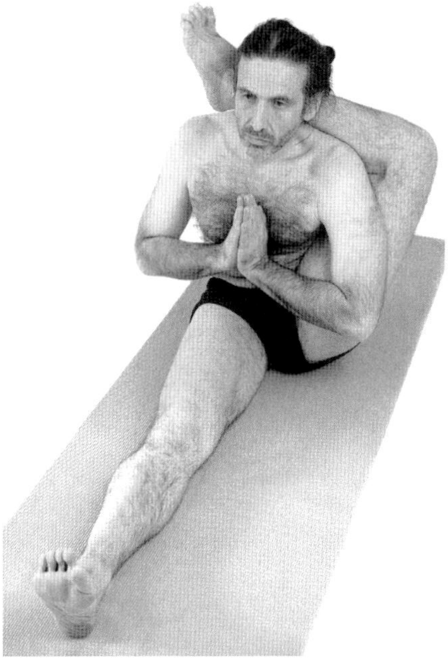

Eka Pāda Śīrṣāsana

Skandāsana

Bhairavāsana

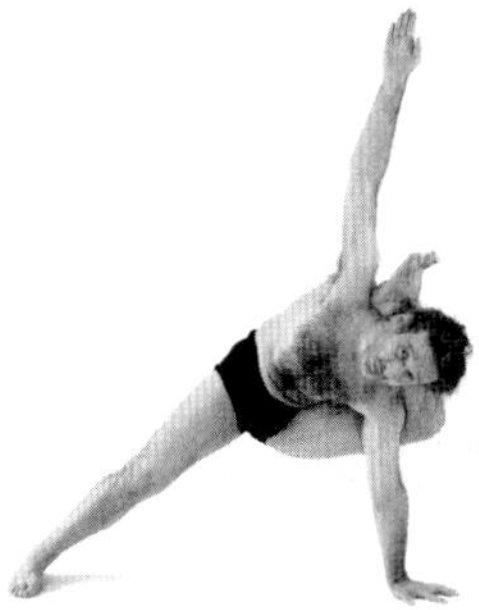

Kāla Bhairavāsana ...

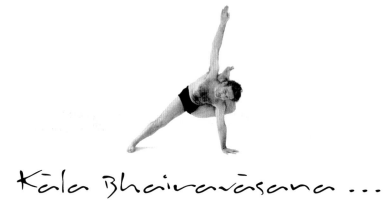

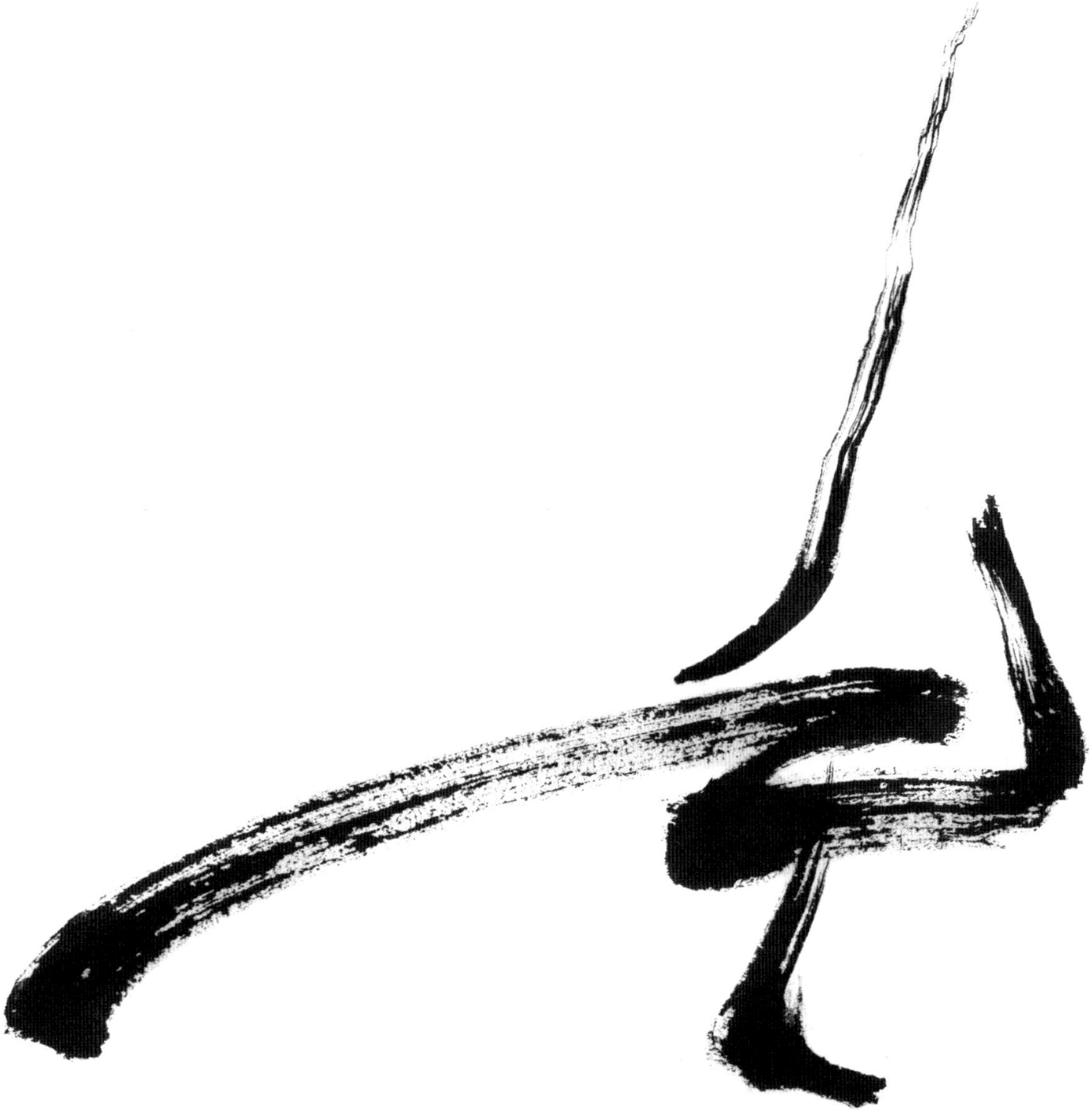

• Kāla Bhairavāsana: The Engulfing of Time

The past and future can only be actualised in the present, and the present can only exist through spatio-temporal localisation. What enables these three times to be actualised is Presence, as Consciousness, which devours them (Kāla Bhairava).

"He (Bhairava) shines on those whose mind is intensely attached to the contemplation known as 'engulfing of time' (kālagrāsa) and who exhaust the substance of time, which sets the constellations into motion."
ABHINAVAGUPTA, TANTRĀLOKA I, 96-100

• Cakorāsana: The Bird that Savours the Moon's Rays

The fullness of Consciousness can be sensed in the diversity of all manifestations and expressions. The wonder of this foreboding becomes the food of this soaring ascent as the moon's rays take us to the moon.

• Eka Pāda Śīrṣāsana in Marīcyāsana: Throwing Yourself into the Monster's Mouth

Practice awakens ever more subtle contractions. We voluntarily put ourselves into situations that are barely supportable in order to explore the various faces of our agitation, which appear and disappear in the background of Consciousness.

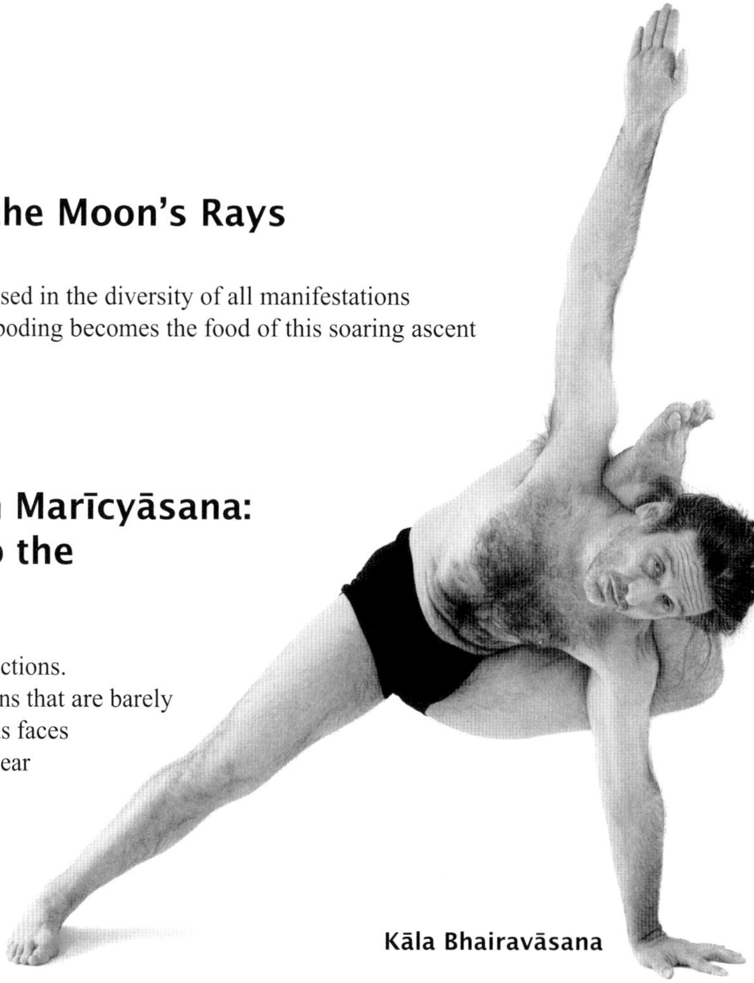

Kāla Bhairavāsana

"Having fixed one's eyes on a particular object, one should slowly withdraw the gaze from it, as well as the knowledge of that object along with the thought of it. Then, O Goddess, one becomes an abode of the void."

Vijñāna Bhairava 120

"When one perceives a particular object, other objects gradually appear as if void. Meditating on this void in the mind, one attains peace, even when the object is still perceived."

Vijñāna Bhairava 122

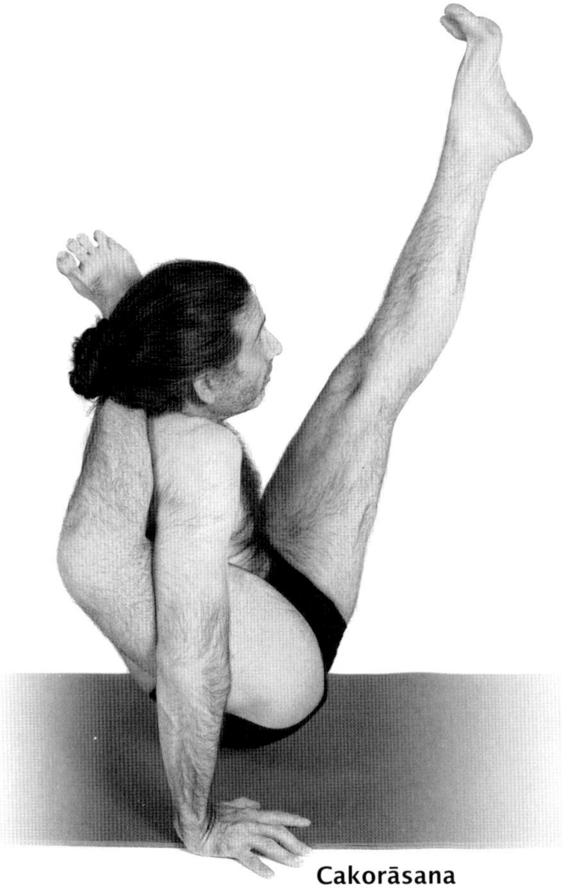

Cakorāsana

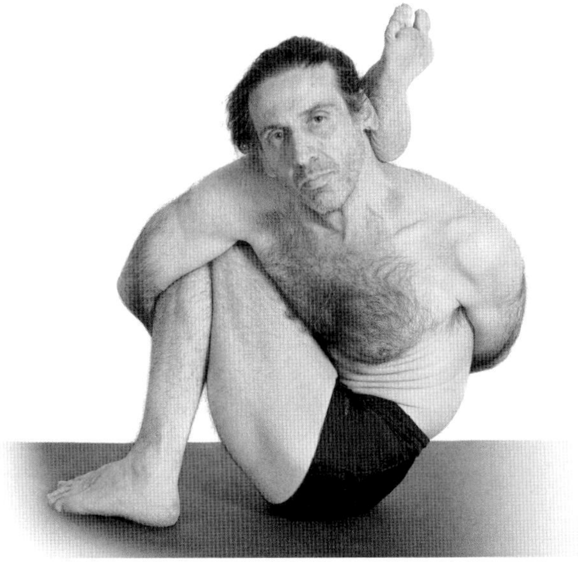

Eka Pāda Śīrṣāsana in Marīcyāsana

*"Towards whichever object the mind moves,
one should withdraw it from there at that very moment.
By thus leaving it without support,
one will become free from mental agitation."*

VIJÑĀNA BHAIRAVA 129

• Durvāsāsana: Holy Rage

In mythology, the sage Durvāsa is famous for his fits of anger. What can be said of this anger? It is said that the wisdom of the Bhairava Tantra was lost at the advent of kali yuga. All that remained were progressive doctrines and bargaining rituals, which were merely the praise of bourgeois values. And so Śiva decided it was time to chase the traders from the temple. He appeared as Shrīkaṇṭha and once again revealed the non-dual teachings to the sage Durvāsa. Whenever Durvāsa opened his mouth, all that came out was the holy rage of non-duality that reduced the mind's sand castles to nothingness.

• Ṛcīkāsana: On the Wisdom of Effacement

"Stay inside yourself and show yourself as Nothing. Otherwise you will suffer." HENRY SUSO

From the fire of Brahmā was born Bhṛgu, who taught Bharadvāja about the birth of the Pañcabhūta. From Bhṛgu was born Cyavāna, 'the one who fell from the womb', and whose brilliance reduced to ashes the demon that had abducted his mother. From this brilliance was born Ūrva, a hermit known as the radiant one; his radiance blinded the kṣatriya kings. Ūrva fathered Ṛcīka, the expression of light itself, which he passed on to his wife and mother-in-law in two forms: the first like the brilliance of brāhmaṇa (brahmatejas) and the second like the brilliance of warriors (kṣātratejas). Legend tells that his wife, Satyavatī, wanted a child. She also asked that her mother could bear children. He gave her two rice balls. Into the one for his wife he had breathed the brilliance of brāhmaṇa, and into the other the brilliance of kṣatriya. But destiny would decide differently. Satyavatī ate the rice ball full of kṣātratejas (Brahmānda Purāṇa, chapter 57). This is how Viśvāmitra came to be born from the brilliance of warriors. Ṛcīka is the grandfather of Paraśurāma.

प

Pa

mind (manas)

The labials,
from PA to MA,
says the Tantrāloka,
come from the power
of awakening
or unfolding,
that is, from
the phoneme U.

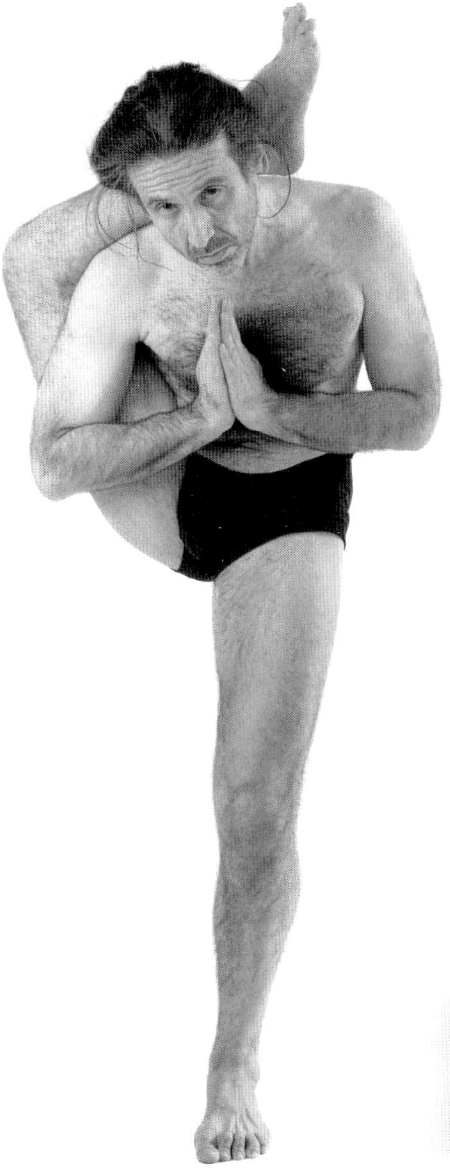

Durvāsāsana

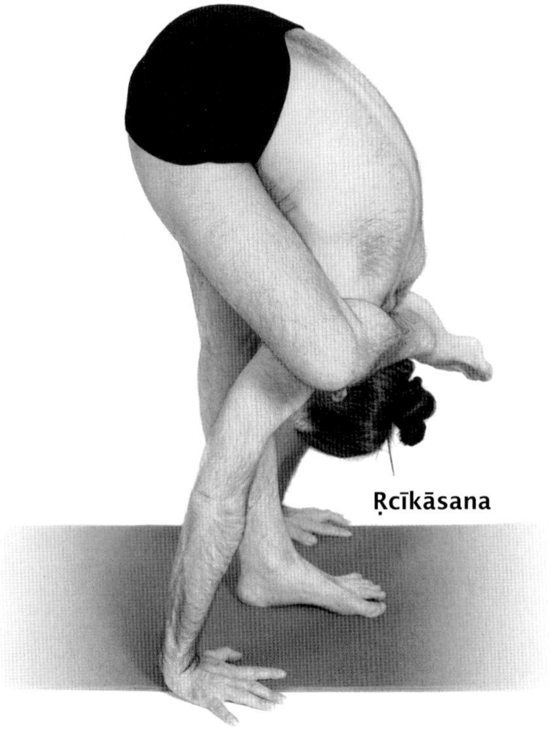

Ṛcīkāsana

Contemplating the Intuitive Landscape

> *"Looking at the clear sky one should fix one's gaze without blinking and make one's body motionless. In that very instant, O Goddess, one attains the Divine nature."*
> VIJÑĀNA BHAIRAVA 84

• Yoga Nidrāsana: Dissolution of the Phenomenal World

At the far edges of hell (pātāla) resides a manifestation of Lord Viṣṇu dominated by darkness (tamas). He is known as Ananta or Saṅkarṣaṇa (the resorber; according to the Padmapurāṇa, one of the twenty-four main forms of Viṣṇu), and is characterised by the unification of subject and object. (BHAGAVATAPURĀṆA V, 25.1)

"In the primordial waters, Hari lies down on Śeṣa, his eyes closed in yogic sleep." BHAGAVATAPURĀṆA III, 11.31

Viṣṇu lying down represents the sleep of reintegration (yoganidrā), during which, at the end of the cosmic cycle, the power of cohesion rests upon the serpent (Śeṣa), symbolising the infinite (ananta) and representing the remnants of resorbed universes. We all long for this rest, as it is said:
"Not only have we found nothing substantial during our erring ways, but we have worn ourselves out. O You, who sleeps on the ocean, you resorbed the entire universe into you during your yogic sleep. You thus know the true nature of everything, since you have taken rest in your Essence. A tired person will have an almost envious reverence for one who is resting. So homage to you, Essence of this universe."
ABHINAVAGUPTA, DHVANYĀLOKALOCANA 3, 43B

In āsana practice, the Viṣṇu mudrā is performed by spreading certain regions or by lying down in infinity. In Yoga Nidrāsana, the organs of action, which are primarily conditioned for survival, are coiled into the back and vanish. The gaze (dṛṣṭi) is placed in contemplation of the external sky, which echoes the sky of Consciousness. A lotus sprouts from Viṣṇu's navel, representing the seed of the next universe. This universe is nothing other than Viṣṇu's cosmic dream.

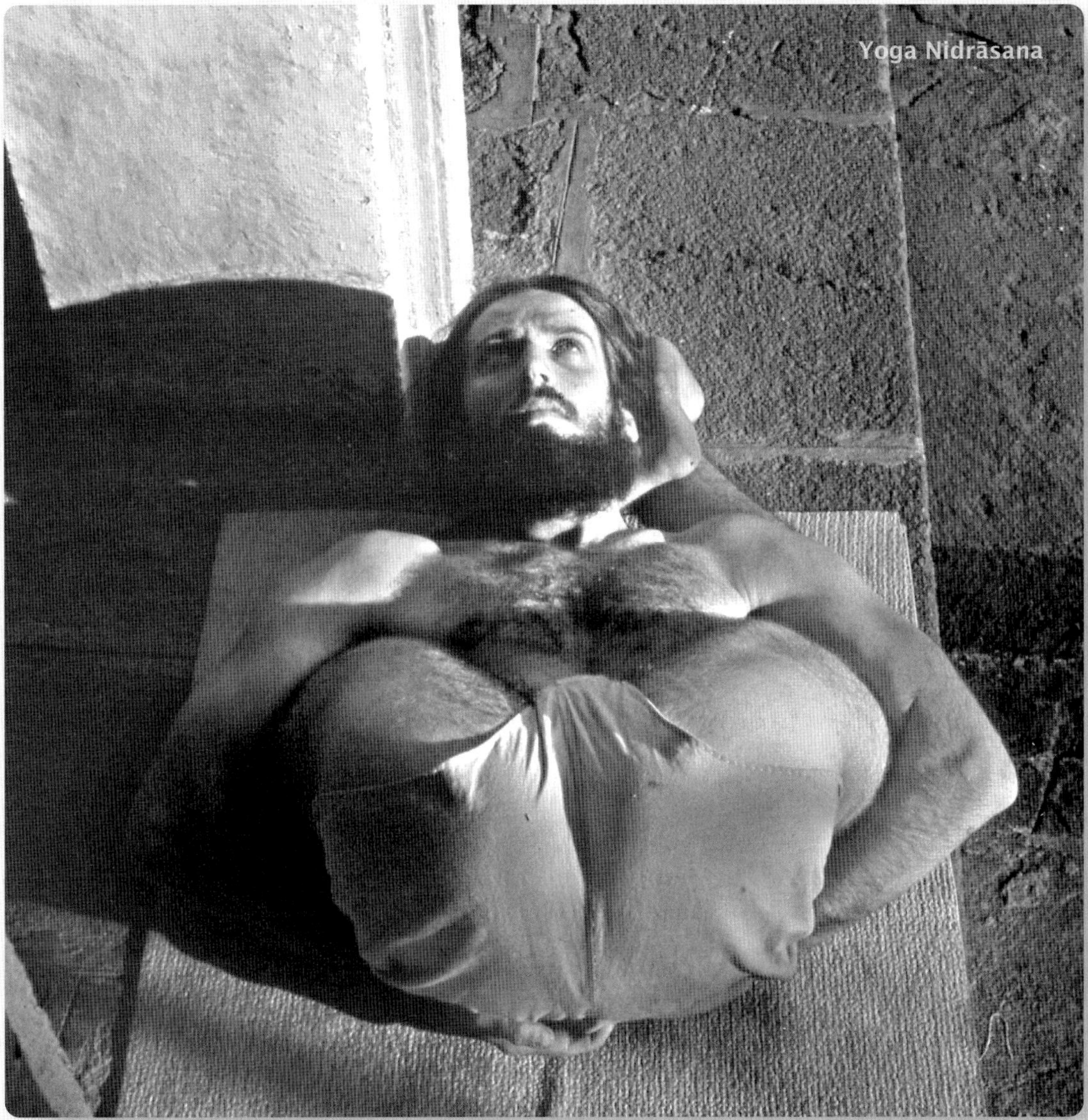

Yoga Nidrāsana

"One should cast one's gaze on an open stretch of land devoid of trees, mountains, walls, etc. When the state of the mind is fixed there, then the fluctuating thoughts dissolve by themselves."

Vijñāna Bhairava 60

• Supta Pādāṅguṣṭhāsana 1: On the Incarnation of the Infinite in the Lower Back

In the gradual approach of this āsana, a simple variation is used where one leg remains straight and the other is bent against the abdomen. A variation where both legs are bent against the abdomen is also used. They are known as wind liberating āsana (Pavanamuktāsana). The preliminary actions in the sacred art of yoga place stress on cleansing movements that free the apānic region, and which favour the flow of exhalation and the discharge of toxins. These toxins are found in the form of wind in the intestines, but also as contractions in the lumbar area.

In its final form, this āsana cleanses the back of the legs, freeing the pelvis and lower back.

The World's Navel: Abdominal Toning Āsana

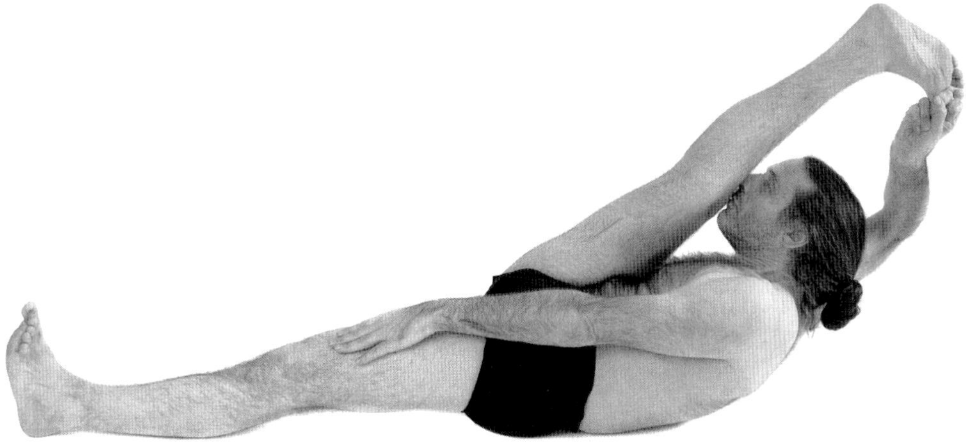

Supta Pādāṅguṣṭhāsana

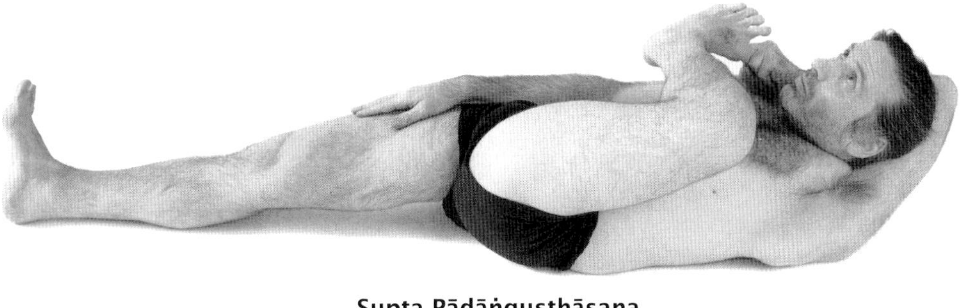

Supta Pādāṅguṣṭhāsana

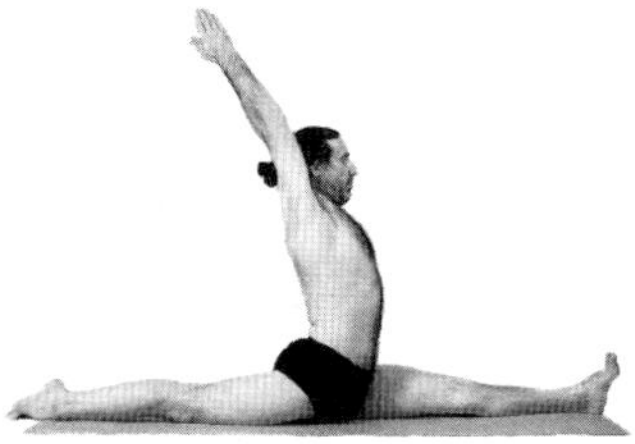

Hanumànàsana ...

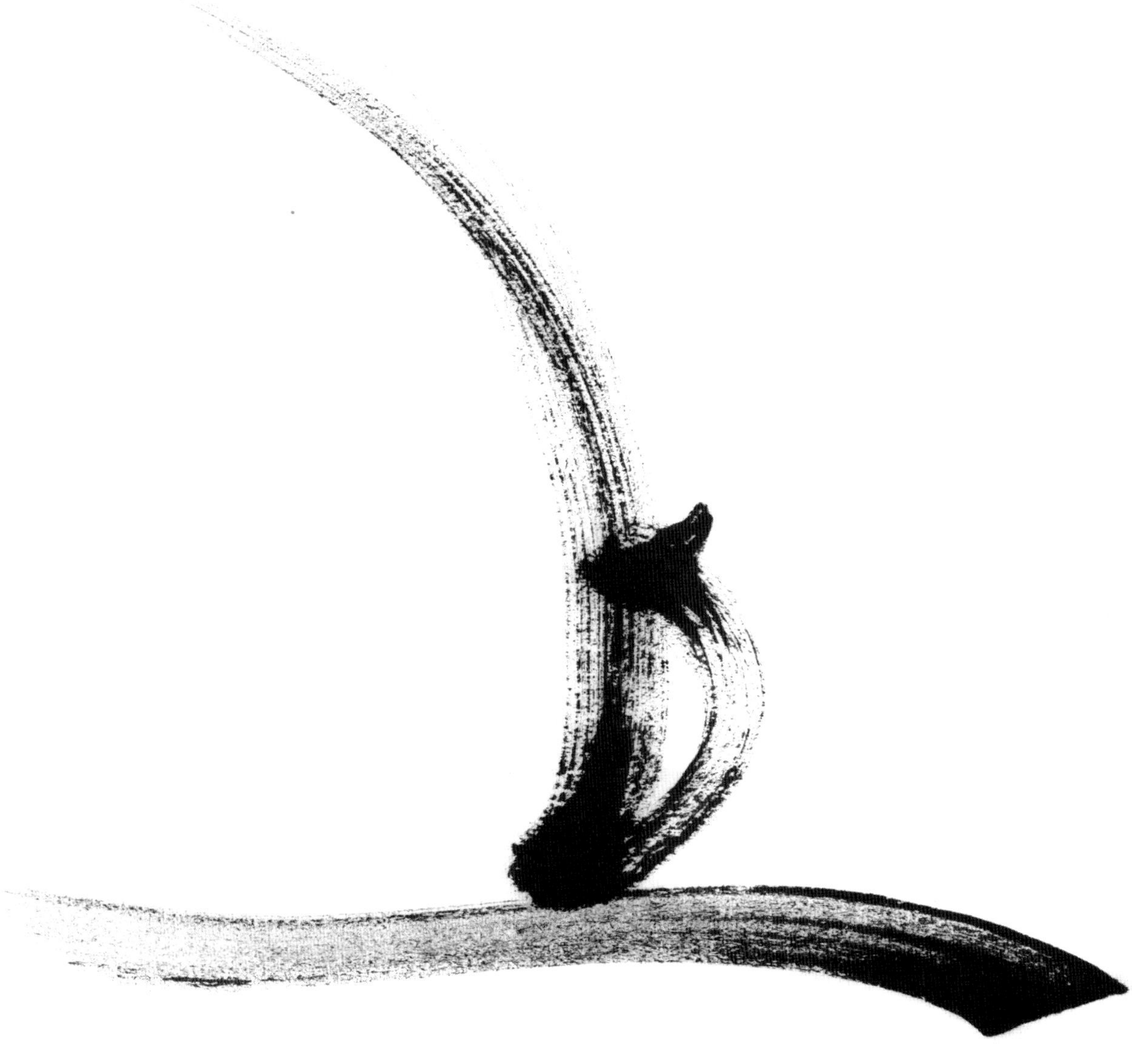

• Hanumānāsana: The One Seated on the Top Lip

"Śiva took the form of Māruti (Hanumān) to serve Hari (Rāma) who himself adored Rāmeśvara, who was no other than Śiva." Śiva Cālīsā

Hanumān, which signifies 'the one with strong jaws', is the incarnation of strength. He is recognised as being Mahā Rudra. There are eleven rudra, who are the incarnations of Śiva's power. One of these incarnations is Hanumān. Hanumān's strength has several expressions. Not only is he famous for his physical feats, but he was also an expert in arts such as music and poetry. He had mastery over grammar and possessed esoteric knowledge of the alphabet, making him a powerful speaker. But he is also 'the one who grants the grace of aṣṭāṅgayoga', as he himself is the supreme yogi.

Although the mysterious Hanumān had this incredible power, he revelled in Rāma's service. According to the laws of the world, those who are powerful are never servitors. For Hanumān, all his powers* were the opportunity to worship the Absolute.

'Ha' is the first syllable of Hanumān. It is transformed by the anusvāra into the seed syllable HAṂ, which represents Hanumān. The bīja HAṂ symbolises sky or space. When we add the sound 'RA', which represents fire (agni), the bīja is transformed into HRAṂ. When the energy of Śakti or Devī is unfolded, then the bīja is transformed into HRĪM. These three bīja are considered powerful formulas of protection or destruction, and are especially used with Hanumān. There are also a group of five bīja specific to Hanumān: HSPHRĒM, KHPHRĒM, HSRAUM, HSKHPHRĒM, HSAUM. When the formula 'hanumate namaḥ' is added, it becomes the mahāmantra of Hanumān.

Another meaning of his name is 'the one seated on the top lip'. This region is known as the dvādaśānta (12 fingers in front of the nose) or outer heart, where exhalation dies and external air becomes inhalation. It is the privileged place for observing the breath. Hanumān, son of Vāyu, is the deity presiding over prāṇāyāma. It is Hanumān that allows the inseparability of Rāma (puruṣa) and Sītā (prakṛti) to be recognised. When an idol of Hanumān is installed in a temple it must be represented holding a vajra in one hand, and his feet must give the impression that they are tearing up the ground (Agnipurāṇa, chapter 5). When the Rāmāyaṇa is read in temples, a seat is always placed for Hanumān. As soon as Rāma's name is pronounced, Hanumān is there!

* **The eight powers** *(aṣta siddhi) in the Śaivāgama non-dual approach are seen as being identical to Bhairava, who is our true nature. They are therefore not intended to control, dominate or manipulate a world that is external to us.*

Animā: *to assimilate all manifestation with divine Consciousness, which is our own essential nature.*

Laghimā: *to reduce to nothingness all notions of diversity.*

Mahimā: *the sense of the omnipresence of the divine.*

Prāpti: *to reside in one's true nature.*

Prākāmya: *to see the various expressions of reality and of the world as the joyful play of the divine.*

Vaśitva: *non-separation with all that exists.*

Iśatva: *to reside continually in divine Consciousness.*

Yatrakāmāvasāyitva: *the unfolding of the energy of will (icchāśakti) that characterises Śiva as being our own nature.*

On the Contemplation of Extremes: Āsana of Adoration to Gods and Goddesses

"Hail Hanumān, the ocean of knowledge and goodness, Hail Kapīśa, by whom the three-fold world is luminous."

TULSĪDĀS HANUMĀN CĀLISĀ 1

फ

Pha

principle of individuation (ahaṃkara)

"In the same way on a dark night, at the beginning of the dark fortnight, while meditating on the darkness, one attains the nature of Bhairava."

VIJÑĀNA BHAIRAVA 87

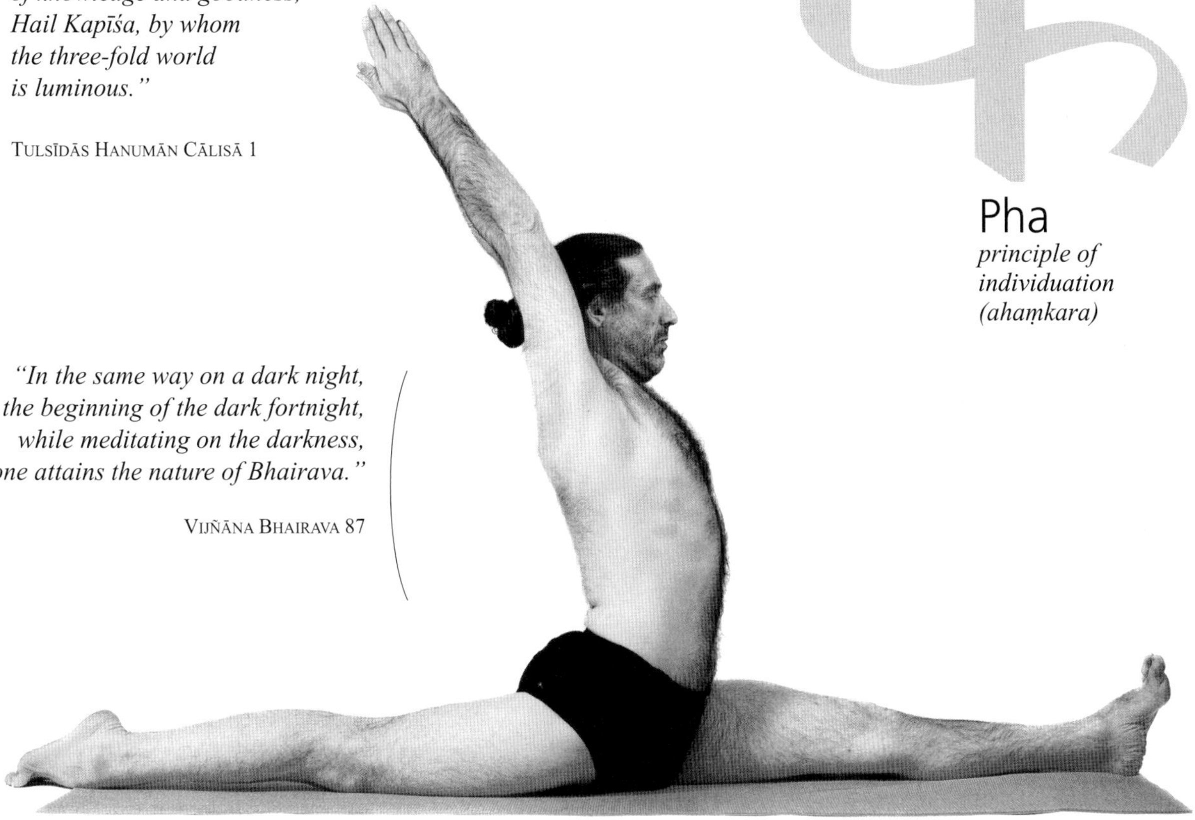

Hanumānāsana

"By standing above a deep well or any abyss
and fixing one's eyes on the bottom,
one becomes completely free from thoughts,
and immediately the mind will certainly be dissolved."

VIJÑĀNA BHAIRAVA 115

• Supta Trivikramāsana: Nowhere To Go

The three worlds are circumscribed by the three steps of Viṣṇu Trivikrama, like three mad strides of the energy that creates, measures, conquers and transcends both the visible and invisible. Māyā comes from the root MĀ, meaning 'to measure'. The crazy wager and function of Viṣṇu (from the root VIṢ vyāptau, to spread out, to pervade) is to measure the immeasurable, which becomes space-time.

"Viṣṇu is truly the sacrifice, by striding (vikrama) he obtains for the gods that all-pervading power which now belongs to them. By the first step he gained the same earth, the second the aerial expanse, and by his last step, the sky."
ŚATAPATHABRĀHMAṆA 1-9, 3-9

Even if we could cover the three worlds, we would only encounter the measurable. The true sacrifice is to abandon all this to that by which we are able to know ourselves in these three worlds or states.

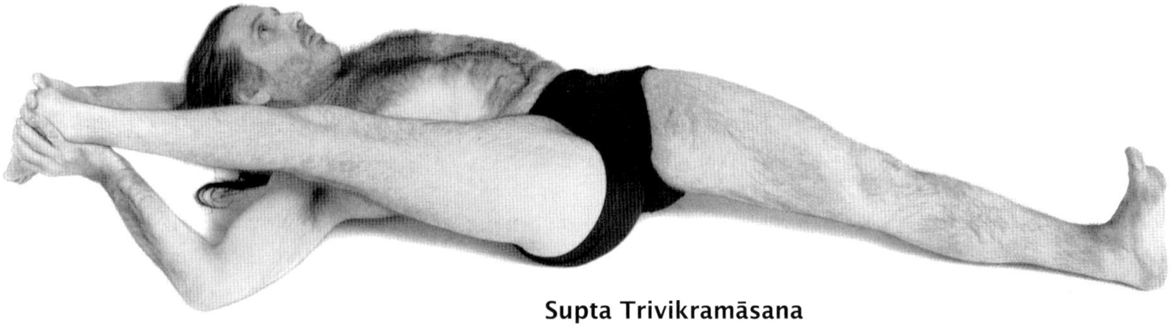

Supta Trivikramāsana

"While looking at a particular space the mind should abandon the thought of all remembered objects and thus making the body free from all support, the Lord reveals Himself."

VIJÑĀNA BHAIRAVA 119

• Bharadvājāsana 2: The Back of the Belly

The meaning of this name can be found in the Bhāgavatapurāṇa: *"I protect even those who are not my sons. I protect my disciples. I protect the deva and the brāhmaṇa. I protect my wife. And all of this I do with ease, this is why they call me Bharadvāja."*

Bharadvāja is one of the seven ṛṣi who represent the seven stars of the Great Bear. The cosmic maṇḍala is found in the body, and the universe is nothing other than the Lord's body. Āsana thus enable certain constellations and their savours to be explored. Bharadvāja, the protector, cleanses and frees the dorsal and lumbar regions.

• Marīcyāsana 3, Marīcyāsana 4: Viṣṇuloka

In these two variations, Marīci continues his work of cleansing the abdominal region.

"Viṣṇuloka is located in the abdomen. Viṣṇu is its deity and he conducts different functions in the body."
GORAKṢANĀTHA, SIDDHASIDDHĀNTAPADDHATI III, 4

One of the names for Viṣṇu is 'the one who supports and nourishes all living beings' (śarīrabhṛt). Marīcyāsana is hence the avatāra, the descent of Viṣṇu into this region, stimulating the digestive fire, but also cleansing it organically and ensuring the correct working of essential functions such as digestion and assimilation.

Stoking Up the Fire of the Entrails: Lateral Extension Āsana

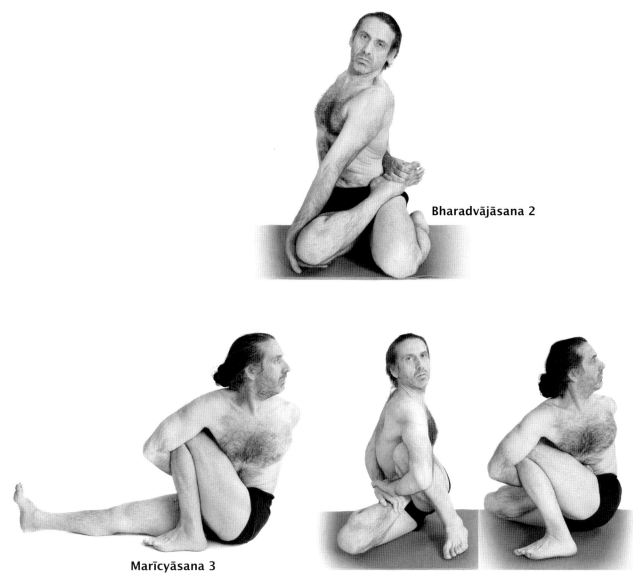

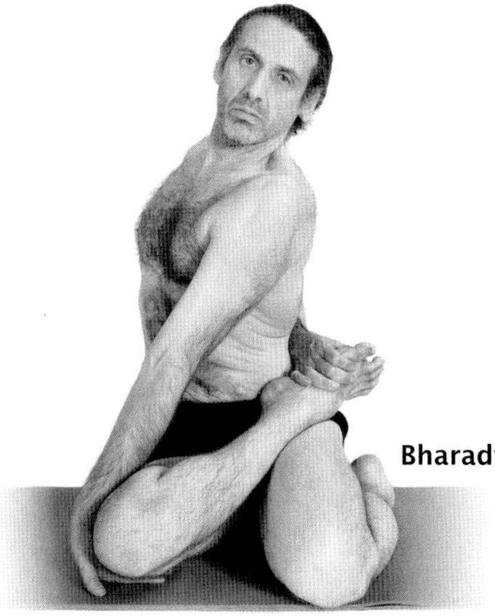

Bharadvājāsana 2

Marīcyāsana 3

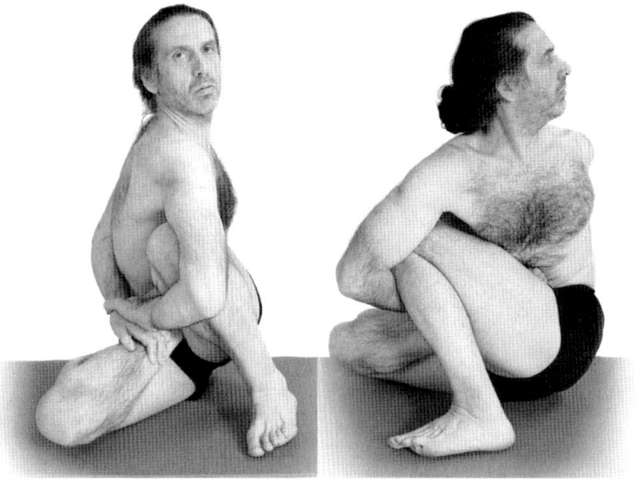

Marīcyāsana 4

Contemplating the Source of Sound (Nādānusandhāna)

> *Tactily contemplate the twelve supports* in which the twelve vowels resonate. Free yourself from objectivity and let the supreme Subject (Śiva) shine forth."*
> Vijñāna Bhairava 30

• Ardha Matsyendrāsana 1 & 2, Paripūrṇa Matsyendrāsana: The Forge

Matsyendranātha had been able to listen to the revelation of the Kula teaching whilst in the fish's belly. The nature of this energy (kula) is revealed in a place of entrails *(see The Great Crematorium: The Belly of the Fish, Chapter 13)*. It is in the organic forge that the fire (jaṭhara agni) and its śakti are incarnated: liver, gall bladder, pancreas and spleen. The Chinese speak of it as the Triple Burner: the above-umbilical burner that transforms, the below-umbilical burner that eliminates and the upper burner that distributes. By being attentive to this constellation, the organs find their radiance and qualities: quality of protection incarnated in the liver, quality of accomplishment in the gall bladder, quality of digestion in the pancreas and quality of transformation in the spleen. It is at the heart of the entrails, at their confluence, that the body itself appears as the organic revelation of a sole and same energy.

• Pāśāsana: The Knot of Space

The fabulous play of Consciousness unfolds a series of contractions, of knots, which only appear limiting through an optical illusion. The first knot, the most subtle, is that of non-completeness (āṇavamala), the second is that of differentiation between subject and object (māyīyamala), and the third is that of activity and illusion of a doer (kārmamala). The knot, the contraction, can only exist by and in space.
"A person who sees objects as his own form is called a pati (master), while one lying under the effects of delusion and seeing objects as different from him is called a paśu (bound being)." Utpaladeva, Īśvarapratyabhijñākārikā III, 2.3

* Janmāgra: organs of generation
Kanda: the bulb
Hṛid: the heart
Tālu: the palate
Lalāṭa: the brow
Śakti: pure energy
Mūla: the root
Nābhi: the navel
Kaṇṭha: the cavity at the back of the throat
Brūmadhya: the point between the eyebrows
Brahmarandhra: the crown of the head
Vyāpinī: the omnipresent

"Contemplate on the beginning
and the end of a letter.
Let the void resonate within you,
and become that void."

VIJÑĀNA BHAIRAVA 40

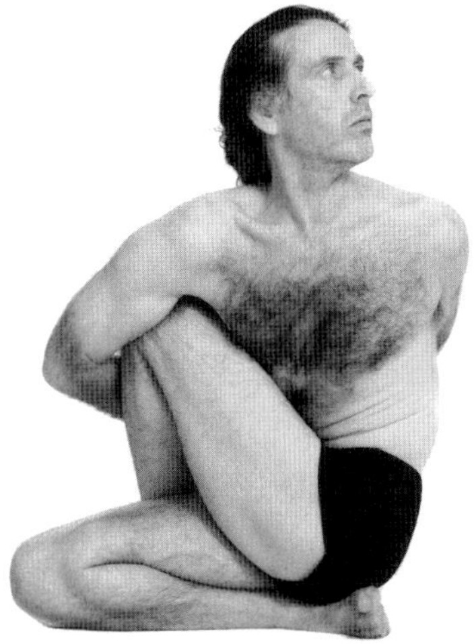

Ardha Matsyendrāsana 1

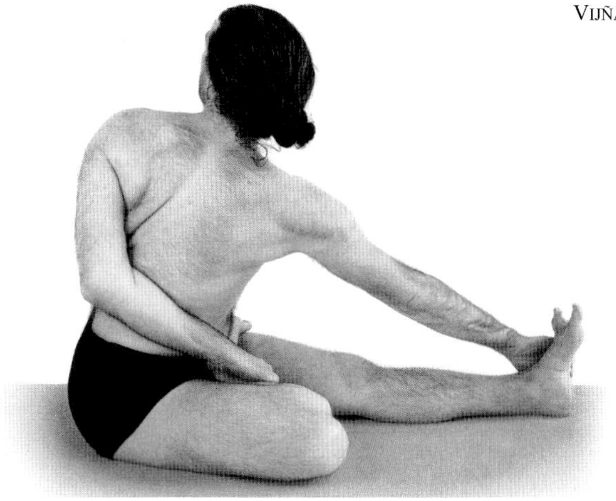

Ardha Matsyendrāsana 2

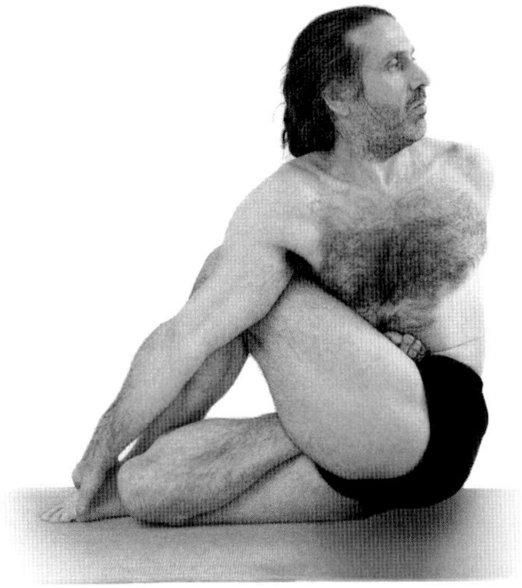

Paripūrṇa Matsyendrāsana

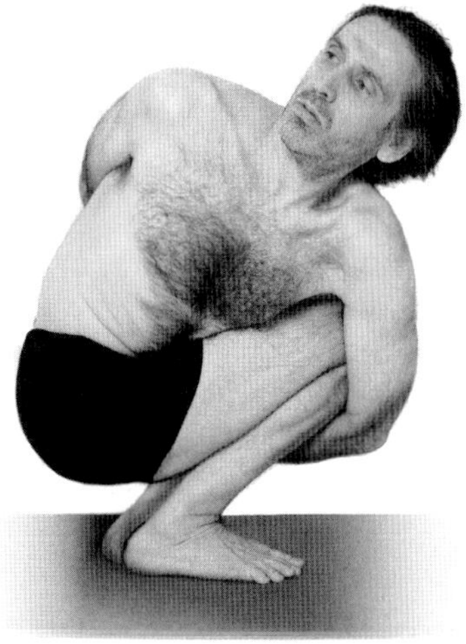

Pāśāsana

Ba

intellect (buddhi)

ब

• Ūrdhva Dhanurāsana: The Backstage of the World

Eastern transmission (pūrvāmnāya), actualised in the anterior side (the east, pūrva) of the body, symbolises the origin, the source. Kuleśvara and Kuleśvarī, the inseparable lords of energy (kula), who represent Śiva and Śakti, are worshiped here.

The back is a part of the body that can never be seen.
This is why backward extensions must be felt rather than expressed.
The other groups of āsana can, to start with, be expressed before later being felt.

Backward extensions put us in contact with this region.
According to Śrī B.K.S. Iyengar, backward extensions are a means of introversion for the yogi.
The backward gaze is not that of the eyes, but of a sensation that does not stop at the periphery, and which makes us sense the background of the body-mind.

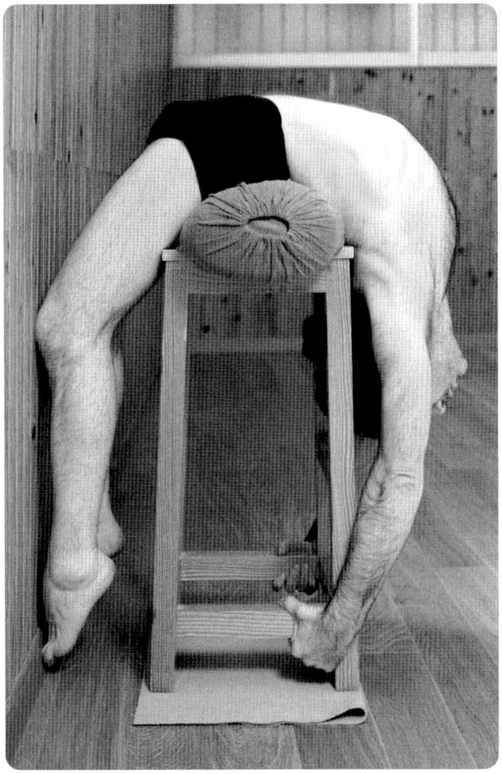

"Closing one's ears and similarly closing the lower opening (the anus), one should meditate on the sound without vowel and consonant. Then one will enter the eternal Brahman."

VIJÑĀNA BHAIRAVA 114

"O Bhairavī, by uttering the praṇava and by meditating on the void at the end of the protracted sound, one attains the state of the Void by means of the Supreme Energy of the Void."

VIJÑĀNA BHAIRAVA 39

The Vision Behind the Gaze, The Back of Creation: Backward Extension Āsana

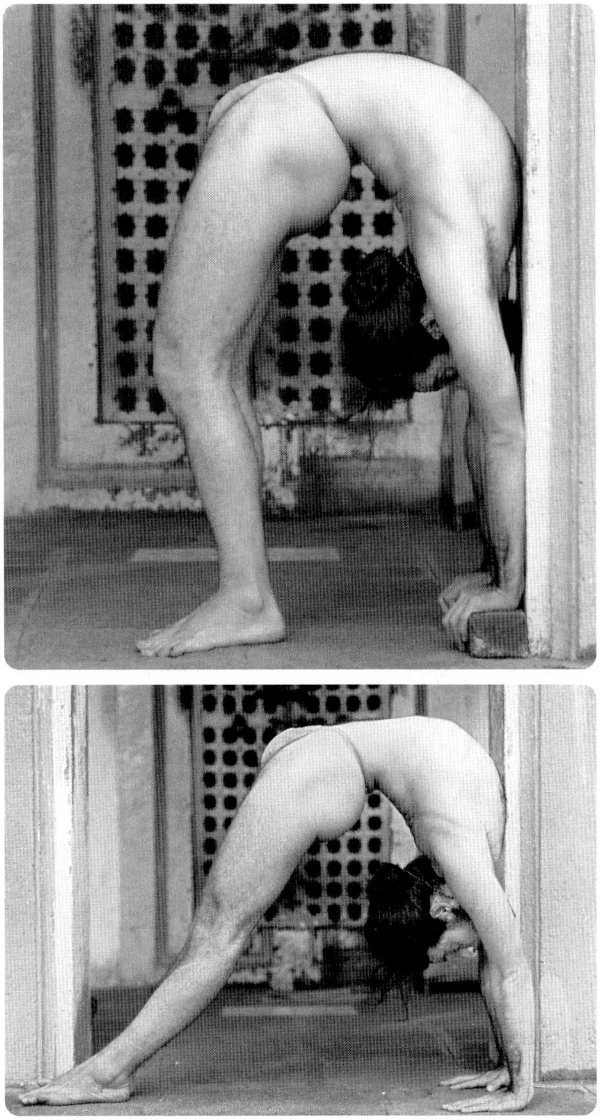

Ūrdhva Dhanurāsana

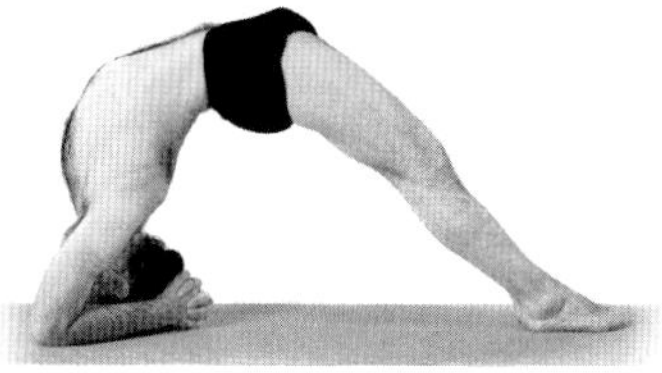

Dwi Pāda Viparīta Daṇḍāsana ...

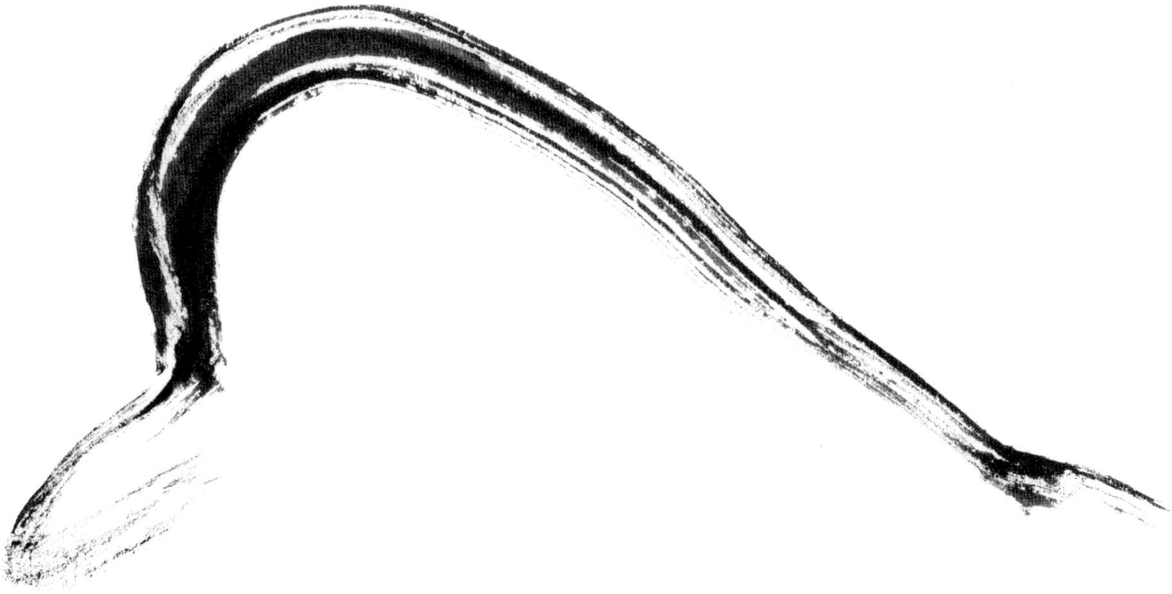

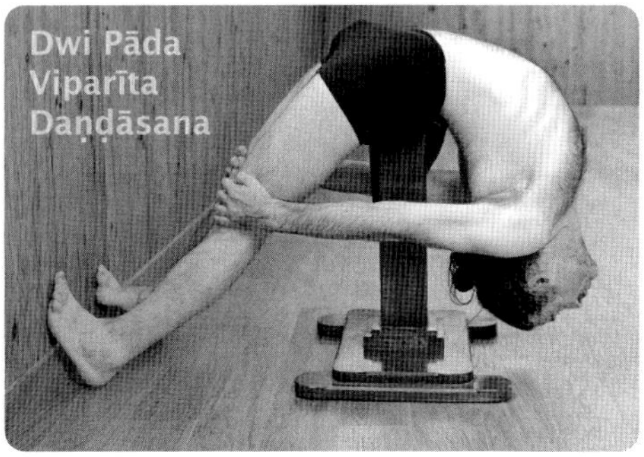

भ

Bha

nature (prakṛti)

• Dwi Pāda Viparīta Daṇḍāsana, Eka Pāda Viparīta Daṇḍāsana 1 & 2: The Ultimate Prostration

That which can be seen, felt or experienced is localised in space-time, which is only a shadow of the Presence that allows its actualisation. Everything that can be accomplished in space-time is merely external prostration and therefore of no importance. It is just a pretext for realising our own fullness.

"I am everything. There is no-one else to bow down before. Realising this is the true prostration to Ātmaliṅga."

Śaṅkarācārya, Nirguṇa Mānasa Pūjā 2

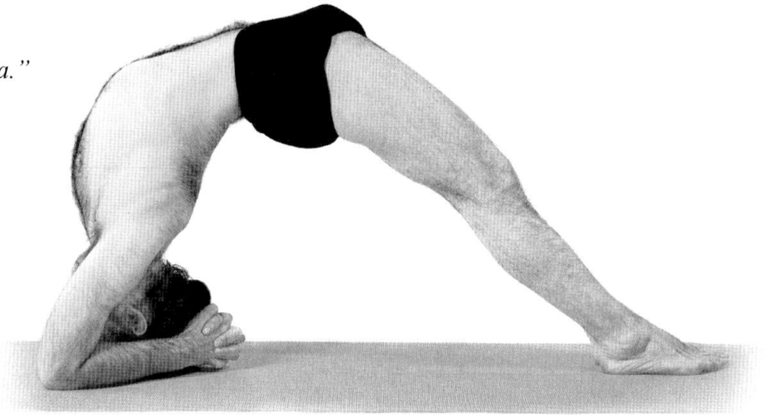

Dwi Pāda Viparīta Daṇḍāsana

"Give yourself to the spontaneous sound,
vibrating without cause in the void of the ear,
uninterrupted like the sound of a waterfall.
In this way, one attains the supreme Brahman."

VIJÑĀNA BHAIRAVA 38

"If one recites the great 'A'-sound without bindu or visarga,
then, O Goddess, the Supreme Lord,
who is a torrent of wisdom, arises at once."

VIJÑĀNA BHAIRAVA 90

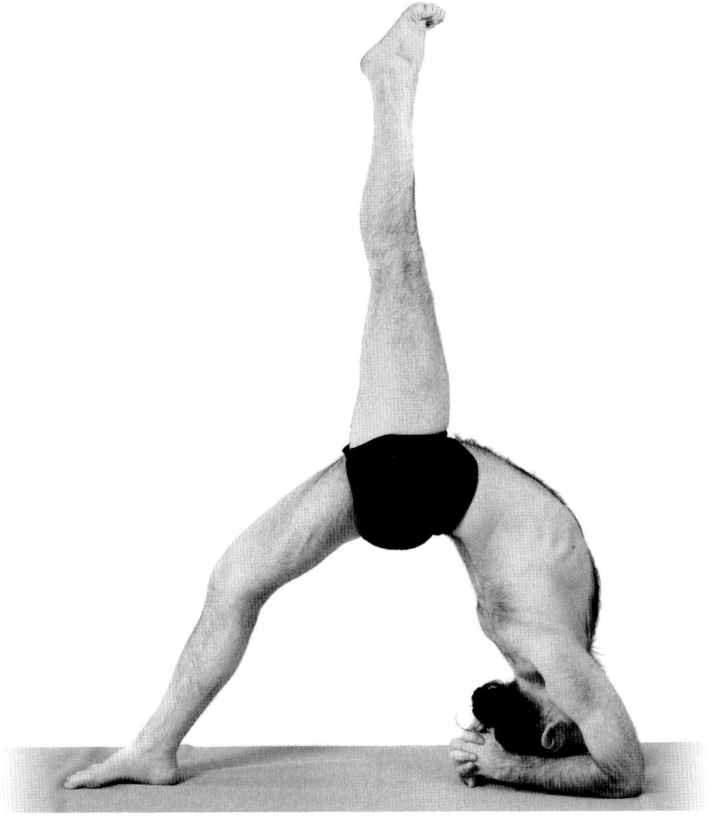

Eka Pāda Viparīta Daṇḍāsana 1

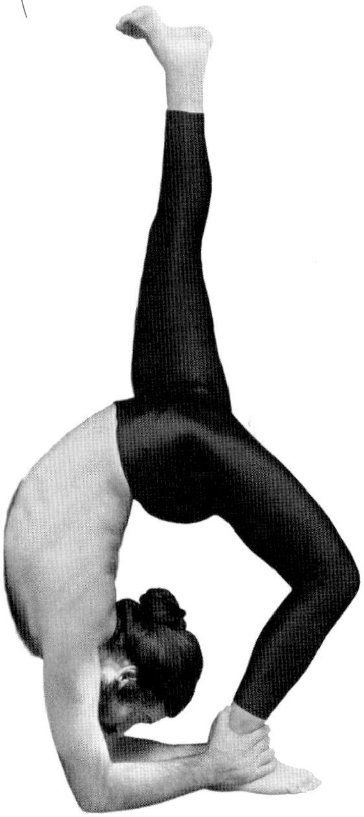

Eka Pāda Viparīta Daṇḍāsana 2

Contemplating the Spontaneous Offering

"True worship does not consist in offering flowers and other substances.
True worship is fixing one's mind in the void of Consciousness, free from dualities.
From this fervour, absorption in Śiva takes place."
VIJÑĀNA BHAIRAVA 147

"Real oblation consists in offering all the elements,
the senses and sense-objects along with the mind into the fire
of the Great Abode of the Void, using awareness as the sacrificial ladle."
VIJÑĀNA BHAIRAVA 149

• Cakra Bandhāsana: The Wheel of Energies Bound in Their Source

This is the etymology of cakra according to Abhinavagupta:
"The term cakra, wheel, is associated with the verbal roots meaning to spread out the essence (kaṣ), to be satisfied in this essence (cak), to break the ties (kṛt), and to act effectively (kṛ). The wheel thus unfolds, is satisfied, breaks off, and has the power to act." ABHINAVAGUPTA, TANTRĀLOKA XXIX, 106-107

The waves of Consciousness unfold according to the five expressions of Lord Śiva: emanation, maintenance, resorption, concealment and revelation. These five expressions are said to take their place within us in a continuous and spontaneous manner. In their solidification phase, they separate the known (prameya), experience (pramāṇa) and the subject that experiences (pramātṛ). In their fluidity phase, they regain their energetic colouration (cakra) as ever increasingly subtle states of Consciousness, corresponding to the movement of resorption of the elements. According to yogic intuition, each of these movements contains all the others and simply expresses the fullness of their source.

"The Goddess takes delight in the ultimate and perfect evidence of Consciousness. May I reside in this intuition free of succession." ABHINAVAGUPTA, KRAMASTOTRA 27

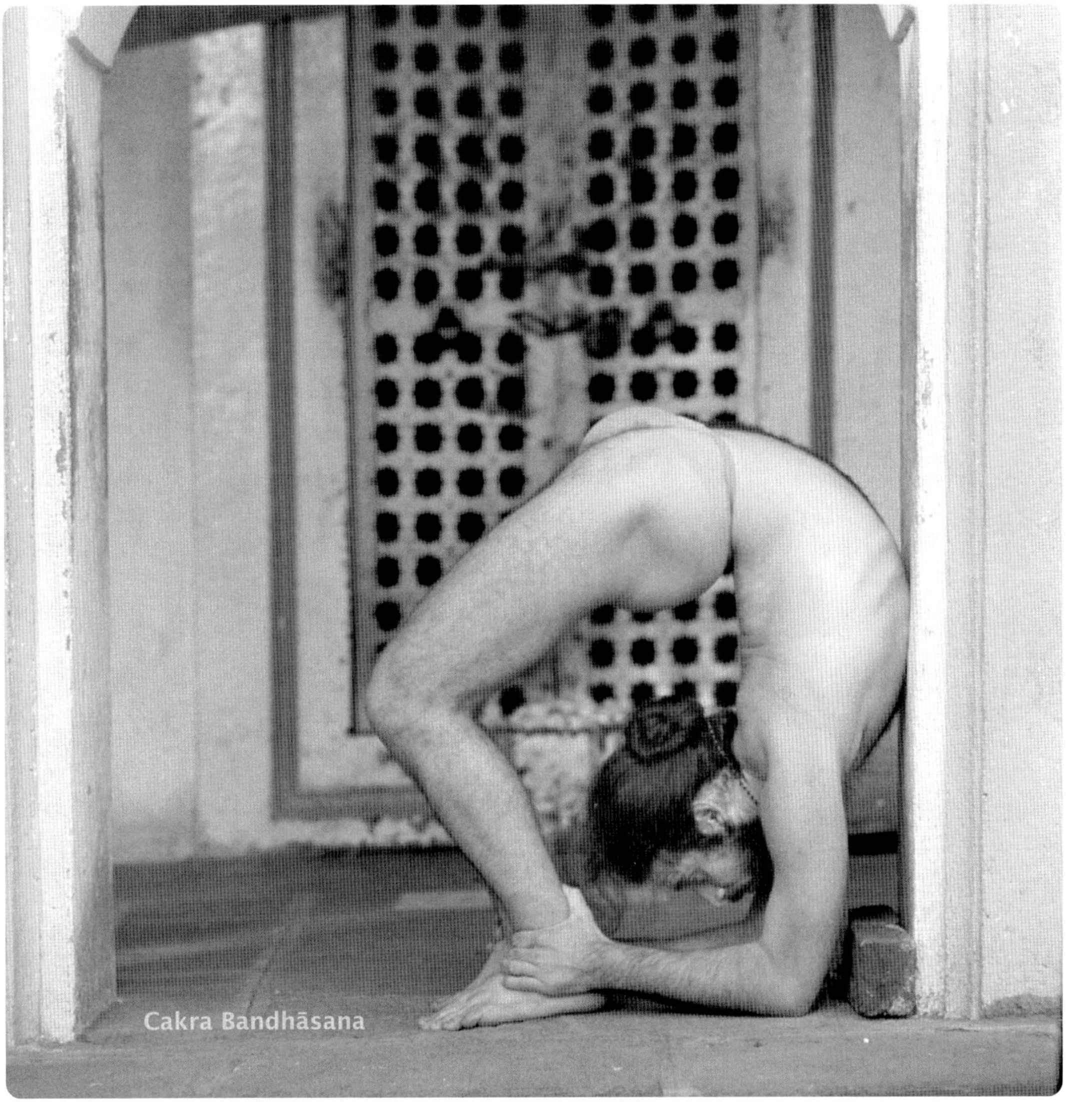
Cakra Bandhāsana

"Consciousness takes on the faces of the worshipper,
worshipping and the worshipped.
Only Consciousness exists.
And this is spontaneous worship."

VIJÑĀNA BHAIRAVA 153

"Reciting and being continuously immersed
in the Great Goddess and being established
in the sacrificial ritual of great bliss,
one is united with this Goddess
and attains union with Bhairava."

VIJÑĀNA BHAIRAVA 155

म

Ma
individual (puruṣa)

• Kapotāsana: The Cooing of the Self

According to tantric classification of phonemes, the guttural KA represents the Earth and is reflected in the intermediary state of sound (parāpara) as KṢA, or the vibratory aspect (śakti) as the eternal Śiva (Sadāśiva). Sadāśiva is the realisation of 'I am the totality of the universe'. The world is no longer objectivised and grasped externally, but appears in our own Presence. This intuition, symbolically actualised by the opening of the chest, imitates the exuberant and vibrant chest of a cooing pigeon (kapota).

The phoneme KA already resonates with the emptiness (KHA) at the centre of the Heart. KHA means the void, the hollow of the axle-wheel which makes the movement of the wheel possible. If the centre of the Heart is empty (kHA) the movement of life is free and smooth, hence su-kha; if it is blocked there is obstruction, hence duḥ-kha.

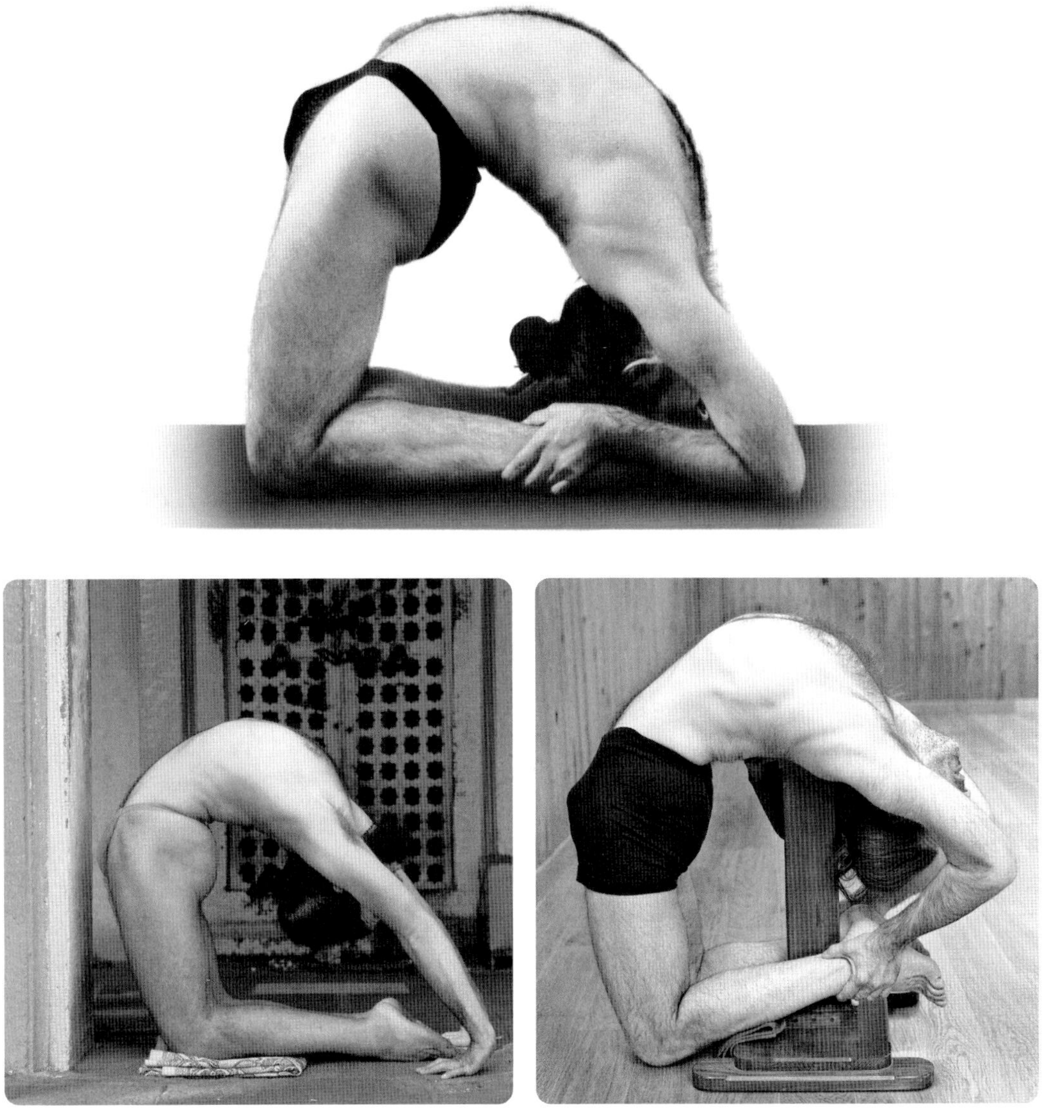

Kapotāsana

Contemplating the Source of Pain

"*If one pierces any limb or part of the body with a sharp needle or any other instrument, then by concentrating on that very point, one attains the pure state of Bhairava.*"
VIJÑĀNA BHAIRAVA 93

"*If one strikes part of the body either deliberately or accidentely, remain at the source of pain and be engulfed by the non-dual state of void, and then the Self shines forth.*"
VIJÑĀNA BHAIRAVA 89

• Eka Pāda Rājakapotāsana 1, 2, 3, 4: On the Variations of Cooing

The variations of these āsana explore the openings of the groins, as well as the unfolding of the chest and its inner spaces, its energies linked to different colourations of the breath, and its associated mental attitudes. In these āsana we become acquainted with supports (ādhāra) and very important prāṇic junctions: the pelvic floor or the support of the base (mūlādhāra), where the fire is lit; the support of the anus (gudādhāra) that, by its contraction and expansion, makes apānavāyu steady; and the support of the genital organs (medhrādhāra) in the secret cave of the bee, which unfolds vajrolī, where the sperm is immobilised and moves upwards. The stimulation and intense irrigation of these ādhāra fills the body with vital energy.

"*Fusion of the thousands of energies perceived in all possible ways into a single energy, such is the supremely free Śiva, whose essence is the upsurge of his own heart.*"
MAHEŚVARĀNANDA, MAHĀRTHAMAÑJARĪ 13

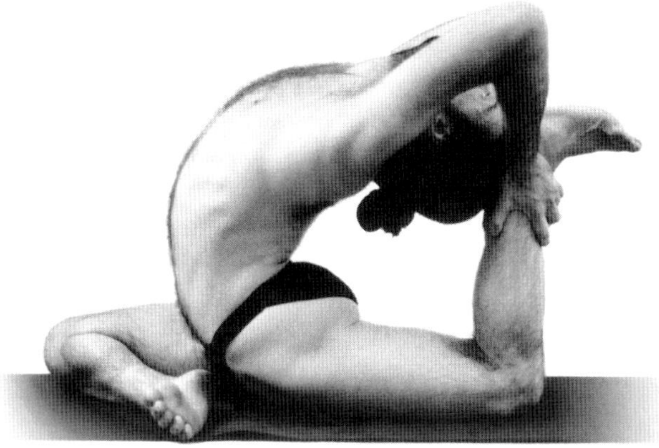

Eka Pāda Rājakapotāsana 1

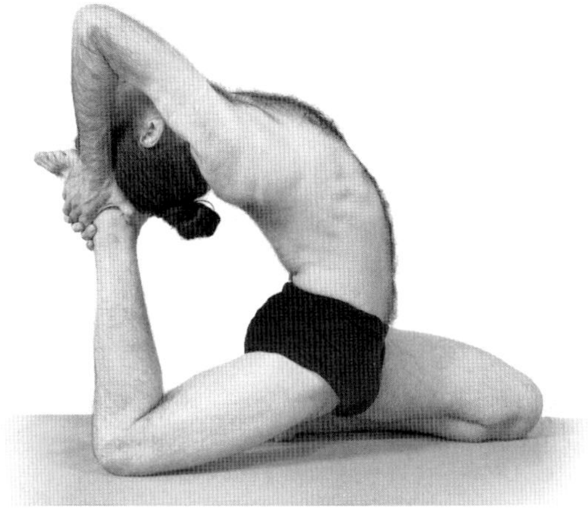

Eka Pāda Rājakapotāsana 3

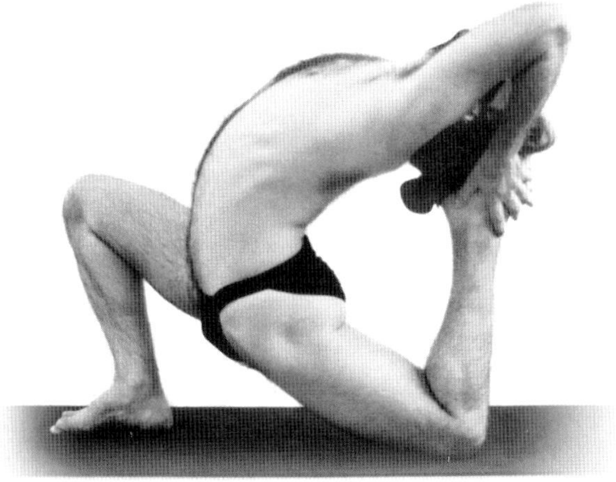

Eka Pāda Rājakapotāsana 2

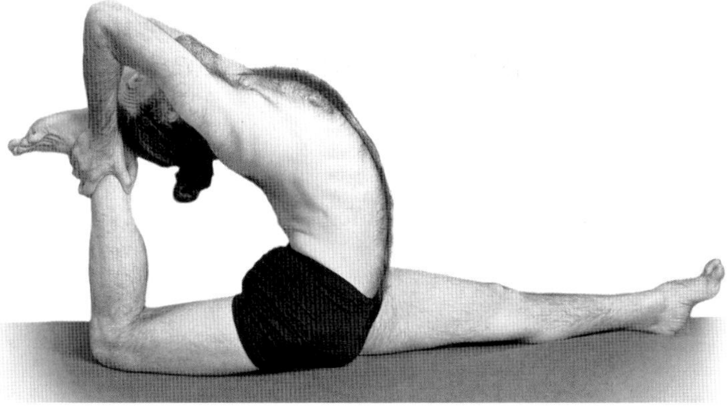

Eka Pāda Rājakapotāsana 4

Contemplating Statelessness

> *At the time of vision of oneness while practising the mudrā Karaṅkiṇī (of death), Krodhanā (of anger), Bhairavī (of fixedness of gaze), Lelihānā (of uninterrupted suction) and Khecarī (of contemplation of space), the pervasiveness of Supreme Consciousness is revealed."*
> VIJÑĀNA BHAIRAVA 77

> *"Seated comfortably, with the sensation the buttocks, hands and feet are unsupported, attain fullness."*
> VIJÑĀNA BHAIRAVA 78

• Bhujaṅgāsana 2: The Venom of Awakening

One of the names of Viṣṇu is Bhujogottama: 'the one who is the supreme serpent'. In the Lakṣmī Tantra there is a description of Śeṣa, the royal serpent (Nāga Rāja), considered to be the son of Śiva: *"His face resembles the full moon, he is crowned with a thousand hoods and his eyes are hazed by intoxication."* In Kashmiri, the word for 'source' is serpent (nāga). Nāga are considered to have been the first inhabitants of this region. It is said that the etymology of Kashmir comes from Kaśyapa, the father of the nāga. Many temples are built close to springs and rivers, and are dedicated to the worship of the nāga. Patañjali is the incarnation of Śeṣa. Śiva wears a cobra around his neck. In yogic practices, the serpent is the rising vertical breath that blazes in the nāḍī of cremation (śmaśāna nāḍī) where differentiations are burnt.

• Rājakapotāsana: When Cooing is Royal Silence

The contact of the feet with the head symbolises the absence of spatiotemporal localisation and succession. The north (head) and south (feet) cardinal points are joined, and the posterior side (west) moves into contact with the anterior side (east). The succession of elements is ended when the brahmarandhra, the upper part of the cranial vault, referred to by Gorakṣanātha as 'the wheel of extinction', representing that which is beyond the elements, and the feet, which symbolise the apānic region in its most dense form, the earth, meet. There never has been time, space or elements.

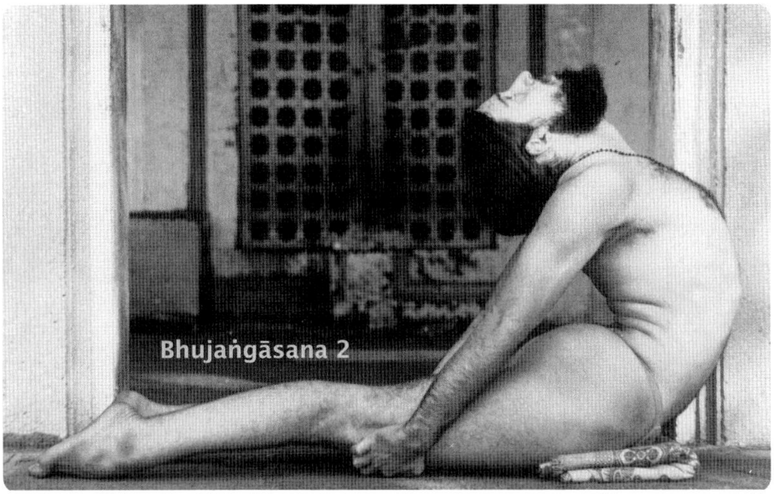

Bhujaṅgāsana 2

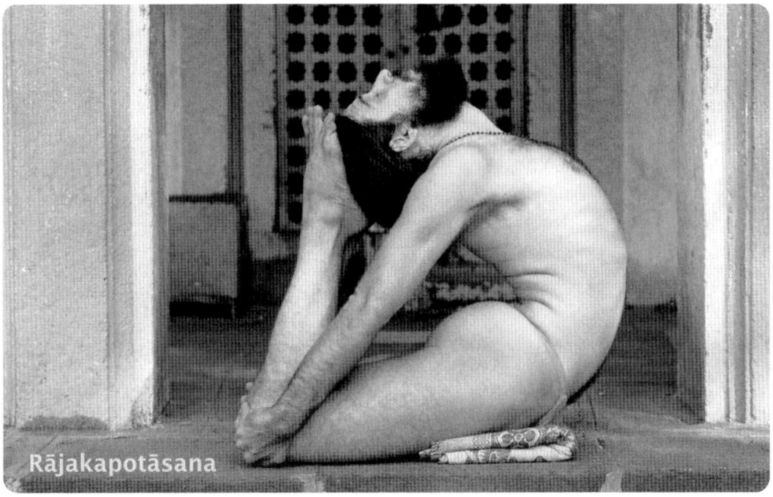

Rājakapotāsana

य

Ya

attachment (rāga)

The junction of the vowel I, the phoneme representing the vital surge or energy of will (icchāśakti), when it joins with the vowel A, the without-equal, gives the sound YA. This junction is characterised by a sharp and swift action. This is the reason this sound is considered to be the seed of wind.

• Vālakhilyāsana: The Messengers of Clarity

They are known as Vālakhilya or Bālakhilya. Some myths say they sprang from the sperm of Brahmā, who could not hold back his seed upon seeing Pārvatī. Others attribute their birth to Santati, the wife of Kratu, one of the seven ṛṣi sires. They number sixty thousand, are the height of half a thumb and are as luminous as the sun. They live as hermits in the sūrya maṇḍala and travel in front of the sun as birds.

When we no longer argue with reality, the luminous scintillations of the sixty thousand hermits, the quiver of clarity, can be sensed at the fringe of events.

"After rejecting the attachment to one's body one should realise: 'I am everywhere' with firm mind and with undistracted vision, then one attains bliss."

Vijñāna Bhairava 104

"One should imagine that there is no internal organ within me consisting of mind. Then owing to the absence of thoughts one will be freed from all thoughts."

Vijñāna Bhairava 94

"All knowledge is without a cause, without a support and deceptive. In reality this knowledge does not belong to anybody. Contemplating in this way, O Dear One, one becomes Śiva."

Vijñāna Bhairava 99

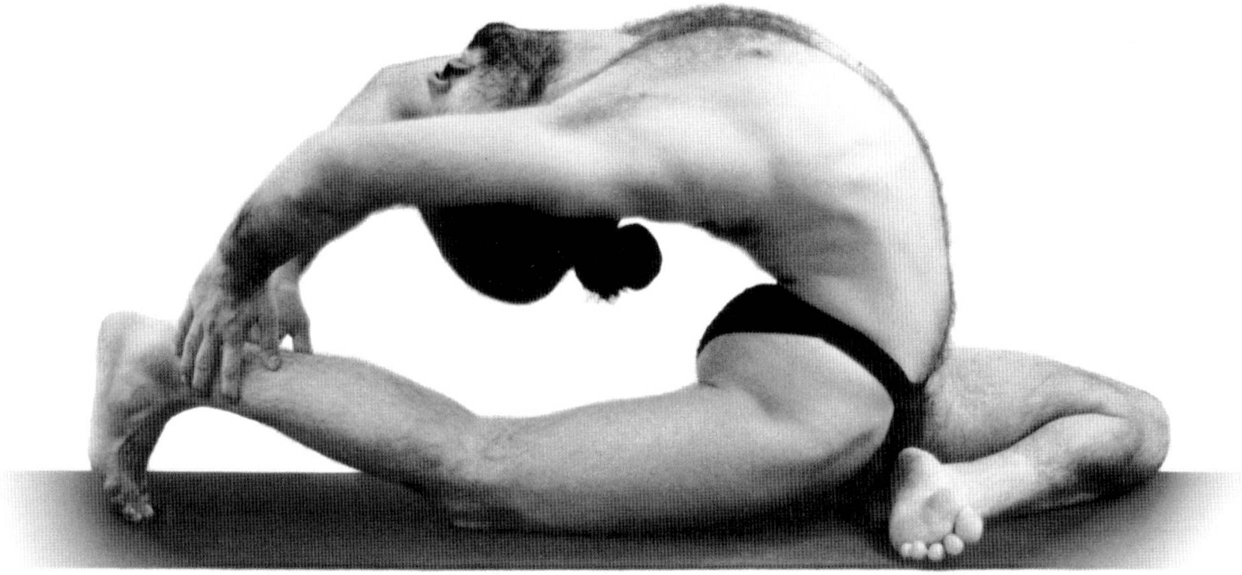

Vālakhilyāsana

Vṛścikāsana 2

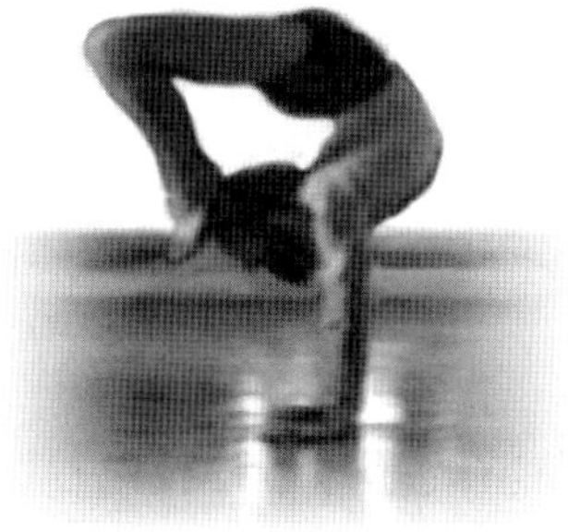

"The One which is characterised as Consciousness is residing in all the bodies; there is no differentiation in anything. Therefore, if a person realises that everything is full of that very Consciousness, he conquers the world of becoming."

Vijñāna Bhairava 100

"If one meditates on the universe as a magic show, or as a painting, or as a moving picture, contemplating on everything in this way, one experiences bliss."

Vijñāna Bhairava 102

• Vṛścikāsana: The Beginning of the Instant

In some āsana, such as the scorpion pose, the feet are in contact with the head. This figure can also be found in other civilisations such as the Olmecs and their Tlatilco acrobat. In his book 'The Art of Yoga', Yogācārya Śrī B.K.S. Iyengar entitles this āsana "Taming one's own pride". The pride of believing we live in separation when everything else in the universe is interdependent, of believing ourself to be body-mind whose apogee is our thinking process, our head. Nisargadatta Mahārāj says that in Marathi, the word for foot signifies the beginning of the instant, where Consciousness gushes forth well before any conceptualisation.

• Gaṇḍa Bheruṇḍāsana: Contemplation of the Dreadful

Bheruṇḍā is one of the eight yoginī who lived as a hermit in the forest, and who looked after the goddess Durgā. They are described as emaciated and ferocious. The term Bheruṇḍā also has the connotation of terrifying. Here, the terrifying face (Gaṇḍa) of the Goddess is contemplated.
The face of the goddess is the absence of our own face. All we think of as being ourselves, from our social mask to our innermost representations and identifications, is wiped away, devoured by this face of darkness. And this is why it is so terrifying!

Vṛścikāsana 1

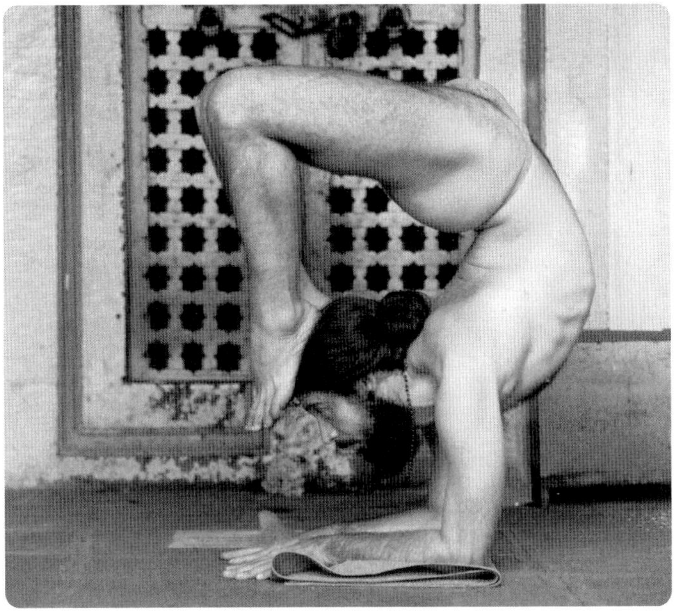

र

Ra
limited knowledge (vidyā)

THE PHONEME RA
IS THE SEED OF FIRE.
IT THEREFORE
HAS THE QUALITY OF
BURNING, BLAZING.

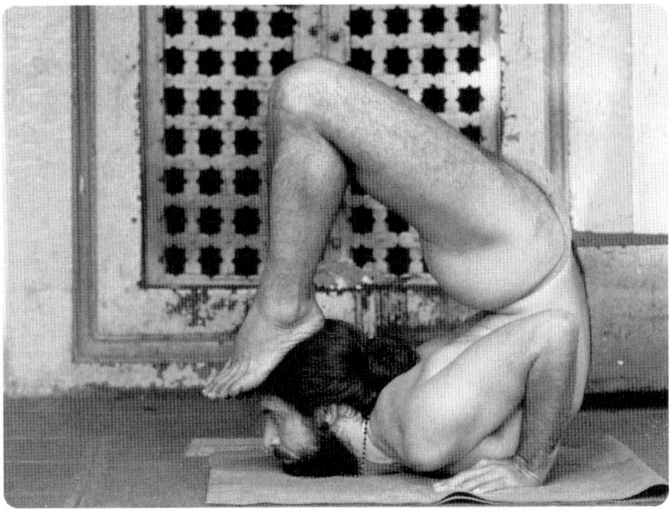

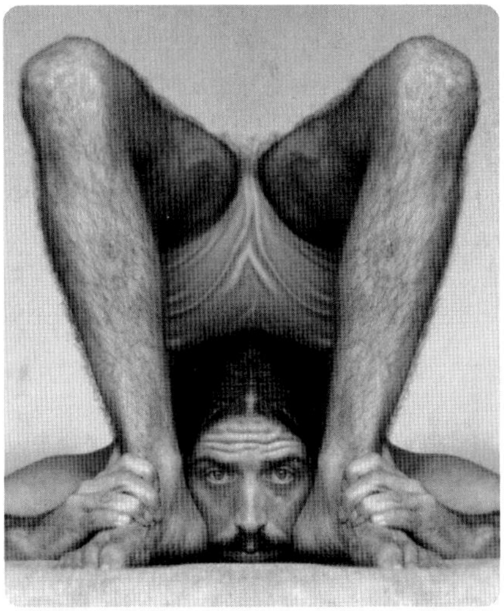

Gaṇḍa Bheruṇḍāsana

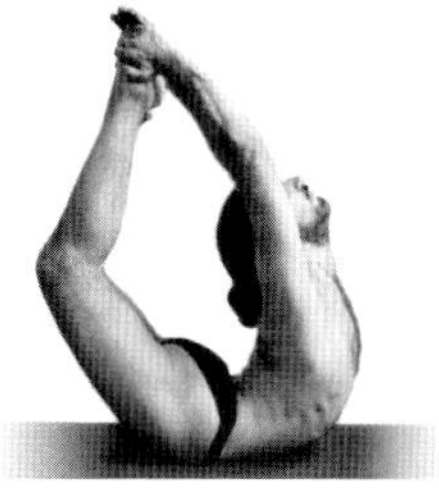

Pādāṅguṣṭha Dhanurāsana ...

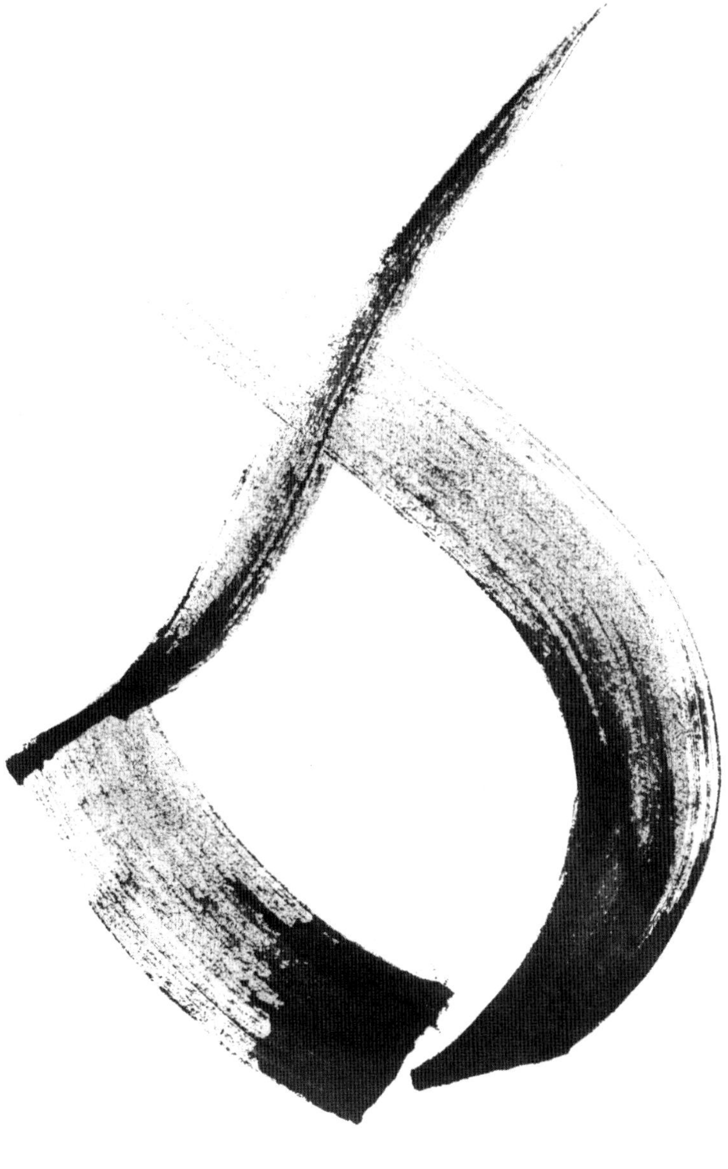

• Pādāṅguṣṭha Dhanurāsana: The Absence of a Target

Wanting to test the skill of his disciples, Droṇa, the famous master of weaponry, summoned them well before daybreak. They knew this place only too well. There was the intimate familiarity of their sweat, their effort, of exercises repeated a thousand times, their pain, their cries and tears mingled with the soil of this arena. It was still dark and cold. Yet they were all there, Kaurava, Pāṇḍava and other princes. They knew they had no chance against Arjuna, but they were ready to prove their superiority over the others. Droṇa was going to test their archery skills. He first called Yudhiṣṭhira.
"Look at the straw bird in that tree. Aim at it and shoot when I give the order."
Yudhiṣṭhira bent the bow, chosen specially for its stiffness, which was an exploit in itself!
"What do you see?"
"I see myself, I see my brothers, I see you, I see the tree and I see the bird."
Droṇa repeated the same question. Yudhiṣṭhira gave the same reply. His arm started to tremble.
Exasperated, Droṇa said to him: *"You are not worthy of shooting. Stand aside."*
Each of the princes was called in turn. All gave a vague reply and were pushed aside in the same way. Then it was Arjuna's turn. He was asked the same question.
"I can see neither you nor the tree. I can only see the bird."
"Describe it to me."
"Impossible. I can only see its eye."
"Shoot."
Arjuna was one with his target. And because there was no longer a target, he could not miss.
Later, before the king and court, Droṇa asked Arjuna to make him a promise:
"If one day we meet as enemies in the battlefield, you must fight me as an enemy."
And this is what happened!

"Freeing the mind of all supports one should not allow any thoughts to arise. Then, O gazelle-eyed Goddess, the state of Bhairava will be attained when the self has merged in the Absolute Self."

VIJÑĀNA BHAIRAVA 108

"Just as waves arise from water, flames from fire and rays from the sun, in the same way the differentiated aspects of the universe have sprung from me, Bhairava."

VIJÑĀNA BHAIRAVA 110

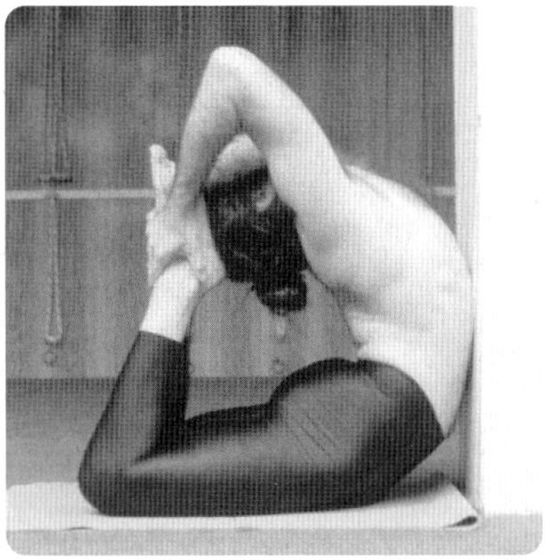

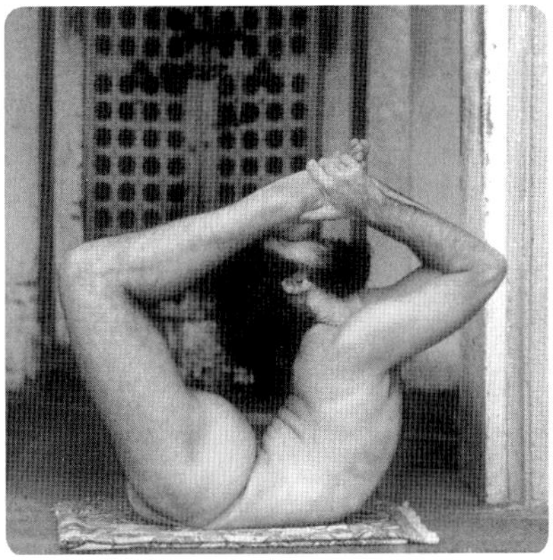

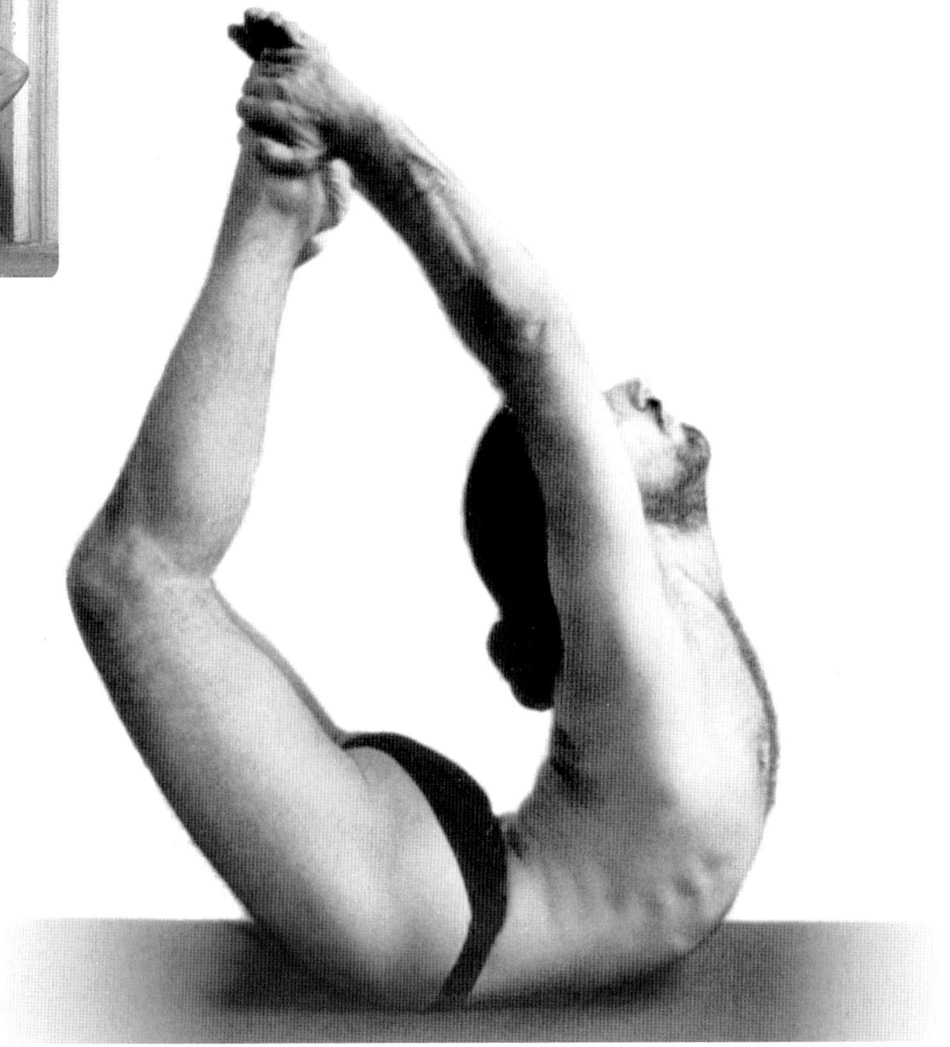

Pādāṅguṣṭha Dhanurāsana

"The reality of Bhairava is present everywhere,
even in common people.
He who knows that nothing exists apart from Him,
attains the non-dual state."

Vijñāna Bhairava 124

• Naṭarājāsana: The Garland of Sounds

In the sound Naṭa there is the phoneme NA, which corresponds to hearing and speech. The phoneme ṬA corresponds to movement and prakṛti. At the end of his dance, Śiva hit his ḍamaru fourteen times thus creating the Maheśvara Sūtra, the womb for the language of the gods (gīrvāṇabhāṣā), the web of the world. Śikṣā is the science of sound and is the first discipline in the Vedāṅga.

According to the Taittirīya Upaniṣad, it has six aspects: syllables (varna), vowels (svara), tempo (mātra), intonation (svarita), diction (sāma) and euphony or harmony between sounds (santāna). The Bhagavad Gītā describes the discipline of speech. Words must not create agitation (anudvegakaram vākyam), they must express truth (satyam), be full of benevolence (priyahitam) and be used to investigate Supreme Reality (svādhyāya).

The first sound in the Māheśvarasūtra is the vowel A. It is said:
"Let the sound A be of the nature of ultimate reality without qualities, and the essence of all things. The sound A leads all the other sounds. It is this sound that illuminates..." Nandikeśvara Kāśikā 3-4

The last sound is 'HA' and ends with the anusvāra (Ṃ), or nasalisation. The phonematic emanation, which is the emanation of the universe, can therefore only be expressed through 'I' (AHAṂ).
"She is known as Mālinī, womb of sounds, where the effervescent and agitated elements mingle. Her beauty is the emission produced by the co-penetration of seeds and wombs, the supreme energy, and She is described as having the universe as her form." Abhinavagupta, Tantrāloka III, 232-233

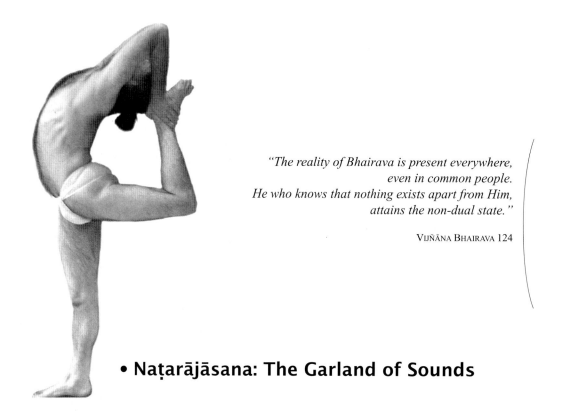

La

limited creativity (kalā)

THE PHONEME LA IS
THE SEED OF THE EARTH.
ITS PREDOMINANT QUALITY IS
THAT OF STABILITY, IMMOBILITY.

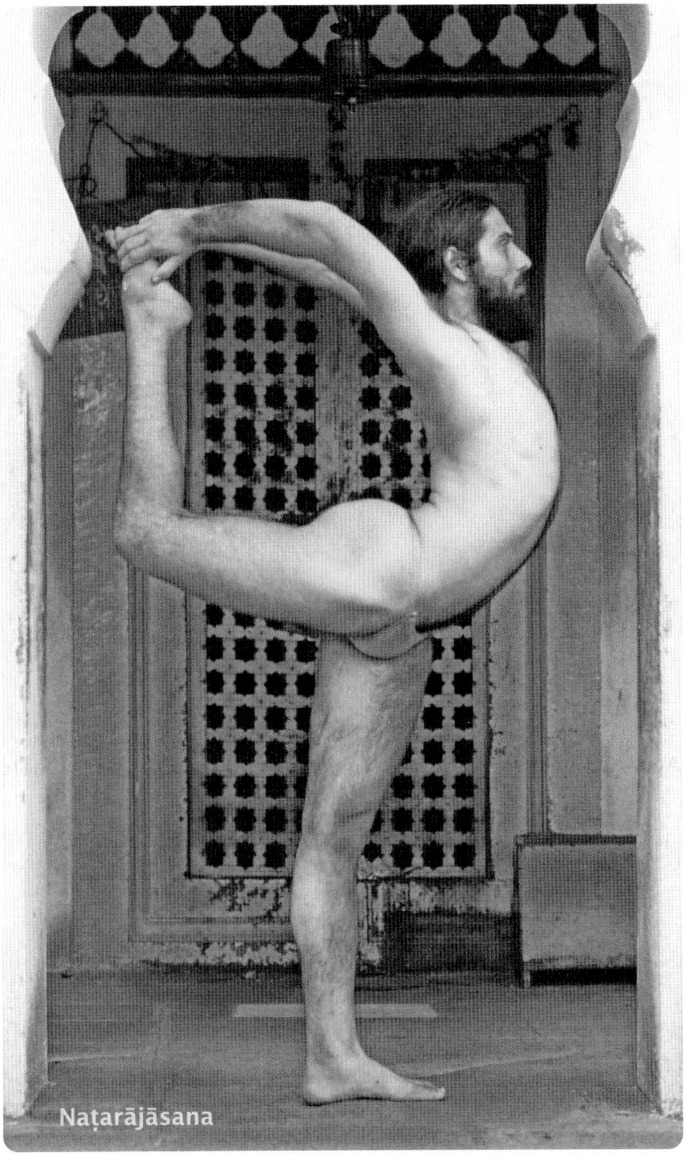
Naṭarājāsana

*"From the sky
of Consciousness
of the Heart springs forth
the dancer Naṭarāja
with his blissful consort,
Freedom, to the delectation
of his devotees who are
thus liberated forever.
Unto that Ānanda Naṭeśa
we do render our
devout salutations."*

ṚBHŪ GĪTĀ I, 2

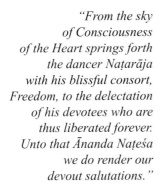

"All this universe is without reality, like a magic show,
for what reality is there in a magic show?
By firmly thinking in this way, one obtains peace."

VIJÑĀNA BHAIRAVA 133

"How can the immutable Self have any knowledge or activity?
All external objects depend on our knowledge of them.
Therefore this world is void."

VIJÑĀNA BHAIRAVA 134

• Śīrṣāsana: Opening of Hearts

All āsana put us into contact with very important junctions where our psychophysical reality is woven and knotted (granthi). Inverted āsana have a privileged action on these regions. Śīrṣāsana opens the pelvic and thoracic diaphragms that unfold mūlabandha and uḍḍiyānabandha. Breathing patterns can be explored in the apānic and samānic regions. Rope Śīrṣāsana enables profound contemplation of these geographies.

"The sun devours all the nectar flowing from the moon, the celestial beauty.
When no more remains, the body decays.
Yet there exists a divine remedy to seal the sun's lips.
Theoretical study of millions of instructions is of no use.
It must be learnt directly from a guru.
When the navel is above and the palate below, then the sun is below the moon.
This is the inverted āsana (Viparīta Karaṇī), and can only be learnt through the instructions of a Guru."

HAṬHAYOGAPRADĪPIKĀ III, 77-78-79

The Seal of Effacement Viparīta Karaṇī Mudrā: Inverted Āsana

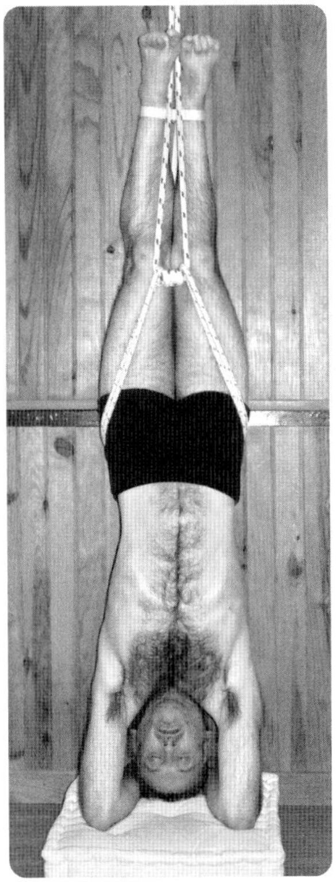

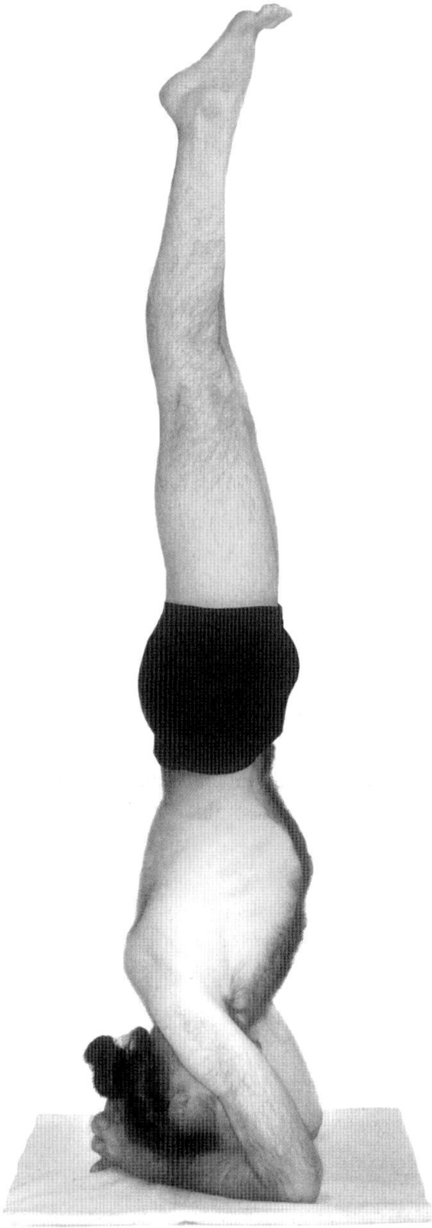

Śīrṣāsana

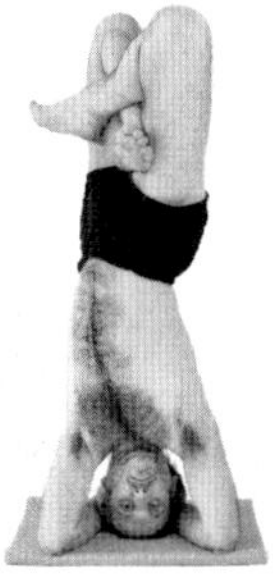

Pārśva Ūrdhva Padmāsana ...

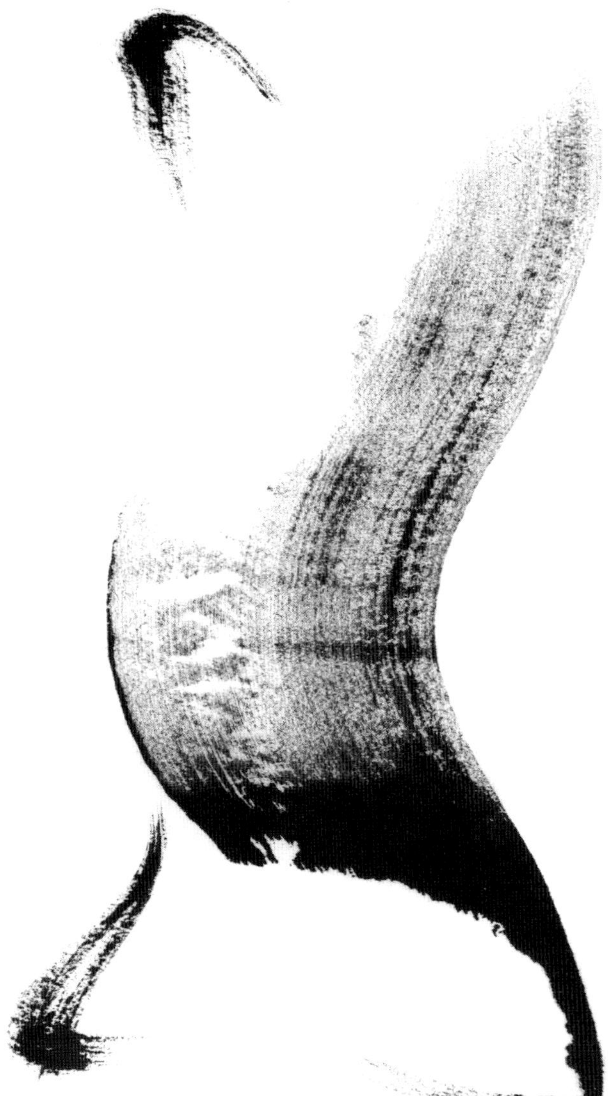

"There is neither bondage nor liberation for me,
they are just like bogies for the fearful.
This world is like a reflection in the mind,
just as the sun is reflected in water."

VIJÑĀNA BHAIRAVA 135

"If one moves round and round with the body
and suddenly falls on the ground, then, when the energy
of agitation comes to an end, the supreme state arises."

VIJÑĀNA BHAIRAVA 111

• Eka Pāda Śīrṣāsana, Pārśva Śīrṣāsana, Parivṛttaikapāda Śīrṣāsana, Pārśva Ūrdhva Padmāsana in Śīrṣāsana: Cleansing and Rinsing of Hearts

The variations of Śīrṣāsana, and especially those in Padmāsana, intensify the rinsing action of the abdominal and pelvic cavities. When this region is explored a knot is revealed, a solidification that contracts our perception into name and form (nāma, rūpa). Here, the senses become agents of separation and agitation (indriya vṛtti). This knot is known as Brahmā Granthi and is located in the mūlādhāra cakra.

In the Yoginīhṛdaya, it is said:
"As for the granthi, it is as though the universe has been threaded upon it, like a precious stone threaded onto a string."
PŪJĀSAṂKETA 91-93

"This worship must come to fruition by penetration of Consciousness, blazing through the twelve knots..."
PŪJĀSAṂKETA 135

व

Va

limitation of time
(māyā kāla)

THIS PHONEME
COMES FROM THE ENERGY
OF AWAKENING U
AND THE WITHOUT-EQUAL A.
IT IS THE SEED OF WATER AND,
ACCORDING TO THE TANTRĀLOKA,
CAUSES EMANATION TO RAIN DOWN.

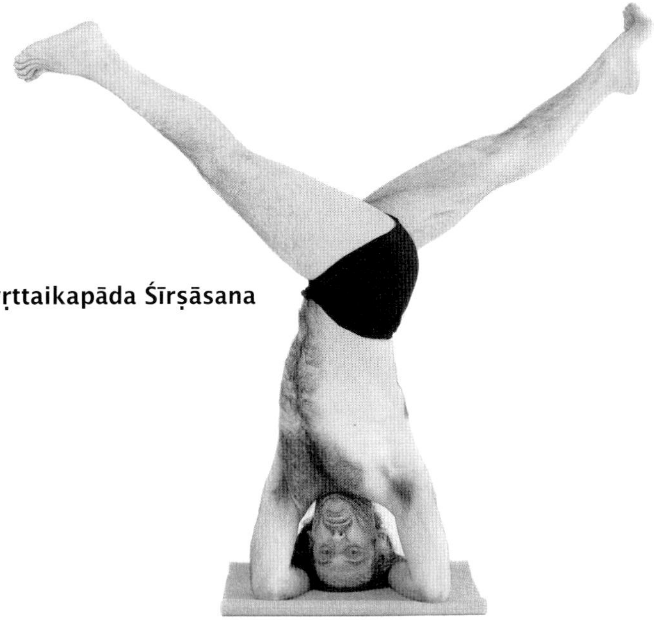

Parivṛttaikapāda Śīrṣāsana

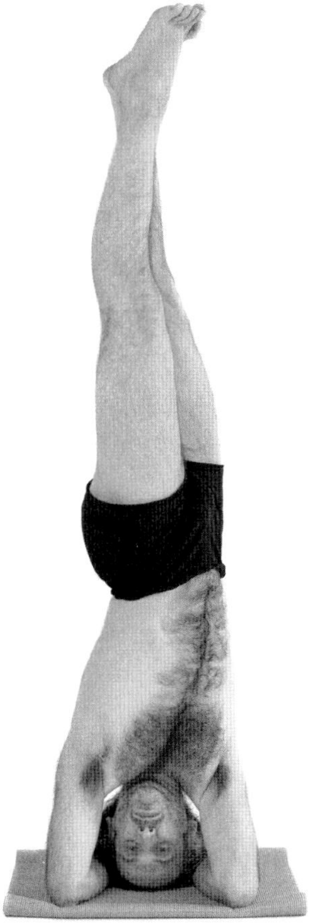

Pārśva Śīrṣāsana

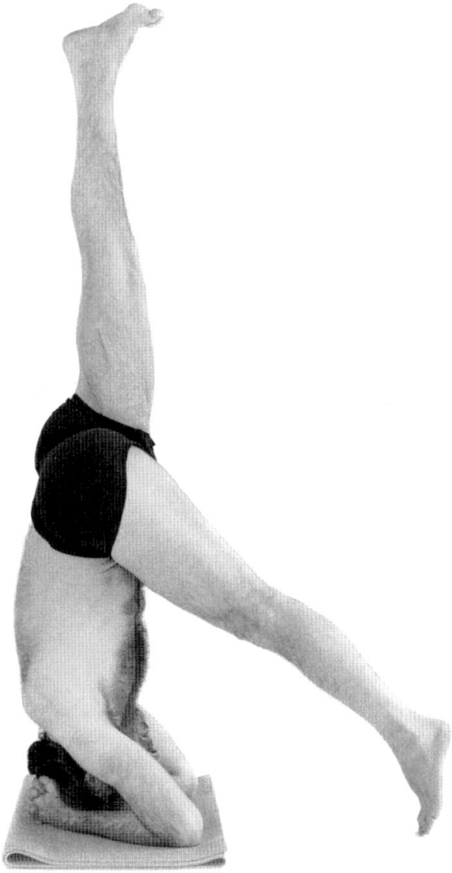

Eka Pāda Śīrṣāsana

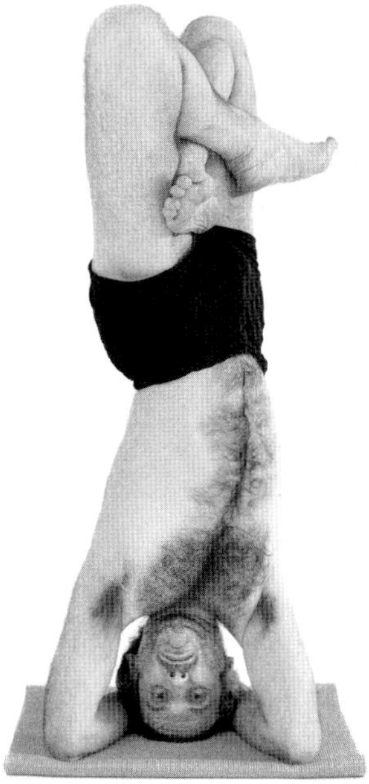

Pārśva Ūrdhva Padmāsana in Śīrṣāsana

• Sarvāṅgāsana, Halāsana: Totality of the Terrain and the Prāṇic Plough

In Sarvāṅgāsana and Halāsana the vocal diaphragm is explored. The entire area of the shoulders, neck, upper part of the head, and throat are released, thus allowing jālandharabandha to unfold.

In these āsana, as well as in Śīrṣāsana, there is a shift from frontal brain or verbal perception, which dissects the world into categories, to the much more holistic perception of the primitive or back brain. They thus participate in cerebral integration, where there is harmony of perception between the two hemispheres and the so-called internal and external realities.

When doing Sarvāṅgāsana on a chair, the space of the chest becomes vast. The dorsal region is fully alert and supports the breastbone. There is a feeling of fullness in the armpits. Supported Halāsana lets us connect with the ease in the lower back. Since the thighbones are supported, the lower back becomes very passive, almost meditative. Here the abdomen takes on a very specific shape. It becomes possible to contemplate the abdominal cavity and the moving back of the abdomen towards the spine, creating a movement of resorption that is very pacifying. In this āsana, the breathing very quickly becomes cellular, almost foetal, as though still bathing in the amniotic liquid.

The configuration of these two āsana done with support allows the jālandharabandha to unfold spontaneously, and the frontal region of the head is able to surrender completely into the space of the heart. *"The three binds are achieved with ease, spontaneously, and thus the functions of the mind go into a state of suspension."* (Haṭhayogapradīpikā I, 42)

"Knowledge illumines everything in this world;
and the Self is the one who illumines. Since they have the same nature,
knowledge and the known should be contemplated as one."

Vijñāna Bhairava 137

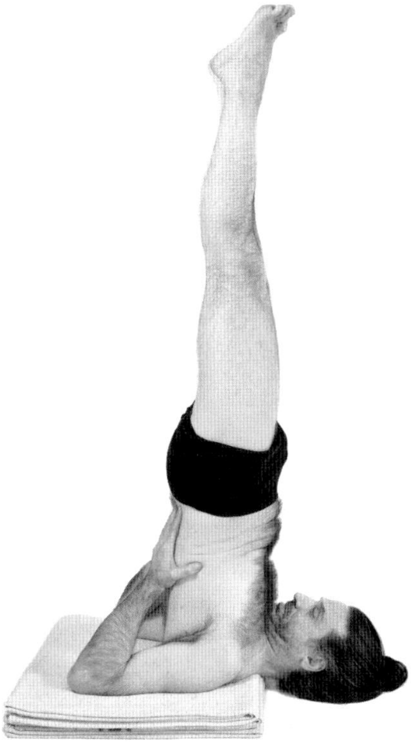

Sarvāṅgāsana

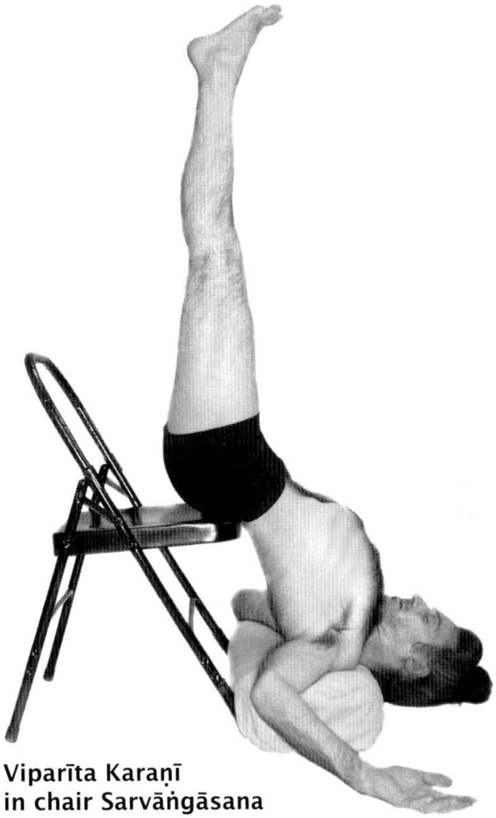

Viparīta Karaṇī
in chair Sarvāṅgāsana

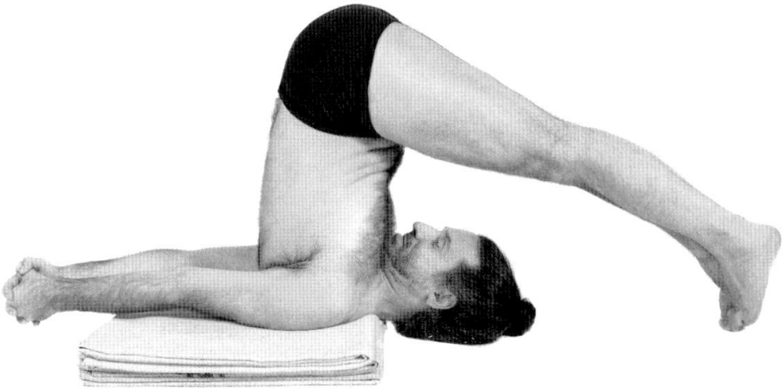

Halāsana

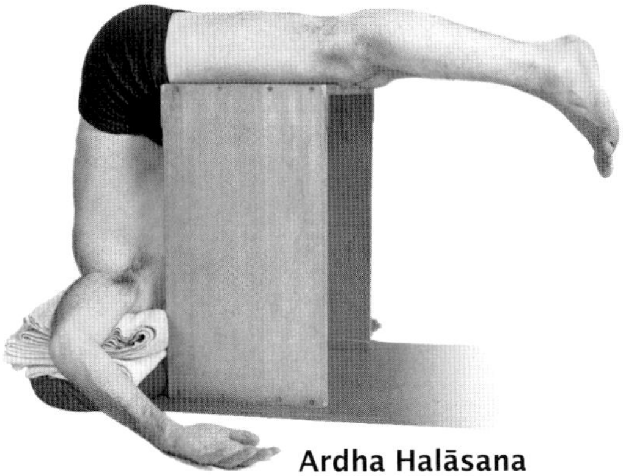

Ardha Halāsana

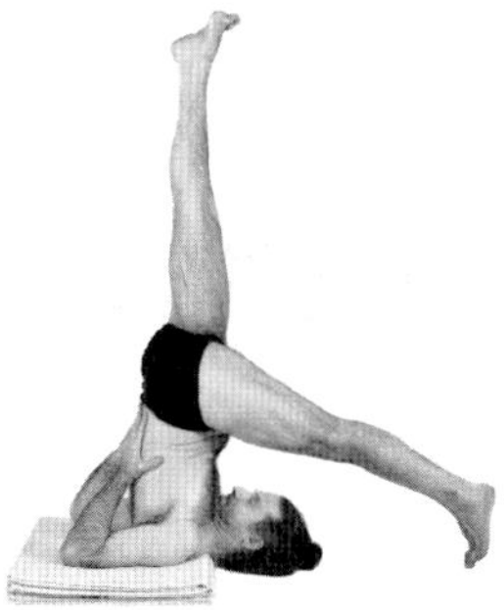

Eka Pāda Sarvāṅgāsana ...

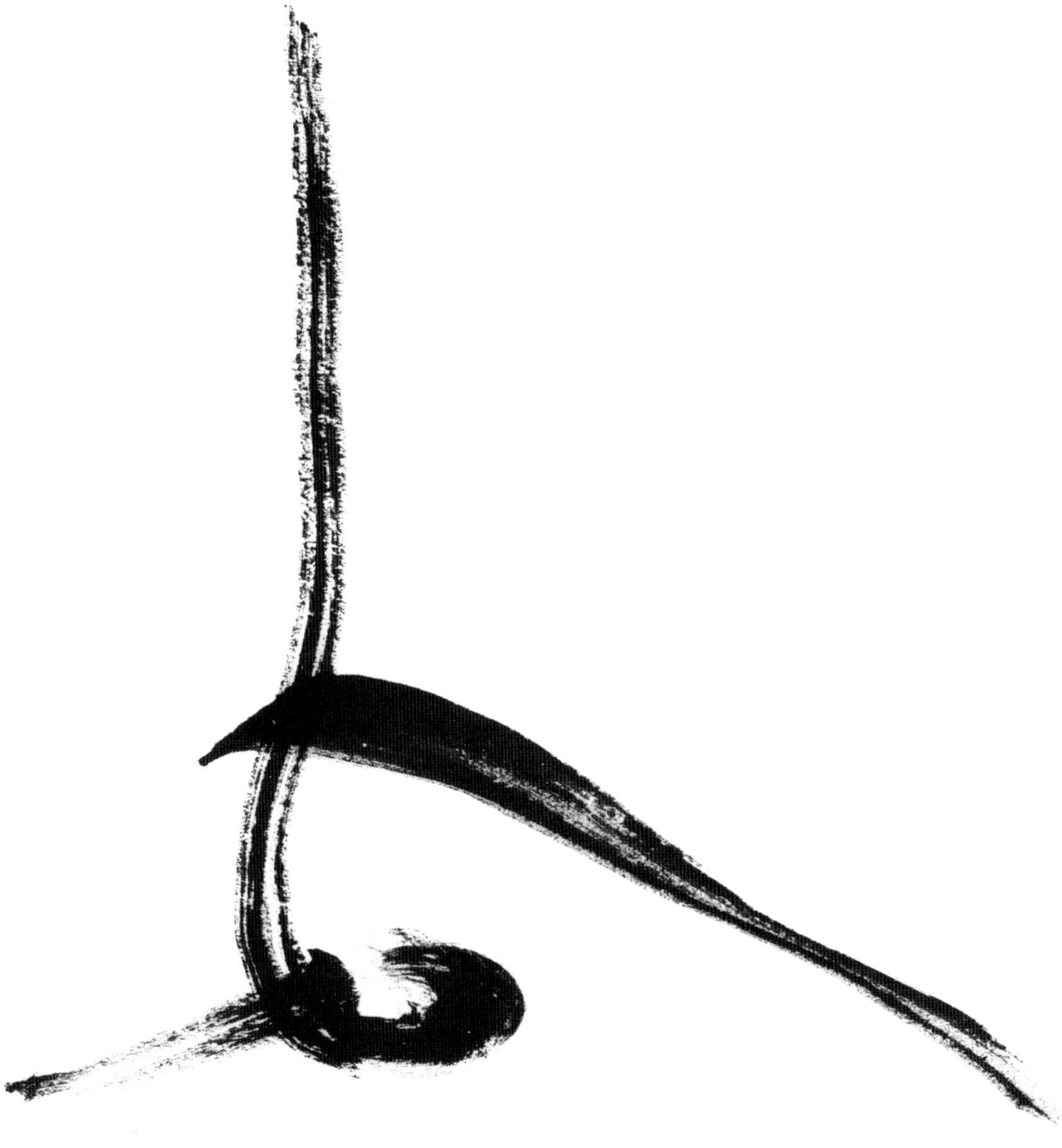

श

Śa

pure knowledge (śuddavidyā)
Balance of 'I am this'
and 'this I am'

"The spontaneous awareness of being is the supreme practice.
That which resonates spontaneously in the space
of the heart is the only mantra."

Vijñāna Bhairava 145

• Eka Pāda Sarvāṅgāsana, Pārśva Sarvāṅgāsana, Ūrdhva Padmāsana in Sarvāṅgāsana, Piṇḍāsana in Sarvāṅgāsana: Cutting the Throat's Knot (Viṣṇu Granthi)

These variations, like those of Śīrṣāsana, cleanse the abdominal and pelvic cavities. Sarvāṅgāsana, Halāsana and their variations of intensification are a contemplation of the throat's knot (Viṣṇu Granthi), where named reality solidifies, actualised by the gushing forth of bodily speech (vaikarī) and concept.

There are two worlds, or planes of Consciousness, located in the region of the throat. At its base is the eternal Śiva (Sadāśiva), ocean of subjectivity of the 'I'. The waves of this ocean are the universe. At the centre of the throat lies the world of Nīlakaṇṭha, or 'the one with the blue throat'. Nīlakaṇṭha is an auspicious form of Śiva whose function is to protect. When the asura and deva churned the primordial ocean a terrible poison was produced. Śiva drank it. Pārvatī (Śakti) squeezed Śiva's throat (jālandharabandha) to stop the poison reaching his stomach. This is why his neck is blue.

"The eighth (ādhāra) is the support at the throat. The breath must be stopped at the root of the throat by means of the chin. The vital energy (vāyu) in Iḍā and Piṅgalā then becomes stable."

Gorakṣanātha, Siddhasiddhāntapaddhati II, 17

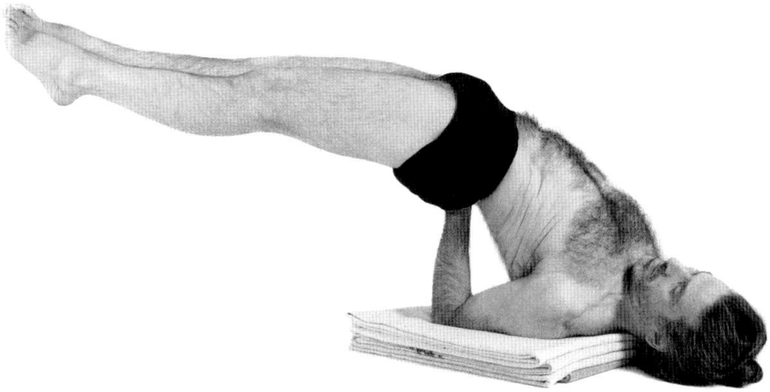

Pārśva Sarvāṅgāsana

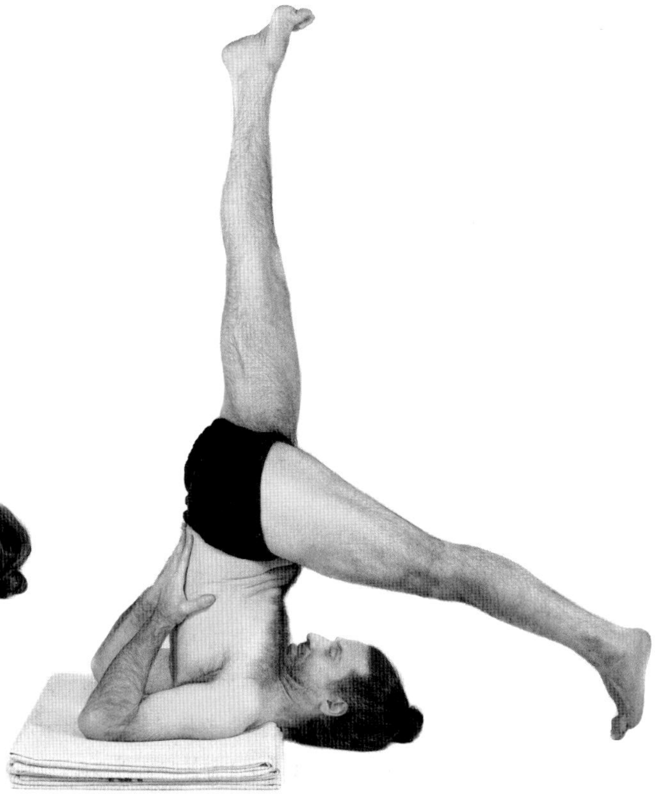

Eka Pāda Sarvāṅgāsana

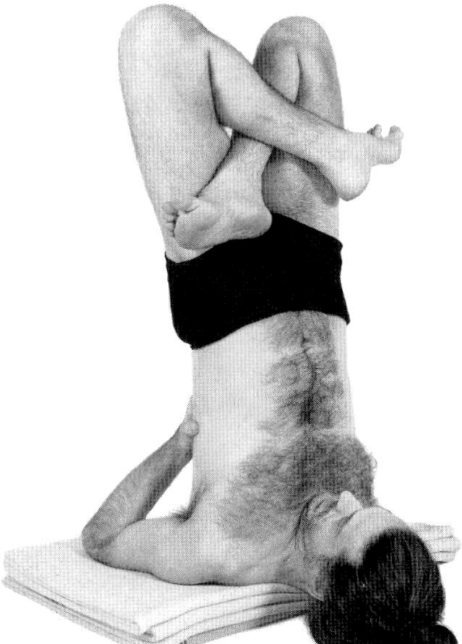

Ūrdhva Padmāsana in Sarvāṅgāsana

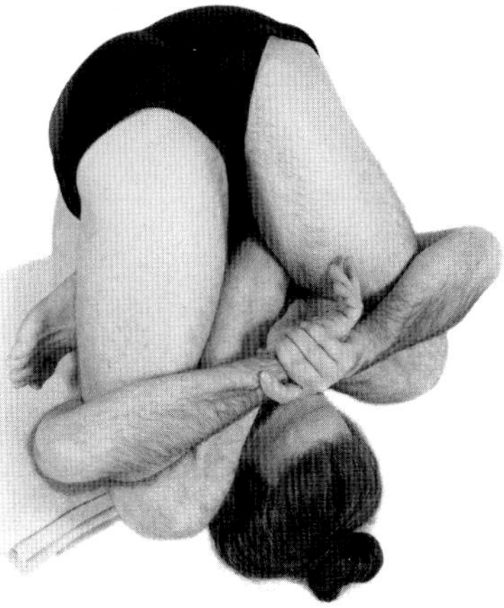

Piṇḍāsana in Sarvāṅgāsana

• Setu Bandha Sarvāṅgāsana: Bridge and Fluvial Confluence

This āsana is also known as the unfolded or dancing peacock (Uttāna Mayūrāsana). It is told in the Uttara Rāmāyaṇa how the peacock obtained its beauty. At the head of his army of rākṣasa, Rāvaṇa wanted to subject all the other kings to his authority. At the foot of Mount Uśīravīra he set his heart on subjugating a king engaged in ascetic practices. The gods were present to receive their offerings. Upon seeing Rāvaṇa they camouflaged themselves. Indra took on the form of a peacock. It is said that Indra was smitten with this bird. *"Until now you have been blue. From now on your feathers will take on different colours. I shall also give you my thousand eyes. You will be immunised against all disease. Whoever kills you will perish quickly. You will dance at the start of the rainy season. Everyone will welcome you with joy and wonder."*

Indra is known as 'the one with immense power', 'sovereign of the heavens', and also 'the one who gives rain', the symbol of fertility and food. His father is Dyauṣ Pitṛ, the sky, and his mother Pṛthivī, the earth. He is also holder of the thunderbolt. All these qualities are found in the attitude of the peacock, Uttāna Mayūrāsana. In the Vijñāna Bhairava, it is said: *"By meditating on the five voids of the senses, which are like the various colours of the peacock's feathers, the yogi enters in the Heart of the absolute Void."* (Śloka 32)

Setu Bandha is the action of unfolding various bridges between the gross and subtle bodies. Their junction is the diaphragm. The diaphragm becomes a heart which, when fully open, favours the flow of emotions. Without this flow, the energy of emotion becomes the thought of emotion, emotivity. In this āsana another solidification is encountered, which too is called Viṣṇu Granthi, the knot of the heart. It is here we create strategies aimed at emotionally reassuring ourselves, as well as the desire to organise and maintain the resulting structures through traditions and rituals.

In Setu Bandha Sarvāṅgāsana we learn how to unfold the three bandha: Mūlabandha, Uḍḍiyānabandha and Jālandhara-bandha. Jālandharabandha unfolds spontaneously when a support is used. The opening of the chest allows the frontal brain to be pacified. Here, we encounter another knot, Rudra Granthi, located between the eyebrows. It is here time contracts through Iḍā and Piṅgalā, the lunar and solar paths. Supported Setu Bandha Sarvāṅgāsana enables in-depth contemplation of the flow of the vāyu and of their different locations and confluences. In Uttāna Padma Mayūrāsana, ablutions are done in the fish's belly. *"Where both currents gather in the lake of the fish's belly, simply bathing there ensures liberation."* (Kṛtyakalpatara, Tīrthavivecanakāṇḍa, Commentary on the Liṅga Purāṇa)

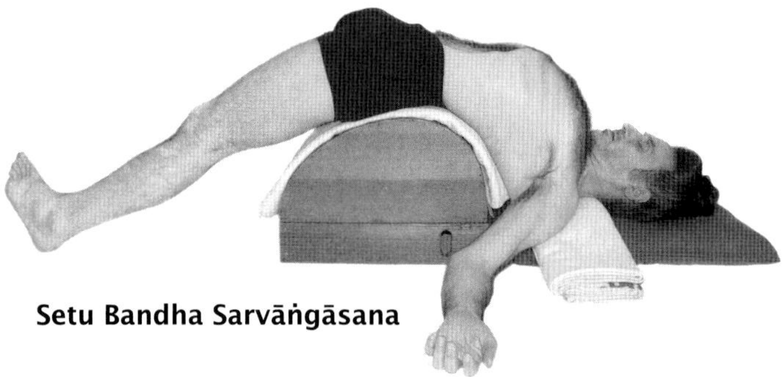

Setu Bandha Sarvāṅgāsana

"O Dear One, when the mind,
the individual consciousness,
the vital energy and the limited self,
when these four have disappeared,
then the nature of Bhairava appears."

Vijñāna Bhairava 138

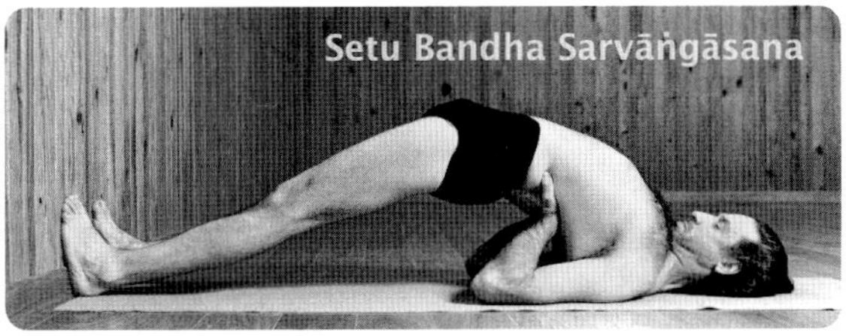

Setu Bandha Sarvāṅgāsana

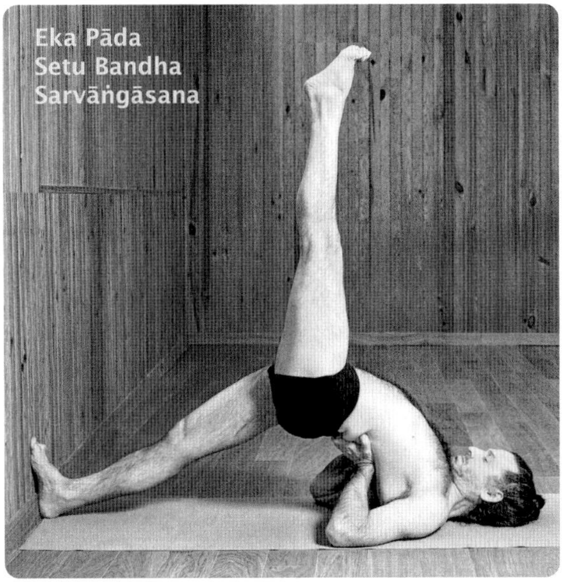

Eka Pāda
Setu Bandha
Sarvāṅgāsana

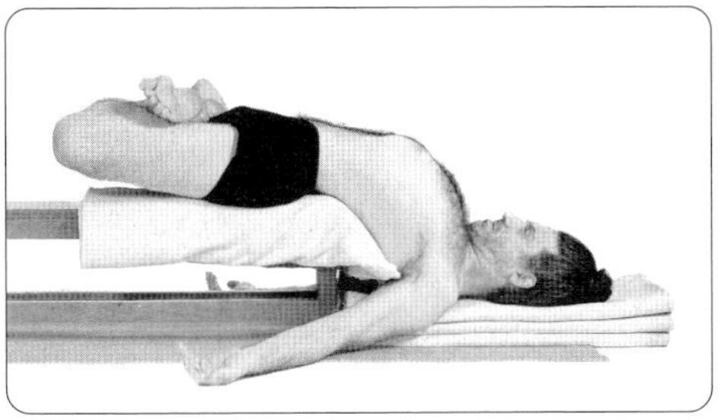

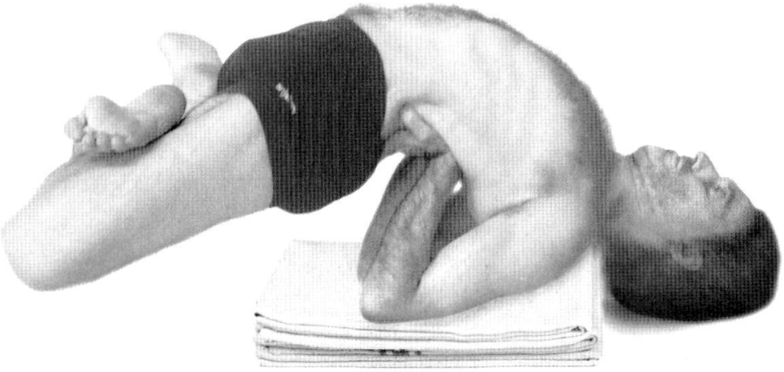

Uttāna Padma Mayūrāsana

"When Consciousness awakens to itself
and is full of its own awareness and vitality,
it unfolds the universe, its own reflection.
We call it Mudrā as it delights and unfolds the universe."

YOGINĪHṚDAYA I, 56

"That which blossoms out"

Abhinavagupta defines mudrā (mud: joy, ra: to give) as that which reflects our own nature in the body itself. *"That which blossoms out"* is the etymological meaning of the Sanskrit word 'hasta' (hand). This blossoming takes on the multiple forms of creation and is codified in a set of gestures and attitudes. In scriptures pertaining to dramaturgy, no less than 115 mudrā are described! These mudrā are merely reminders of different energies.

"Wherever the hands go, the eyes follow; attention is wherever the eyes are.
The energy unfolds wherever attention blossoms, and with it the vibrant rapture."
NĀṬYA ŚĀSTRA

They are grouped according to the use of two hands (saṃyutahasta) or one hand (asaṃyutahasta). There are gestures used by gods and goddesses (devatāhasta), the different positions of the hands suggesting the ten incarnations of Viṣṇu (daśāvatārahasta), nine deities of the constellations (navagrahahasta) and eight guardians of the cardinal directions (dikpālakahasta). Each finger becomes the incarnation of an elementary, energetic or divine quality. The different positions of the fingers are thus an evocation of these different qualities. The thumb corresponds to the element of fire, the index finger to the element of air, the middle finger to the element of ether, the ring finger to the element of earth, and the little finger to the element of water. When the thumb is joined to the tip of a finger, the corresponding element is stabilised. When the thumb touches the base or root of a finger, the corresponding element is increased. When the tip of a bent finger touches the base of the thumb and the thumb folds and presses lightly on the same finger (as in Sūrya Mudrā), then the corresponding element is decreased.

Several mudrā and their respective evocations are given in the following pages.

The Great Astonishment: Mudrā

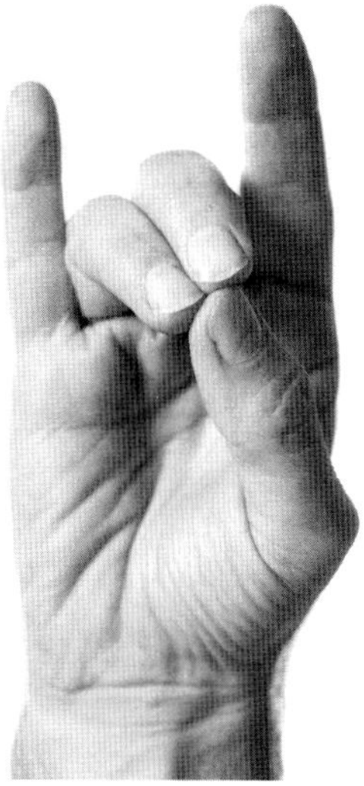

Apāna Mudrā
evocation of apānavāyu

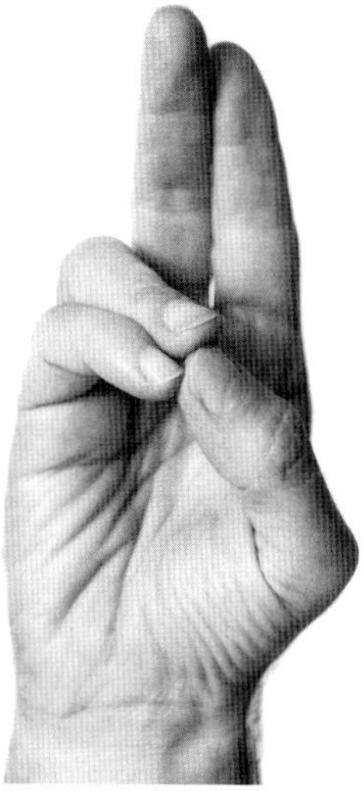

Prāṇa Mudrā
evocation of prāṇavāyu

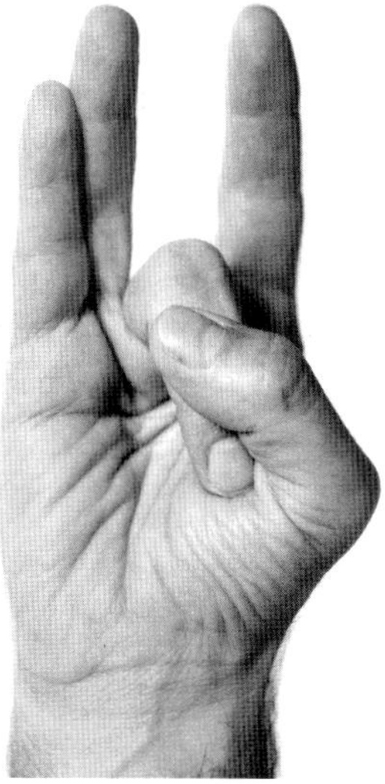

Śūnya Mudrā
evocation of the element of space

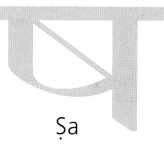

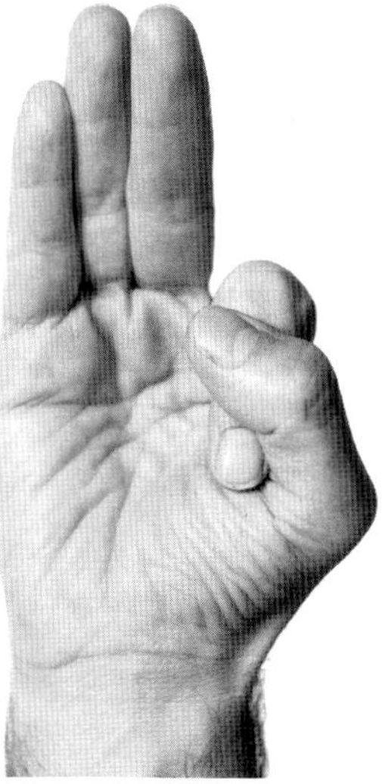

Vāyu Mudrā
evocation of the element of air

ष

Ṣa

The Lord as subjectivity, turned outwards.
The universe is the expansion of my subjectivity (Īśvara)

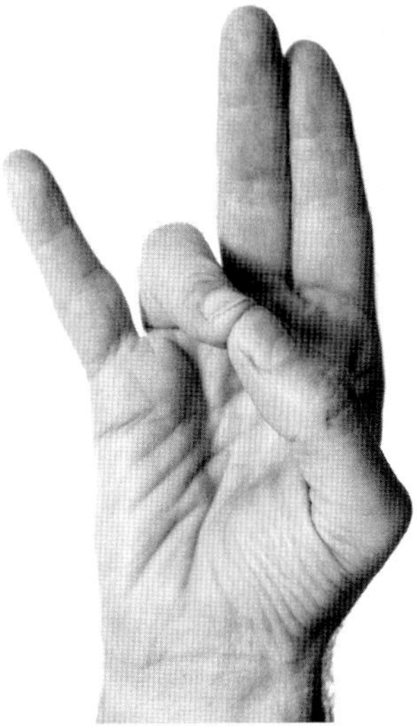

Pṛthivī Mudrā
evocation of the element of earth

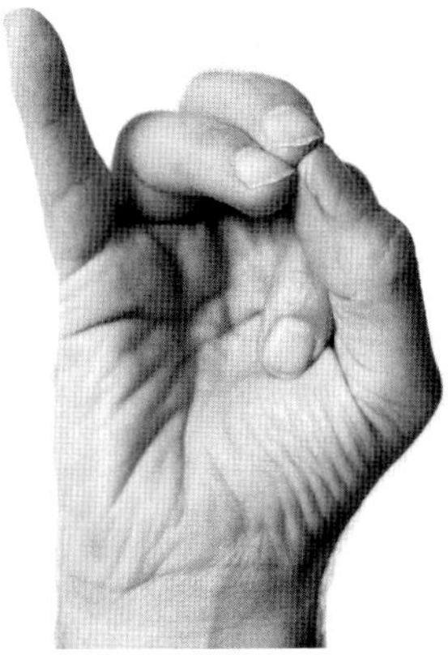

Mṛtsanjīvinī Mudrā
evocation and protection
of the heart

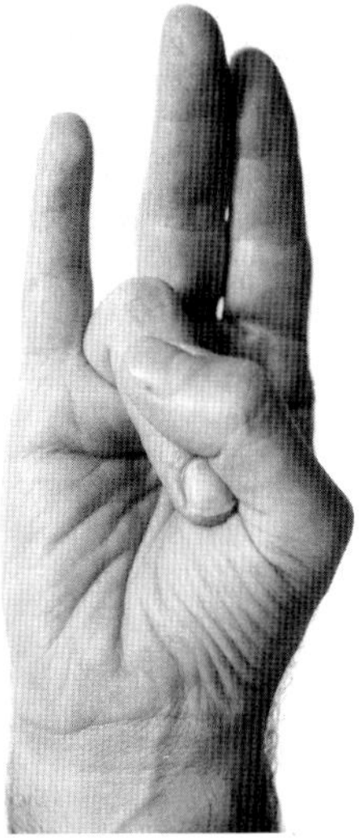

Sūrya Mudrā
evocation of the sun

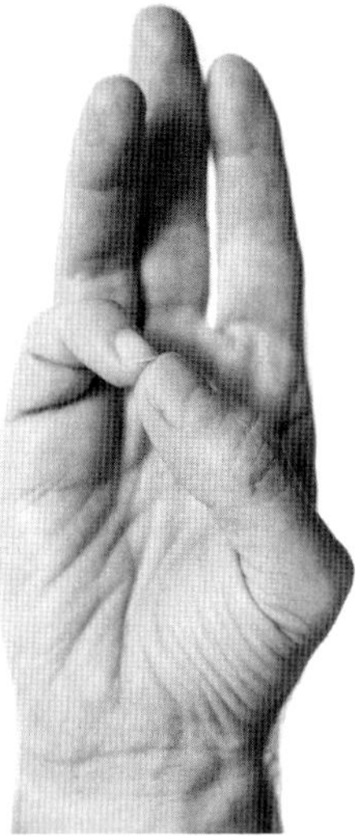

Varuṇa Mudrā
evocation of the element
of water through its guardian deity

Surabhi Mudrā
evocation of the celestial cow
(one of the most important of the
24 mudrā that must be performed
before reciting the Gāyatrī Mantra
and performing the eight mudrā
that follow its recitation)

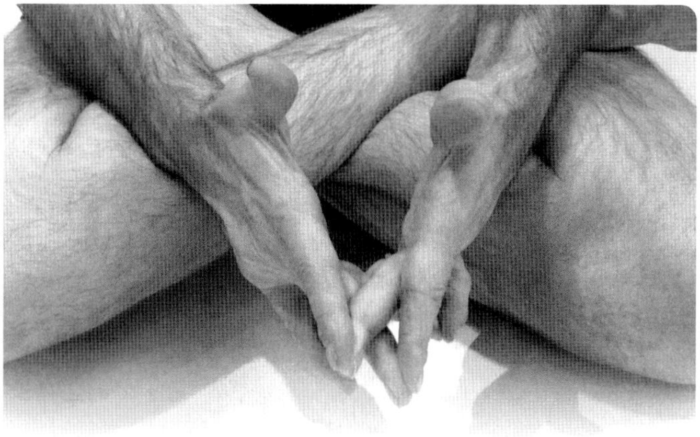

Liṅga Mudrā
"This liṅga, through the union of the seed and the womb, radiates beauty, is the heart of the yoginī and generates an inexpressible Consciousness."
ABHINAVAGUPTA, TANTRĀLOKA V, 121

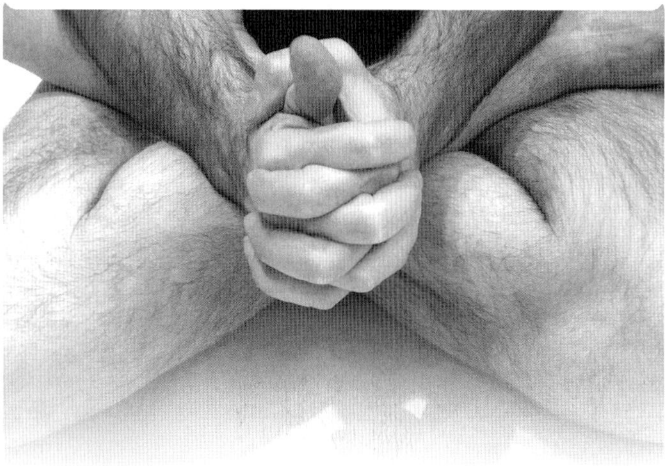

Yoni Mudrā
evocation of the womb
"The lord calls this central wheel 'the mouth of the yoginī' since from her the transmission of the spiritual lineage is founded, and from her one obtains Knowledge. She is beyond duality, cannot be described and as such, it is said, moves from mouth to mouth. Since she is our own Consciousness, how can we describe her?"
ABHINAVAGUPTA, TANTRĀLOKA XXIX, 124-125

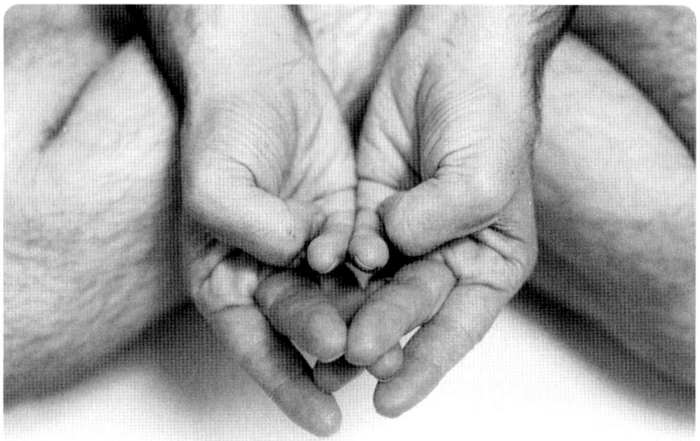

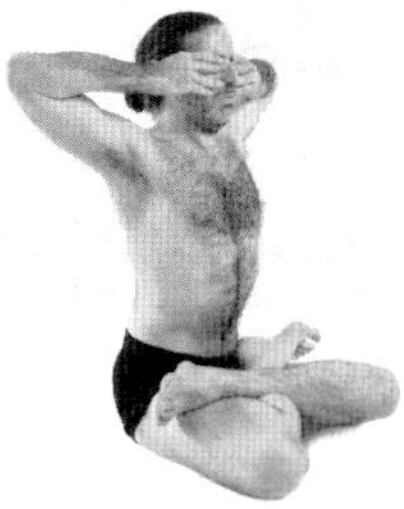

ṣaṇmukhī mudrā ...

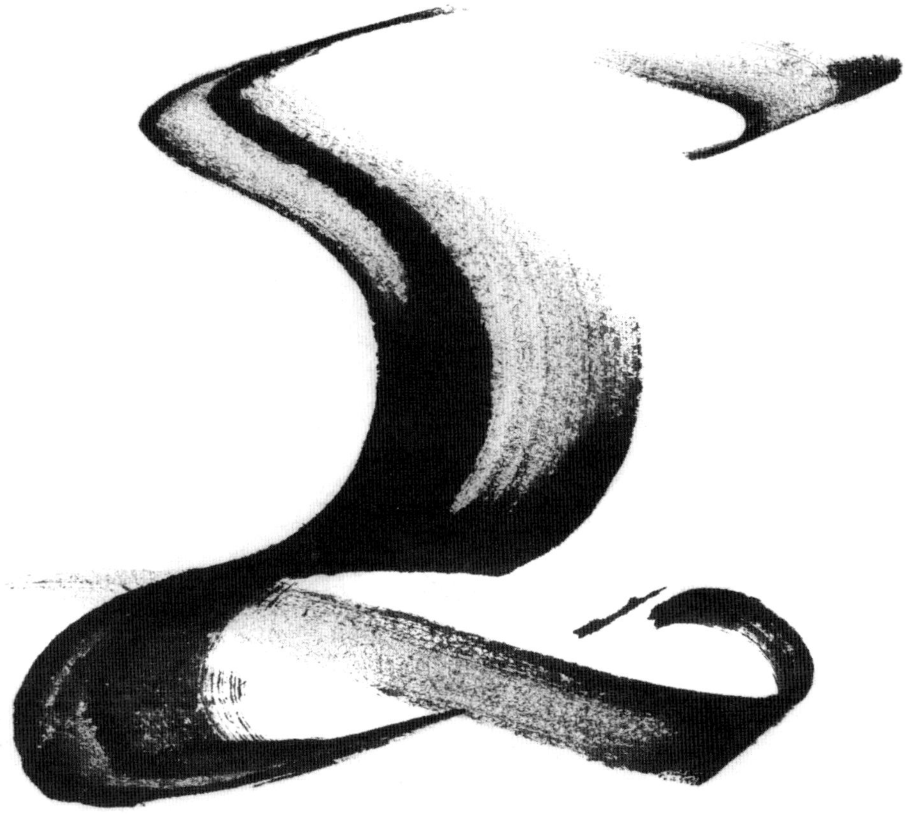

"At the time of making assertions like 'I am' or 'This is mine',
remain at the source of their expression, in the pure
vibration of 'I', and be peaceful."

VIJÑĀNA BHAIRAVA 131

• Ṣaṇmukhī Mudrā: Facelessness

"The resonance that is heard is that of the unstruck sound." HAṬHAYOGAPRADĪPIKĀ IV, 100

It is known as the mudrā of effacement, the seal of facelessness (Parāṇmuhkī Mudrā), of the womb (Yoni Mudrā) and of the auspicious one (Śambhu Mudrā). According to the Gheraṇḍasaṃhitā, it is secretly guarded by the Tantra and is not revealed like the Veda, Śāstra and Purāṇa, which are only courtesans. What is this secret that is nothing but the evidence of our absence as an image and of our presence in this absence? Are we able to see our own face? The eyes freeze what is perceived in a shape and the ears imprison it in a name. When we can neither see nor hear, we are then able to listen to the inner resonance (nādānusandhāna). All yoga techniques are fundamentally ways of listening to this sound, this resonance. The resonance of form (rūpa) takes us back to the vibration (nāda), which takes us back to undifferentiated Consciousness (bindu).

"Oh Mother, the entire body and all its organs, both inside and out,
You lead them all to the void of Consciousness. Such is for us the seal (mudrā)." CIDGAGANACANDRIKĀ

• Mahā Mudrā (mud: joy; rā: to give): The Seal of Joy, The Kiss of Death

"Having closed the throat in Jālandharabandha, the vāyu must be held in a rising fashion.
Like a coiled snake when struck by a rod suddenly straightens itself out like a stick, the Śakti too,
which was coiled, suddenly becomes straight. Then the state of death is known in the two nāḍī."
HAṬHAYOGAPRADĪPIKĀ III, 10-11-12

At the origin of the various sealing techniques is the intuition that everything reflecting our primordial nature in the body is a mudrā. The idea of being happy is fundamentally a bourgeois idea to create a world in which there is no sadness or pain. The tension in our societies is not surprising since their citizens live with the illusion of a paradise that never materialises. There is always something missing. The Mahā Mudrā replaces happiness, and that which appears to be its opposite, in a joyful vision that encompasses them both. In mudrā, the real and the body are one. There is only the body of reality.

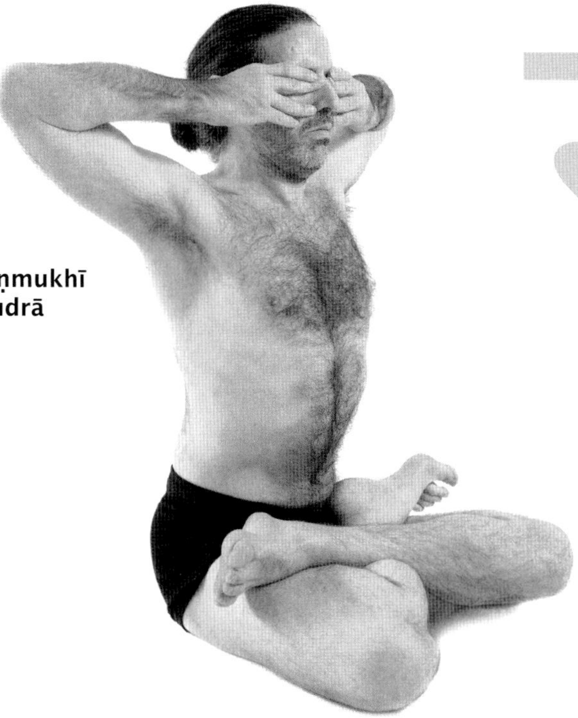

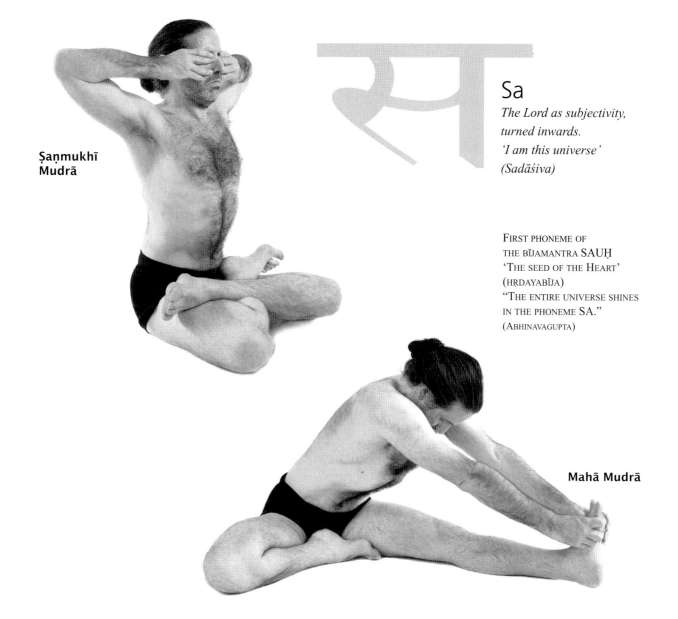

Ṣaṇmukhī Mudrā

स

Sa

The Lord as subjectivity,
turned inwards.
'I am this universe'
(Sadāśiva)

First phoneme of
the bījamantra SAUḤ
'The seed of the Heart'
(hṛdayabīja)
"The entire universe shines
in the phoneme SA."
(Abhinavagupta)

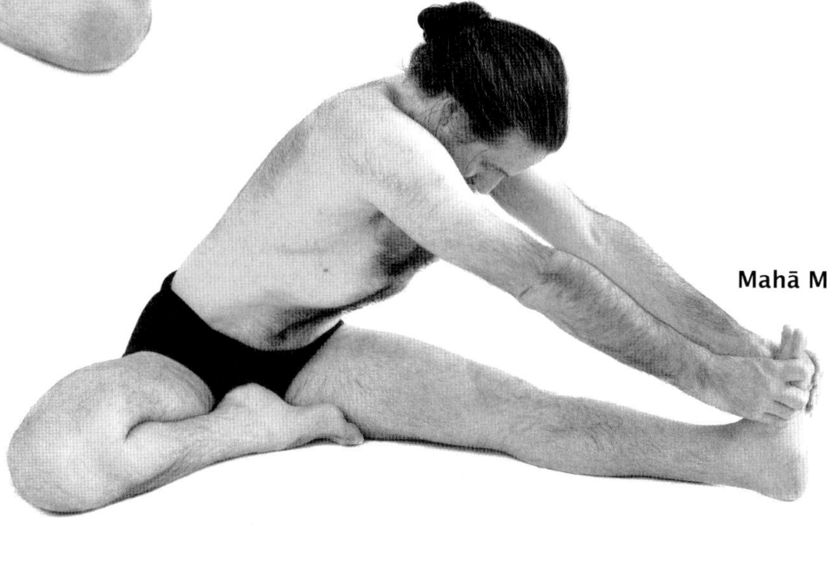

Mahā Mudrā

*"The exhaled breath murmurs 'Sa', and the inhaled 'Ha'.
This threnody Soham is repeated endlessly. And so this chant of the Goddess
is recited effortlessly, and is difficult only for the foolish."*
VIJÑĀNA BHAIRAVA 155-156

*"The exhaling breath (prāṇa) should ascend and the inhaling breath (jīva)
should descend, both forming a visarga consisting of two points.
Their state of fullness is found by fixing them in the two places of their origin."*
VIJÑĀNA BHAIRAVA 24

*"O Bhairavī, by focussing one's awareness on the two voids at the end of the internal
and external breath, thereby the glorious form of Bhairava is revealed through Bhairavī."*
VIJÑĀNA BHAIRAVA 25

*"The Energy of Breath should neither move out nor enter; when the centre unfolds
by the dissolution of thoughts, then one attains the nature of Bhairava."*
VIJÑĀNA BHAIRAVA 26

*"When the Energy of Breath is retained either outside or inside,
at the end of this practice the peaceful state is revealed by means of Śakti."*
VIJÑĀNA BHAIRAVA 27

*"Contemplate the breath like a wave of light rising up from your base (mūlādhāra)
and which dissolves into the upper confluence (ūrdhvadvādaśānta: brahmarandra).
Then the state of Bhairava will awaken."*
VIJÑĀNA BHAIRAVA 28

*"By the coming together of the two breaths, at the extreme point, either within or outside
the body the yogi becomes capable of experiencing the rise of the knowledge of harmony."*
VIJÑĀNA BHAIRAVA 64

*"Closing all the openings of the senses, by the slow upward rise of the Energy of Breath,
one feels a sensation like the movement of ants. At that time the supreme joy is revealed."*
VIJÑĀNA BHAIRAVA 67

A certain silence is needed to observe one's respiration become breath, as well as to observe its colourations. The mind's hunger and thirst must become silent. Āsana have prepared the different regions and spaces of the body, first by their awakening and then by their resorption. They enable the body's constellations to be seated in their source. Observing the breath in its different patterns becomes a three-savoured offering to Consciousness. There is the savour of vacuity with exhalation, the savour of 'I am-ness' with inhalation, and the stability of these states during retention.

The Sacrifice of Breath: Prāṇāgnihotra

"The dissolution of the phenomenal world is called exhalation, the realisation of 'I am' is called inhalation, and the stability of this state is retention. This is the essence of prāṇāyāma for the sage, whilst for the fool it is only torture to the nose."
Śaṅkarācārya,
Aparokṣānubhūti 119-120

"Kālī, who devours Time (Kālasaṃkarṣiṇī) and who dwells at the tip of the nose, is constantly measuring inhalations and exhalations, thus enticing the three-fold time at the bottom of the heart. With the inhalations she induces it to enter, by suspending the breath she controls it, and with the exhalations she consumes it. By rising up the vertical breath she finally devours it completely, in an instant. This power of will, who is called Supreme, who awakens the three energies of will, knowledge and action, is worthy of worship as she devours all the vital breath, which is the foundation of time."

Abhinavagupta quoting a Tantra
Tantrāloka XV, 336-338

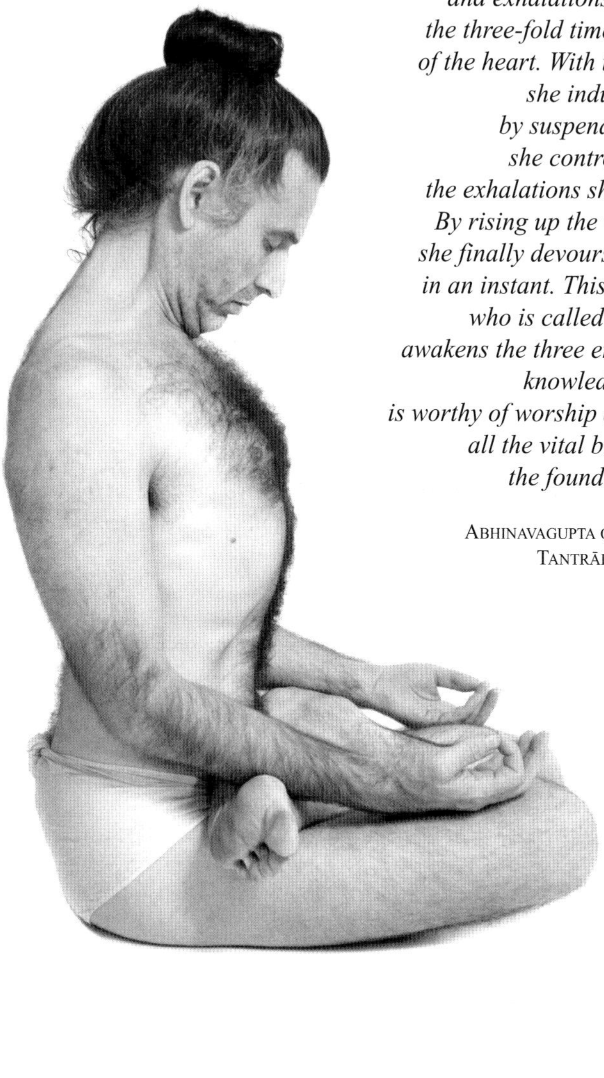

Ha

Pure subjectivity as 'I' (Śakti)
Condensed aspect of the Visarga
symbolising the energy
of the Without-Equal

ह

क्ष

Kṣa

union of two consonants animated by A, the Absolute (anuttara Śiva) and the visarga, the supreme energy (Śakti)

THIS PHONEME THEREFORE SYMBOLISES THE INDISSOLUBLE UNION OF ŚIVA- ŚAKTI (ANĀŚRITAŚIVA: ŚIVA WITHOUT-RELATION, OR TRANSCENDENT VACUITY. "THE GOD OF GODS, ANĀŚRITA, WHOSE POWER BLAZES WITHIN HIM LIKE A THOUSAND MILLION SUNS." ABHINAVAGUPTA, TANTRĀLOKA VII, 397B-399)

"O gazelle-eyed Goddess!
All we can cling to will leave us.
There is nothing we can hold on to.
We must leave behind all we know.
Life itself will abandon us.
There is no substance to any of that.
Give yourself to the sole priority,
that which remains
after everything has disappeared."

VIJÑĀNA BHAIRAVA 160

In essence, Śavāsana cannot be practised because the background cannot be objectivised.

In this 'corpse' āsana, tranquillity (śāntarasa) is left to emerge by rehearsing, or imitating, the dissolution (laya) of the body's psychosomatic sheaths. This dissolution is actualised by exhaling the totality of embodiment, thus imitating the ultimate exhalation and incubating death. It is therefore a lyrical reminder of this emotion. For technical details on how to perform this dissolution and how Śavāsana becomes an act of worship of the absolute, refer to chapter 30 of 'Light on Prāṇāyāma'.

Śiva serves as a seat for the supreme Goddess. He is known by the name of 'the great departed one'. He represents Sadāśiva. The word 'prahasantam' (smiling) has been used for Sadāśiva in order to show his joy in serving as a seat for parā, the transcendental Śakti. Although he is a pure element of subjectivity, he too must die.

In the Paramārthasāra, Abhinavagupta says: *"The body may suffer from loss of memory, paralysis, coughing and other pains, but this is our sort as long as there is a body. But even amidst distractions and in death, he who remains at his source is never abandoned by the effusion of the Self."* (94-95)

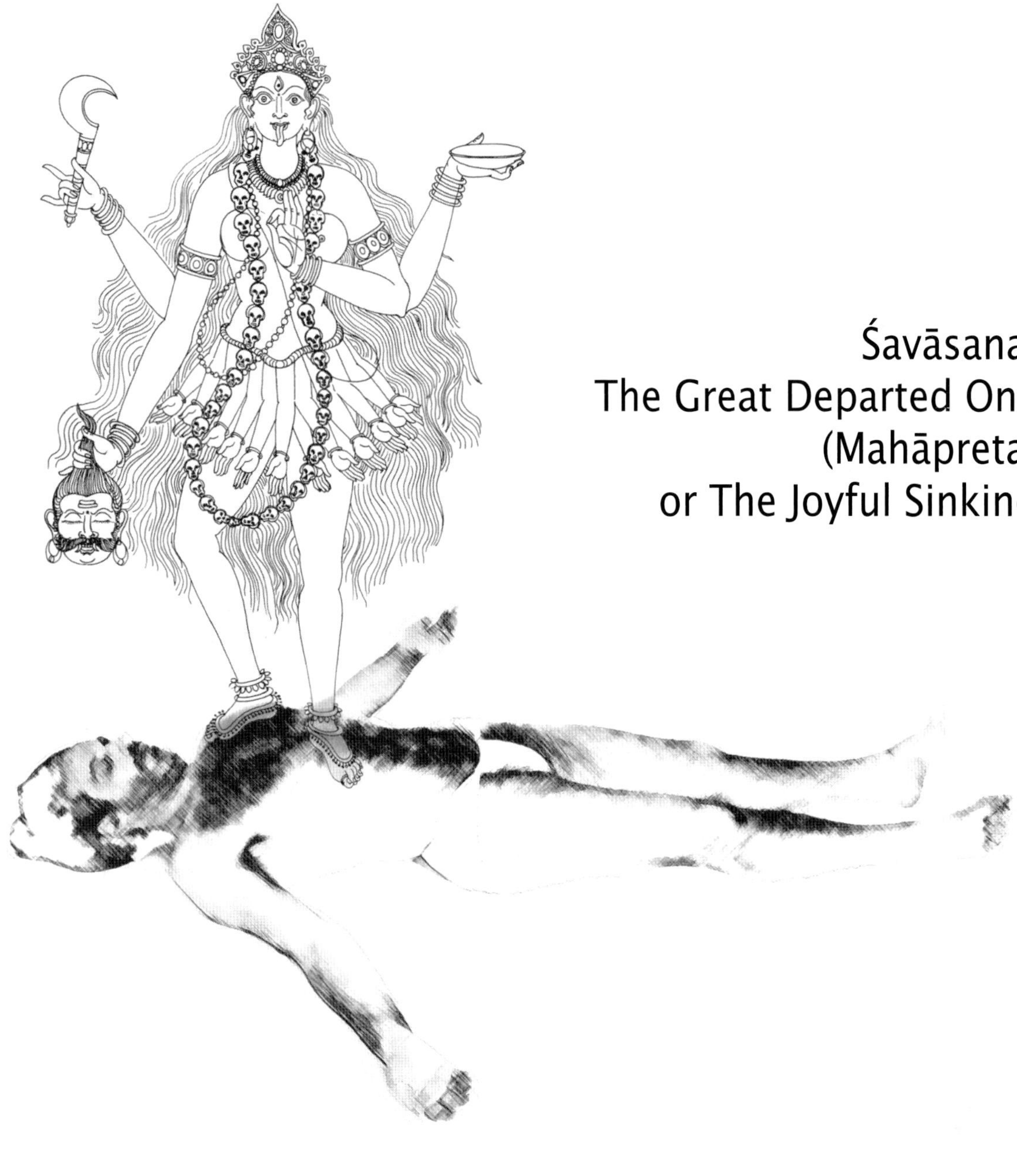

Śavāsana: The Great Departed One (Mahāpreta) or The Joyful Sinking

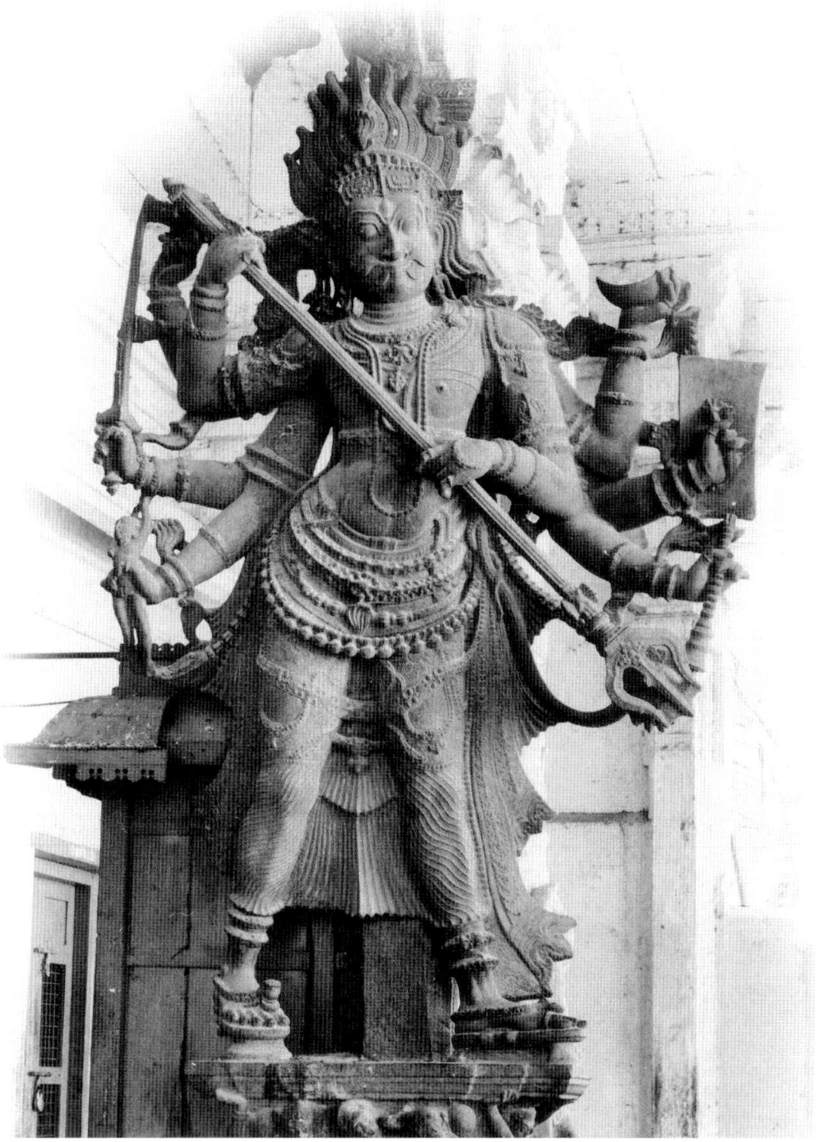

Bhairava *16th century*
(Kāśī Viśvanātha Temple, Tamil Nadu)

Epilogue

The Sinking of Contemplation Itself

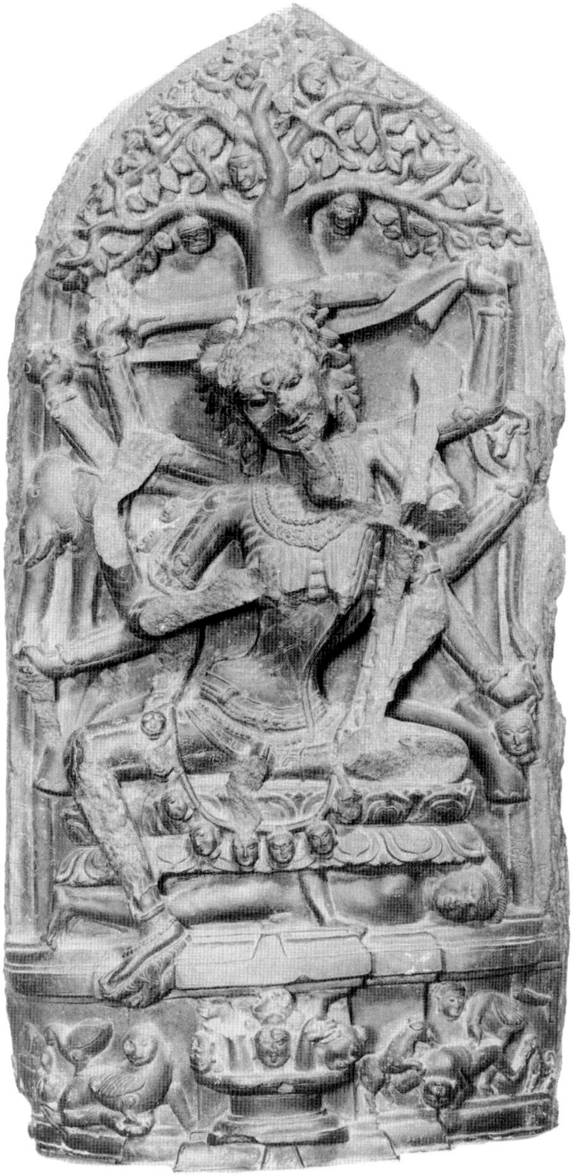

Cāmuṇḍā *12th century*
(Bengal, New Delhi National Museum)

It would have been enough to read just the first chapter (Confessions of Ignorance) and Abhinavagupta's Hymn that follows. All of life's events awaiting a child can be sensed on his face, and in the last moments of existence, all circumstances find their rightful place and return to the child's face. It cannot be any other way. Everything else is just to pass time. And can we even speak of events, time, succession or immediacy? We have worn out all concepts, especially that of being a separate entity, in the different circumstances of our lives until the point where they are discarded of their own accord. All that remains is the evidence of the non-event of 'what I am', which can be sensed from 'what I am not'. Abhinavagupta was one of the most brilliant sages of India, or, as Kṣemarāja says: *"The glorious Abhinavagupta, the best among the venerable, great Śaiva teachers."* I pay homage to him by quoting this hymn.

Eight Echoes of the Unsurpassable (Anuttarāṣṭikā)

Abhinavagupta

(Translated from Sanskrit by Bettina Bäumer)

There is no need of spiritual progress, nor of contemplation, disputation or discussion, nor meditation, concentration nor even the effort of prayer. Please tell me clearly: What is supreme Truth? Listen: Neither renounce nor possess anything, share in the joy of the total Reality and be as you are.

In reality no world of transmigration exits, so how can one talk about 'humans in bondage'? To try to liberate one free already is futile, for he was never in bondage. All this just creates a delusion like that of the shadow of a ghost or a rope mistaken for a snake. So neither renounce nor possess anything. Enjoy yourself freely, resting in your self, just as you are!

What words can describe the Unsurpassable? In the Absolute can there be any distinction between the worship, the one who worships and the object of worship? How and in whom can there be spiritual progress? What are the degrees of absorption? Illusion itself is ultimately the same as non-dual Consciousness, all being the pure nature of the Self, experienced by oneself, so have no vain anxiety.

This bliss is not comparable to that which is experienced through riches or wine or even union with the beloved. The dawning of that Light is not to be compared with the light of a lamp or that of the sun or moon. The joy that is felt when one is freed from the burden of accumulated differences can only be compared to the relief felt while setting on the ground a heavy weight. The dawning of the Light is like finding a lost treasure: the state of universal non-duality.

All states of mind like love and hatred, pleasure and pain, arising and disappearing, to you appear distinct. They are, however, part of the universal body, their nature is not separate. Whenever you observe any one of them arising, at once become aware of their oneness: contemplate in them the form of pure Consciousness. Filled with this contemplation, will you not experience joy?

The non-existent suddenly is brought into existence; such are always the states of being in this world. How, being intermingled due to deformation of the intermediate state, can they possess any reality? How to find reality in the unreal, unstable, in multiplicity of worldly things, a dream's confusion or in deceptive beauty? Transcend the impurity that causes doubt and fear and awaken!

It is not the Innate being that gives rise to these various states. They appear, created by you. Though unreal, they become real through a momentary confused perception. The glory of this universe is born from your will. It has no other origin. Therefore your glory shines in all the worlds. Though one, You have many forms.

Both the real and the unreal, the simple and the complex, the eternal and the temporal, that which, due to illusion, is impure and also the purity of the Self, all shine in the mirror of Consciousness. All this is seen as having the nature of pure light, as consciousness arises in self-awareness. Recognising your glory rooted in your own experience, share in the universal power of the Lord!

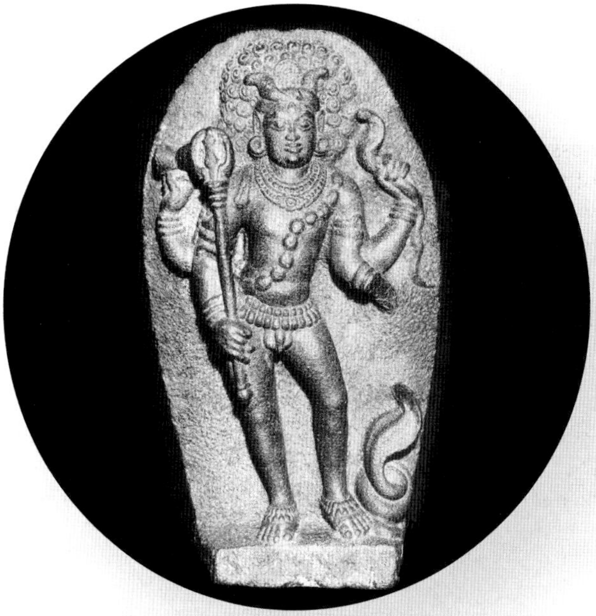

Kāla Bhairava *11th century*
(Begur, Bangalore District, Karnataka, Bangalore Government Museum)

Additional Notes on the
Vijñāna Bhairava

The Vijñāna Bhairava, as its name suggests, is part of the Bhairavāgama that contain the teachings of non-dual Kashmir Śaivism. It is known as the essence of the Rudrayāmala. Along with the Mālinīvijaya and Parātrīśikā it is among the most revered texts of this tradition. Abhinavagupta also refers to it as the Upaniṣad of the mystical teaching of the ultimate reality, Śiva (Śivavijñānopaniṣad). The Śaivāgama usually contain four sections: rituals (kriyā), observances (carya), philosophy (vidyā), and mystical practice (yoga).

The Vijñāna Bhairava is only concerned by the last section that sets out yoga practice. It takes the form of a dialogue between Śiva and Śakti, or Bhairava and Bhairavī. Although Bhairavī has heard the Rudrayāmala and the Trikabheda, which contains the essence of Tantra, she still has questions about the nature of Śiva. She therefore asks him to clarify her doubts. He replies with 112 instructions, traditionally referred to as 'instructions on the changeless' (nistaraṅga upadeśa, see śloka 139).

Apart from the great beauty of the text, these instructions cover everything known and all that supports the known. Hence, each experience, from the most trivial to the most subtle, can become a contemplation of our essence. Each and everything happens at the source of attention, mirror of our true nature. In each of these instructions can be found the heart of the nature of Bhairava, which is described in the following terms by Abhinavagupta in his Tantrāloka: *"I manifest this universe in the space of my Consciousness, I am the creator having the nature of all things."* (III, 283-285)

Some of the translations of the Vijñāna Bhairava are taken from 'The Practice of Centring Awareness' (Swami Lakshman Joo) and others are my own translations, which are often extrapolations. They are intimately linked to my own Yoga practice. I therefore ask for the indulgence of Sanskritists and academicians who will no doubt find them fanciful. I hope I have not strayed too far from their original meaning. Readers who wish to deepen their knowledge of the text in a more classical way with the Sanskrit may refer to the book 'The Practice of Centring Awareness' with a commentary by Swami Lakshman Joo and translated by Bettina Bäumer, or to the book by Jaideva Singh, without forgetting the version by Lilian Silburn (in French).

About the Calligraphies

The End of Postural Obsession

Photographs of āsana are almost always caricatures and inappropriate.
Taken literally, a photograph freezes us in the restriction
of a bodily corset that has achieved something.
This 'something' thus becomes an end, an aim.
Hence the expression: the final pose we should aim for.

A photograph is unable to describe the ritual of consecration
and its different bodily, respiratory and mental attitudes
(kriyā, mudrā, bhāva) that unfold in the instant.

An āsana does not fall into the realm of the visible.
The different bodily, respiratory and mental attitudes,
as well as their interaction, cannot be captured by a photograph.
As the fox says in Saint-Exupéry's The Little Prince:
"It is only with the heart that one can see rightly;
what is essential is invisible to the eye."
A photograph can be nothing more than a pointer
to ever vibrating iconic archetypes.

This is why some of the photographs are accompanied
by calligraphies, reminding the reader that a surge, or stroke
of energy, precedes the body and its aptitudes.

What we are able to do
or not do is therefore
of no importance.

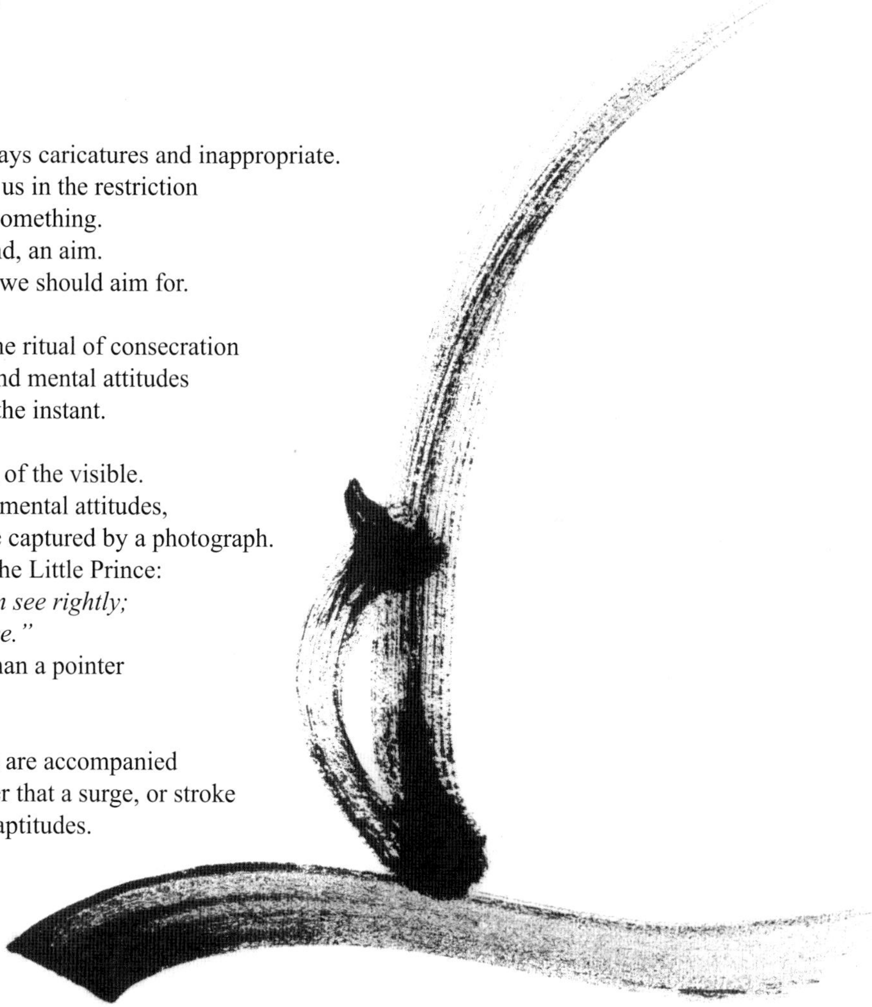

On Painting by the Monk 'Bitter Pumpkin'

The Single Brushstroke

In ancient times there were no Rules. The primordial Unity was still resting in its own essence. But as soon as activity became fragmented, the Rule was established. The Rule, based on the Single Brushstroke, is the source and origin of all things manifest, of all things visible and invisible.

Upon what is this Rule of the Single Brushstroke based?

The foremost Rule, which thus includes all other possible rules, resides in Non-Rule.

Painting emanates from the mind. Whether it is landscapes, people, animals, rivers, trees, houses or gardens that have to be painted, without the Single Brushstroke, it will not be possible to transmit the beauty, scale or essence of the multiple aspects of creation.

There is always a first step to even the longest of journeys.

And so the thousands of millions of brushstrokes all start and end with this Single Brushstroke.

By means of this Single Brushstroke, an artist is able to capture the essence, even of immense things. The clear vision of the mind leads the brush to the source of All things.

If the wrist is not free and light, mistakes will be made, which will lead to a multitude of other mistakes.

The brush must turn and fly in wide and circular movements, stopping abruptly and starting again smoothly; acting in all directions, creating all shapes and figures, angles and circles, pits and humps. It must move fluidly like water, shoot up like a flame, with spontaneous energy, without the slightest effort.

The omnipresent mind renders the Rule omnipresent, making all representations possible: mountains and rivers, trees, people and animals, birds, buildings, fishponds and terraces. Their infinitely diverse appearances, essence and innate character will all be captured, whether painted from life or from the imagination, whether suggesting an ambiance or painting precise strokes.

Although the narrow-minded might not grasp its fullness, such a painting reflects the mind's unity.

Unity has become multiplicity. In the same way, the foremost Rule was established, and from the Unique Brushstroke came the infinite creation.

This is the reason it is said:

"This is my way, that of the Unique,
source of the manifold."

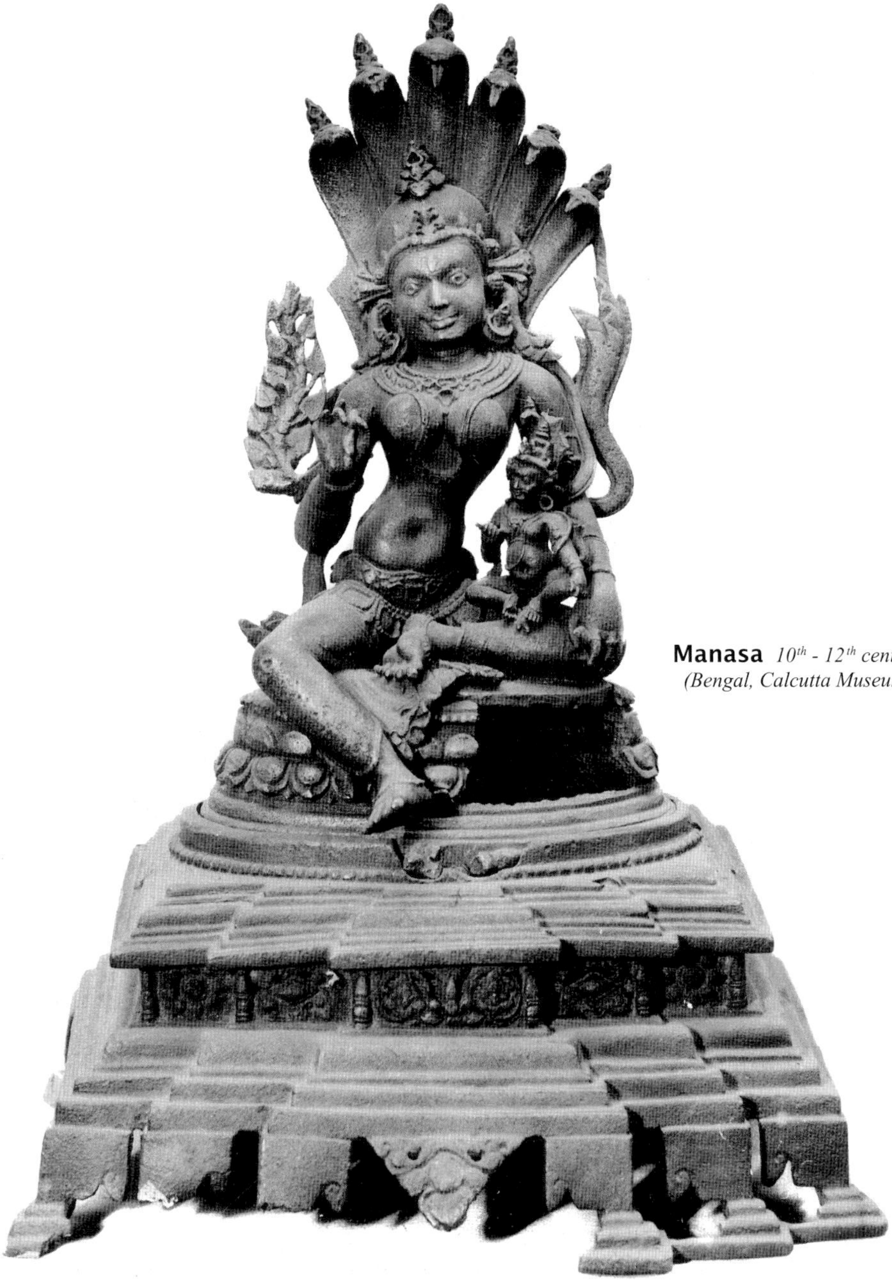

Manasa *10th - 12th century*
(Bengal, Calcutta Museum)

A Brief Bibliography
of Kashmir Śaivism and of Yoga According to the Teachings of Yogācārya Śrī B.K.S. Iyengar

Kashmir Śaivism

Śivasūtra: "The supreme Awakening" with the Commentary of Kṣemarāja, Swami Lakṣhman Joo, Universal Śaiva fellowship

Śivasūtra: The Yoga of Supreme Identity, Jaideva Singh, Motilal Banarsidass Publishers

The Aphorisms of Śiva: The ŚivaSūtra with Bhāskara's Commentary, the Vārttika, Mark S.G. Dyczkowski, SUNY Press

Spandakārikā with the Spandanirṇaya: The Divine Creative Pulsation, Jaideva Singh, Motilal Banarsidass Publishers

The Stanzas on Vibration: The Spandakārikā with Four Commentaries, Mark S.G. Dyczkowski, Dilip Kumar Publishers

Vijñāna Bhairava: The Practice of Centring Awareness, Swami Lakshman Joo, Indica Books

Vijñāna Bhairava or Divine Consciousness, Jaideva Singh, Motilal Banarsidass Publishers

Pratyabbhijñāhṛdayam: The Secret of Self Recognition, Jaideva Singh, Motilal Banarsidass Publishers

Iśvarapratyabhijñākārikā of Utpaladeva: Verses on the Recognition of the Lord, B.N. Pandit, Motilal Banarsidass Publishers

Iśvarapratyabhijñākārikā of Utpaladeva with the Author's Vṛtti, Raffaele Torella, Motilal Banarsidass Publishers

Iśvarapratyabhijñāvimarśinī of Abhinavagupta: Doctrine of Divine Recognition, K.C. Pandey, Motilal Banarsidass Publishers

Bhāskarī: An English Translation of the Iśvarapratyabhijñāvimarśinī in the Light of the Bhāskarī, K.C. Pandey. Motilal Banarsidass Publishers

Śivastotrāvalī of Utpaladeva: A Mystical Hymn of Kashmir, D.K. Printworld

Paramārthasāra of Abhinavagupta, B.N. Pandit, Munshiram Manoharlal Publishers

Paramārthasāra of Abhinavagupta, D.B. Sensharma, Motilal Banarsidass Publishers

Parātrīśikāvivaraṇa of Abhinavagupta: A Trident of Wisdom, Jaideva Singh, Motilal Banarsidass Publishers

Gītārtha Saṃgraha: Abhinavagupta's Commentary on the Bhagavad Gītā, Boris Marjanovic, Indica Books

Tantrāloka of Abhinavagupta, Luce dei Tantra, Raniero Gnoli, Adelphi

Dhvanyāloka of Ānanavardhana with the Locana of Abhinavagupta, Daniel Ingalls, Jeffrey Masson, M.V. Patwardhan, Harvard University Press

Manthānabhairavatantram (Kumārikākaṇḍaḥ): The section concerning the Virgin Goddess of the Tantra of the Churning Bhairava (14 volumes), Mark S.G. Dyczkowski, D.K. Printworld

Virūpākṣapañcāśikā: The Teachings of the Odd-Eyed One, David Peter Lawrence, SUNY Press

Kashmir Śaivism: The Secret Supreme, Swami Lakshman Joo, Sri Satguru Publications

The Awakening of Supreme Consciousness, Swami Lakshman Joo, Ishwara Ashrama Trust and Utpal Publications

Self Realization in Kashmir Shaivism: The Oral Teachings of Swami Lakshman Joo, SUNY Press

The Doctrine of Vibration, Mark S.G. Dyczkowski, SUNY Press

Specific Principles of Kashmir Shaivism, B.N. Pandit, Munshiram Manoharlal Publishers

Śaivāgama and the Kubjikā Tantras of the Western Kaula Tradition, Mark S.G. Dyczkowski, Motilal Banarsidass Publishers

A Journey in the World of the Tantras, Mark S.G. Dyczkowski, Indica Books

The Krama Tantricism of Kashmir, Navjivan Rastogi, Motilal Banarsidass Publishers

The Triadic Heart of Śiva: Kaula Trantricism of Abhinavagupta, Muller-Ortega, SUNY Press

Kuṇḍalinī: Energy of the Depths, Lilian Silburn, SUNY Press

Vāc: The concept of the Word, André Padoux, Sri Satguru Publications

Abhinavagupta: An Historical and Philosophical Study, K.C. Pandey, Chaukhamba Publications

Abhinavagupta, G.T. Deshpande, South Asia Books

Abhinavagupta and His Works, Ahitya Akademi Publications

Śāntarasa and Abhinavagupta's Philosophy of Aesthetics, Masson, Patwardhan, Bhandarkar Oriental Research Institute

The Aesthetic Experience According to Abhinavagupta, Raniero Gnoli, Chaukhamba Publications

The Advaita of Art, Harsha Dehejia, Motilal Banarsidass Publishers

Pārvatīdarpaṇa: An Exposition of Kashmir Śaivism through the images of Śiva and Pārvatī, Harsha Dehejia, Motilal Banarsidass Publishers

Body and Cosmology in Kashmir Śaivism, Gavin D. Flood, Mellen Research University Press

The Tantric Body, Gavin Flood, I.B. Tauris Publishers

The Alchemical Body: Siddha Traditions in Medieval India, David Gordon White, The University of Chicago Press

Iyengar Yoga

Light on Yoga, B.K.S. Iyengar, George Allen & Unwin Publishers

Light on Prāṇāyāma, B.K.S. Iyengar, George Allen & Unwin Publishers

Light on the Yoga Sūtras of Patañjali, B.K.S. Iyengar, Harper Collins Publishers

Light on Life, B.K.S. Iyengar, Rodale Publishers

The Tree of Yoga, B.K.S. Iyengar, Fine Line Books

70 Glorious Years of Yogācārya B.K.S. Iyengar, Light on Yoga Research Trust

Yogapuṣpañjali, Light on Yoga Research Trust

Iyengar: His Life and Work, Timeless Books

Aṣṭadaḷa Yogamālā (Volumes 1-8), Yogācārya B.K.S. Iyengar, Allied Publishers

Yoga: A Gem for Women, Geeta S. Iyengar, Allied Publishers

Yoga in Action for Beginners, Geeta S. Iyengar, YOG Publishers

Basic Guidelines for Teachers of Yoga, B.K.S. Iyengar & Geeta S. Iyengar, YOG Publishers

Alpha & Omega of Trikoṇāsana, Prashant Iyengar, YOG Publishers

Chittavijnana of Yogasanas, Prashant Iyengar, YOG Publishers

Vārāhī *12th century*
(Kalleśvara Temple, Karnataka)

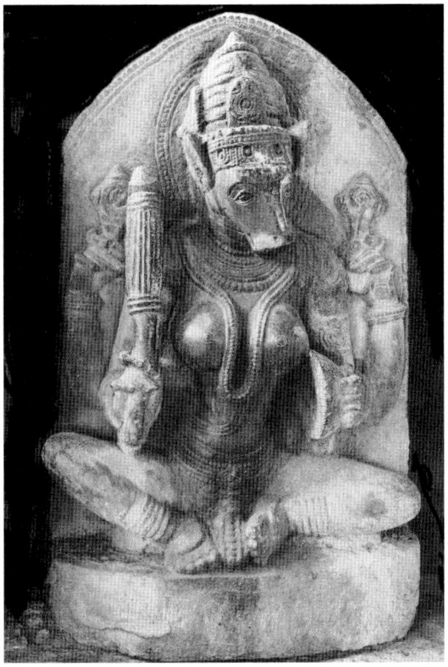

Table of Contents

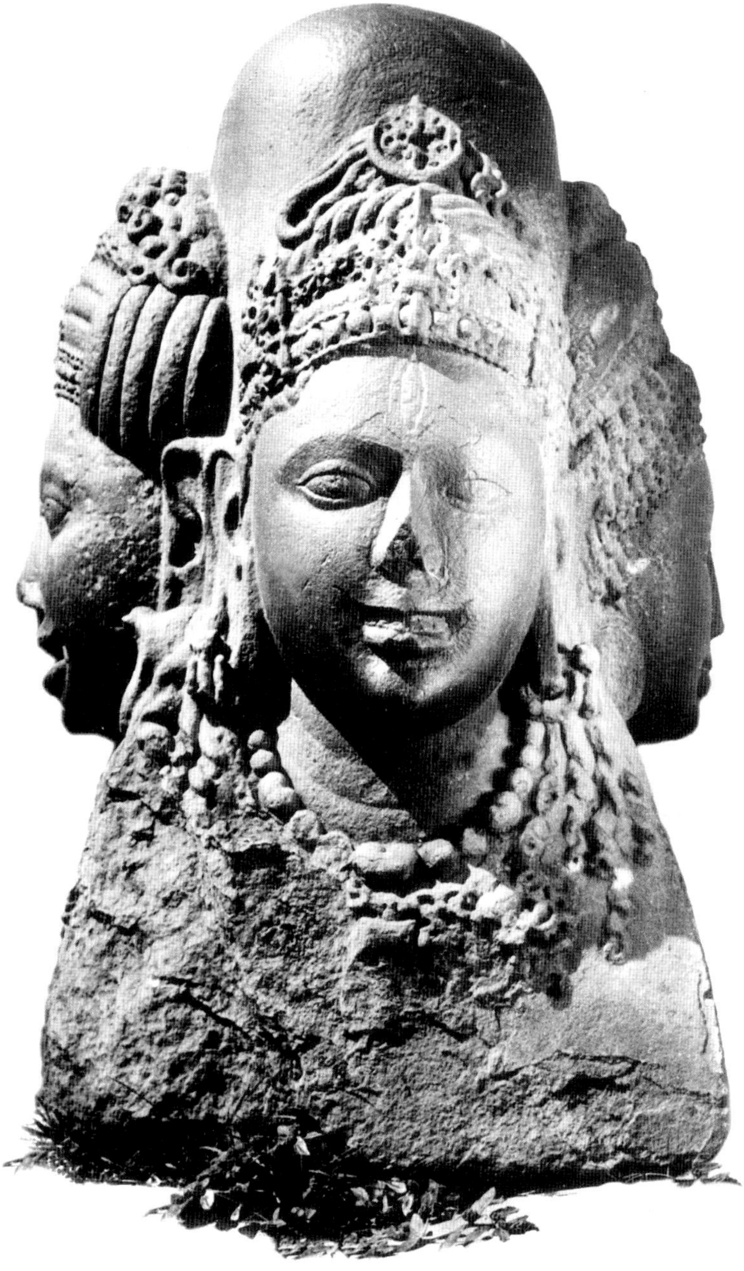

Śiva Liṅga Caturmukha *5th century*
(Pārvatī Temple, Nachna Kuthara, Madhya Pradesh)

अहं

AHAṂ

'I' as pure subjectivity

The first phoneme of the Sanskrit alphabet is the vowel 'A'. It is said: *"Let the sound A be of the nature of ultimate reality without qualities, and the essence of all things. The sound A leads all the other sounds. It is this sound that illuminates..."* (NANDIKEŚVARA KĀŚIKĀ 3-4)

The last phoneme is 'HA' and ends with the anusvāra (Ṃ), or nasalisation. The phonematic emanation, which is the emanation of the universe, can therefore only be expressed through 'I' (AHAṂ).
'AHAṂ' symbolises the culmination of Śakti in her expansion.
'A' symbolises unity, undifferentiated Consciousness (anuttara).
'HA' symbolises diversity.
The point above the 'HA' or anusvāra (Ṃ) symbolises unity in diversity.

"Of manifestation, the delightful form of the energy of the natural, innate mantra known as parāvāk (the Supreme divine utterance) is 'I' (AHAṂ)."
ABHINAVAGUPTA, PARĀTRĪŚIKĀVIVARAṆA, JAIDEVA SINGH, PAGE 54

Reading it backwards gives 'MAHA':
"In this immense cavern of Māyā whose heart is full of pure divine wisdom (śuddhavidyā) which is the vast creative movement, the origin of the emergence of the entire universe, the return movement (MAHA) that occurs by its own inherent dynamism of delight is, indeed, a great secret. By means of this secret it is intended to indicate that there is a return movement from objective manifestation indicated by 'MA' (nara) and 'HA' (śakti) towards the essential nature of the Self which ends in the repose of undifferentiated Consciousness indicated by the letter 'A'."
ABHINAVAGUPTA, PARĀTRĪŚIKĀVIVARAṆA, JAIDEVA SINGH, PAGE 54

Acknowledgements

My infinite gratitude to **My Guru**, *without whom this book would not exist. Should this work have any merit, it is the reflection of his presence, teaching and blessing. Anything that is unclear or confused is purely of my own doing.*

My gratitude to **Mark Dyczkowski** *for having helped me to clarify certain concepts, for his encouragement and friendly support during my moments of doubt, and above all for his great simplicity and humility. Whilst looking out over the Ganges and listening to him share his profound and heartfelt knowledge of Tantra that surpasses even his forty years of study, I realised my madness in embarking upon this book. You can find recordings of his teaching of the Trika on his website: http://markdkashi.com.*

The **American Institute of India Studies**, *Center for Art & Archaeology (Gurgaon, Haryana) and particularly the Managing Director Mr Purnima Mehta and the Director Mrs Vandana Sinha for allowing me to use photographs of the statues, as well as for their invaluable help.*

D.K. Printworld Publications *and Dr* **Frederick. W. Bunce** *for allowing me to reproduce certain yantra and deities from his book: An Encyclopaedia of Hindu Deities, Demi-Gods, Godlings, Demons and Heroes.*

Laurent Hodebert *for the studio photographs of āsana.*

Ben Edwards *for the photographs of āsana taken in front of the Kārttikeya temple in Pune, India.*

Master **Tchieko Imamura** *for creating the calligraphies (www.shodo.fr).*

Romio Bahadur Shrestha *for allowing me to use his Kālī painting (http://romioshrestha.com/about-romio.htm).*

My gratitude to **Ian Sanderson** *for having put his life on hold in order to translate this book with great devotion.*

Dominique Smersu *for correcting the Sanskrit.*

Marie Debove *for the magnificent page layout, her patience and constant encouragement. (marie.debove@wanadoo.fr)*

Paul Walker *(www.yogamatters.com) and* **Martin Wagner** *(www.yogawords.com) for accepting to publish this book.*

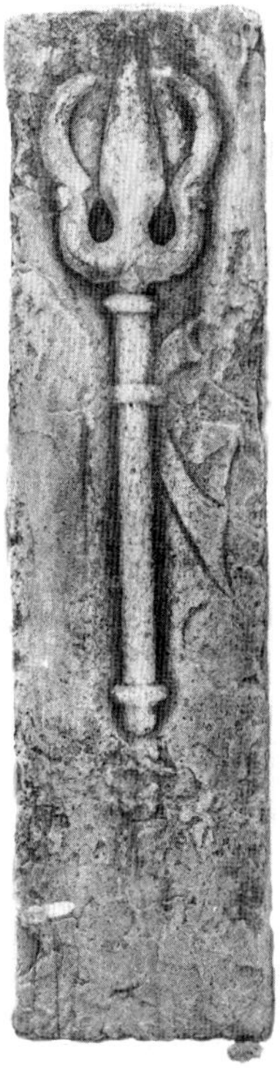